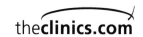

IMMUNOLOGY AND ALLERGY CLINICS OF NORTH AMERICA

Ocular Allergy

GUEST EDITOR
Leonard Bielory, MD

CONSULTING EDITOR
Rafeul Alam, MD, PhD

February 2008 • Volume 28 • Number 1

SAUNDERS

An Imprint of Elsevier, Inc.
PHILADELPHIA   LONDON   TORONTO   MONTREAL   SYDNEY   TOKYO

W.B. SAUNDERS COMPANY
A Division of Elsevier Inc.

Elsevier, Inc., 1600 John F. Kennedy Blvd., Suite 1800, Philadelphia, PA 19103-2899

http://www.theclinics.com

IMMUNOLOGY AND ALLERGY CLINICS	Volume 28, Number 1
OF NORTH AMERICA	ISSN 0889-8561
February 2008	ISBN-13: 978-1-4160-5853-3
Editor: Patrick Manley	ISBN-10: 1-4160-5853-2

The ideas and opinions expressed in *Immunology and Allergy Clinics of North America* do not necessarily reflect those of the Publisher. The Publisher does not assume any responsibility for any injury and/or damage to persons or property arising out of or related to any use of the material contained in this periodical. The reader is advised to check the appropriate medical literature and the product information currently provided by the manufacturer of each drug to be administered to verify the dosage, the method and duration of administration, or contraindications. It is the responsibility of the treating physician or other health care professional, relying on independent experience and knowledge of the patient, to determine drug dosages and the best treatment for the patient. Mention of any product in this issue should not be construed as endorsement by the contributors, editors, or the Publisher of the product or manufacturers' claims.

Immunology and Allergy Clinics of North America (ISSN 0889-8561) is published quarterly by Elsevier Inc., 360 Park Avenue South, New York, NY 10010-1710. Months of issue are February, May, August, and November. Business and Editorial offices: 1600 John F. Kennedy Blvd., Suite 1800, Philadelphia, PA 19103-2899. Customer Service office: 6277 Sea Harbor Drive, Orlando, FL 32887-4800. Periodicals postage paid at New York, NY and additional mailing offices. Subscription prices are $216.00 per year for US individuals, $339.00 per year for US institutions, $105.00 per year for US students and residents, $265.00 per year for Canadian individuals, $142.00 per year for Canadian students, $411.00 per year for Canadian institutions, $283.00 per year for international individuals, $411.00 per year for international institutions, $142.00 per year for international students. To receive student/resident rate, orders must be accompanied by name of affiliated institution, date of term, and the *signature* of program/residency coordinator on institution letterhead. Orders will be billed at individual rate until proof of status is received. Foreign air speed delivery is included in all *Clinics* subscription prices. All prices are subject to change without notice. POSTMASTER: Send address changes to *Immunology and Allergy Clinics of North America*, Elsevier Journals Customer Service, 6277 Sea Harbor Drive, Orlando, FL 32887-4800. **Customer Service: 1-800-654-2452 (US). From outside of the US, call 1-407-563-6020. Fax: 1-407-363-9661. E-mail: Journals** CustomerService-usa@elsevier.com.

Reprints. For copies of 100 or more, of articles in this publication, please contact the Commercial Reprints Department, Elsevier Inc., 360 Park Avenue South, New York, New York 10010-1710. Tel. (212) 633-3813 Fax: (212) 462-1935 e-mail: reprints@elsevier.com.

Immunology and Allergy Clinics of North America is covered in Index Medicus, Current Contents/Life Sciences, Science Citation Index, ISI/BIOMED, Chemical Abstracts, and EMBASE/Excerpta Medica.

Printed in the United States of America.

CONSULTING EDITOR

RAFEUL ALAM, MD, PhD, Veda and Chauncey Ritter Chair in Immunology, Professor, and Director, Division of Immunology and Allergy, National Jewish Medical and Research Center; and University of Colorado Health Sciences Center, Denver, Colorado

GUEST EDITOR

LEONARD BIELORY, MD, Professor of Medicine, Pediatrics, Ophthalmology; Director, Clinical Research and Development; and Director, Division of Allergy, Immunology, and Rheumatology, UMDNJ-New Jersey Medical School, Newark, New Jersey

CONTRIBUTORS

MARCELLA AQUINO, MD, Fellow in Training, Department of Medicine, Division of Allergy, Immunology, and Rheumatology, UMDNJ–New Jersey Medical School, Newark, New Jersey

MARK BALLOW, MD, Chief, Division of Allergy and Immunology, Department of Pediatrics, State University of New York at Buffalo, Women and Children's Hospital of Buffalo, Buffalo, New York

VINCENT BELTRANI, MD, Clinical Professor of Dermatology, Department of Dermatology, Columbia University, New York, New York; Department of Medicine, Division of Allergy, Immunology and Rheumatology, UMDNJ–New Jersey Medical School, Newark, New Jersey

LEONARD BIELORY, MD, Professor of Medicine, Pediatrics, Ophthalmology; Director, Clinical Research and Development; and Director, Division of Allergy, Immunology, and Rheumatology, UMDNJ–New Jersey Medical School, Newark, New Jersey

DAVID S. CHU, MD, Institute of Ophthalmology and Visual Science, UMDNJ–New Jersey Medical School, Newark, New Jersey

PETER C. DONSHIK, MD, Clinical Professor, University of Connecticut Health Center, Farmington, Connecticut

WILLIAM H. EHLERS, MD, Assistant Clinical Professor, University of Connecticut Health Center, Farmington; and Avon, Connecticut

SAMIH ELCHAHAL, MD, Institute of Ophthalmology and Visual Science, UMDNJ–New Jersey Medical School, Newark, New Jersey

MITCHELL H. FRIEDLAENDER, MD, Head, Division of Ophthalmology, Scripps Clinic, La Jolla, California

ANNE-MARIE A. IRANI, MD, Division of Pediatric Allergy, Immunology, and Rheumatology, Virginia Commonwealth University Health System, Richmond, Virginia

JASON JUN, BA, Tufts University School of Medicine, Boston, Massachusetts

ERIC R. KAVOSH, MD, Department of Medicine, UMDNJ–New Jersey Medical School, Newark, New Jersey

MICHAEL A. LEMP, MD, Clinical Professor of Ophthalmology, Georgetown University School of Medicine; and George Washington University School of Medicine, Washington, DC

BELLE PERALEJO, MD, Allergy and Immunology Fellow, Department of Medicine, Division of Allergy, Immunology and Rheumatology, UMDNJ–New Jersey Medical School, Newark, New Jersey

MICHAEL B. RAIZMAN, MD, Associate Professor of Ophthalmology, Tufts University School of Medicine; and Co-Director, Cornea and Anterior Segment Service, New England Eye Center, Boston, Massachusetts

RUDOLPH S. WAGNER, MD, Clinical Associate Professor and Director of Pediatric Ophthalmology, Institute of Ophthalmology and Visual Sciences, UMDNJ–New Jersey Medical School, Newark, New Jersey

CONTENTS

The prevalence of ocular allergy clearly is underappreciated and has been under diagnosed and undertreated. The ocular symptoms associated with the most common ocular allergy conditions, such as seasonal and perennial allergic conjunctivitis, are twice as likely to affect the allergy sufferer rather than nasal symptoms alone. The differential diagnosis of conjunctivitis is quite broad, with the most common forms associated with allergies, infections, and hormones. There are common features and some discerning features that, with a good history and examination, may provide a more focused and appropriate management.

Mast cells have long been recognized for their role in immediate hypersensitivity reactions, by virtue of the presence of high affinity receptors for IgE (FcεRI) on their surface. More recently, mast cells have been postulated to be involved in a variety of chronic inflammatory disorders as numerous mediators released by activated mast cells are characterized. This article summarizes current information on mast cell mediators, heterogeneity, and differentiation, and it reviews studies of mast cells in the normal eye and various ocular disorders.

careful strategy to identify patients with ocular allergy and manage the use of contact lenses in these patients is developed with an emphasis on the avoidance of complications.

Ocular Manifestations of Blistering Diseases

119

Samih Elchahal, Eric R. Kavosh, and David S. Chu

Ocular manifestations are a comorbidity of a group of chronic autoimmune blistering diseases that includes mucous membrane pemphigoid, linear immunoglobulin A disease, epidermolysis bullosa acquisita, and ocular pemphigus vulgaris. Various diagnostic measures differentiate between the diseases and allow for appropriate treatment including a specific selection of immuno-modulatory medications. New treatment modalities offer alternatives that may minimize disease severity and residual tissue damage and may reduce treatment-related complications.

Dermatologic and Allergic Conditions of the Eyelid

137

Belle Peralejo, Vincent Beltrani, and Leonard Bielory

This article reviews the dermatologic and allergic conditions of the eyelid. Topics include various eyelid dermatitis, inflammatory lesions, infections, benign and malignant tumor, urticaria, vascular lesions, and others. Treatment considerations for these conditions of the eyelid are also discussed.

Pediatric Ocular Inflammation

169

Rudolph S. Wagner and Marcella Aquino

Pediatric conjunctivitis often has a benign etiology and a self-limited course. It is common in childhood and may be infectious or noninfectious in nature and acute or chronic in presentation. Infectious causes include bacterial and viral conjunctivitis. Non-infectious causes include congenital nasolacrimal obstruction, ocular allergies, congenital glaucoma, and uveitis. This article reviews the etiology, clinical features, and treatment for pediatric conjunctivitis.

Ocular Allergy Treatment

189

Leonard Bielory

Nonpharmacologic interventions are commonly used as first-line treatment of ocular allergy and include avoidance, cold compresses, lubrication, and the use of disposable daily contact lenses. Pharmacologic management of ocular allergy has increased exponentially over the past decade. Clinically available agents are being expanded to specifically address the various signs and symptoms of inflammation associated with ocular allergy. Immunotherapy has been shown to decrease the sensitivity of the eye 10 to 100 fold and may have an effect for several years after halting of immunotherapy.

FORTHCOMING ISSUES

RECENT ISSUES

VISIT THESE RELATED WEB SITES

Access your subscription at:
www.theclinics.com

ELSEVIER
SAUNDERS

Immunol Allergy Clin N Am
28 (2008) ix–x

IMMUNOLOGY
AND ALLERGY
CLINICS
OF NORTH AMERICA

Foreword

When My Eyes Tear

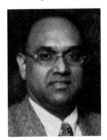

Rafeul Alam, MD, PhD
Consulting Editor

When my eyes tear, I should be sad, but I am not. I am actually irritated because I know my allergies are back. Allergic disorders of the eyes are a common manifestation of environmental allergies and are frequently under-diagnosed. Although the pathophysiology of ocular allergies has many elements that are common to allergic disorders of other organs, there are eye-specific elements that cannot be overemphasized. The importance of Th2 to ocular allergic inflammation is well known. However, the contribution of Th1 cells and their mediators are being increasingly recognized. In this context, it would be interesting to know the role of Th17 and Treg cells in ocular allergic inflammation. The allergen challenge of the eyes and measurement of inflammatory mediators in the tear have produced a wealth of data that has increased our knowledge about the pathophysiology of ocular allergies. Further, the development of an animal model of allergic conjunctivitis has allowed the application of novel investigational approaches as well as the testing of various therapeutic modalities.

To update our readership with the latest progress in ocular allergy, Dr. Leonard Bielory, a recognized leader in the field, has invited an outstanding group of experts. The topics of this issue include not only immunologic disorders of the eyes but also ocular manifestation of dermatologic

0889-8561/08/$ - see front matter © 2008 Elsevier Inc. All rights reserved.
doi:10.1016/j.iac.2007.12.012   *immunology.theclinics.com*

disorders. This update will benefit practicing clinicians from the field of allergy-immunology as well as ophthalmology.

Rafeul Alam, MD, PhD
Division of Allergy and Immunology
National Jewish Medical and Research Center
University of Colorado Health Sciences Center
1400 Jackson Street
Denver, CO 80206, USA

E-mail address: AlamR@njc.org

ELSEVIER
SAUNDERS

Immunol Allergy Clin N Am
28 (2008) xi–xii

IMMUNOLOGY
AND ALLERGY
CLINICS
OF NORTH AMERICA

Preface

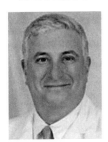

Leonard Bielory, MD
Guest Editor

The eye is probably the most common site for the development of allergic inflammatory disorders, since it has no mechanical barrier to prevent the impact of allergens such as pollen on its surface. Allergists/clinical immunologists frequently encounter various forms of allergic diseases of the eye that present as "red eyes" in their referral practice. However, the eye is rarely the only target for an immediate allergic-type response. Typically, many patients have other combinations of allergic disorders, such as rhinoconjunctivitis, rhinosinusitis, asthma, urticaria, or eczema; there also exists a systemic allergic component. Even so, ocular signs and symptoms can frequently be the most prominent features of the entire allergic response for which these patients come to see their physician.

The treatment of ocular inflammation is perhaps unique in medicine because it initially involved the combination of complex surgical procedures with simple medical management commonly provided by a single medical specialist, the ophthalmologist. The advances in understanding the immunopathophysiology of many ocular disorders have generated the need for a multidisciplinary approach involving various specialists who would cooperatively work together to control inflammation with systemically, topically, or intraocularly therapeutic agents. Over the past 20 years, we have witnessed an astonishing growth in therapeutic advances, ranging essentially from derivatives of simple aspirin to various newly developed biologic immunomodulatory agents, utilizing implantable drug delivery devices that exceed the safety and efficacy of those available for other organ systems, and

0889-8561/08/$ - see front matter © 2008 Elsevier Inc. All rights reserved.
doi:10.1016/j.iac.2007.12.008   *immunology.theclinics.com*

resorting to advanced surgical techniques for the correction of sight-threatening, disease-related complications.

The small compartment that the eye resides in has been commonly considered a disadvantage, but suddenly becomes a huge advantage. The eye itself is not lacking in immunologic complexity, as there appears to be an external conjunctival associated lymphoid tissue system and a paradoxical internal immune system that acts in a manner as a secluded immune compartment. Overall, with the expanding knowledge base, the intricacy of ocular inflammation appears to be becoming ever more manageable and, with the team approach between the ophthalmologist and the clinical allergist/immunologist, the new "immuno-ophthalmology" approach improves patient outcomes.

In this issue of *Immunology and Allergy Clinics of North America*, which focuses on ocular allergy, I have attempted to bring together various topics in anterior ocular inflammation in order to provide the allergist/clinical immunologist a better understanding and to become an active partner in the diagnosis and management of ocular inflammation of the anterior portion of the eye, primarily known as "conjunctivitis."

Acknowledgement

I would like to personally acknowledge Ms. Lynn Baltimore for her invaluable library assistance, and all of the authors for the dedicated efforts in making this issue a reality!

Leonard Bielory, MD
UMDNJ–New Jersey Medical School
90 Bergen Street
DOC Suite 4700
Newark, NJ 07103, USA

E-mail address: bielory@umdnj.edu

ELSEVIER
SAUNDERS

Immunol Allergy Clin N Am
28 (2008) xiii

IMMUNOLOGY
AND ALLERGY
CLINICS
OF NORTH AMERICA

Dedication

To the memories of my father, Max Bielory; my father-in-law, Daniel Gilan; and my brother, Charles Bielory.

doi:10.1016/j.iac.2007.12.010
immunology.theclinics.com

ELSEVIER
SAUNDERS

Immunol Allergy Clin N Am
28 (2008) 1–23

IMMUNOLOGY
AND ALLERGY
CLINICS
OF NORTH AMERICA

Ocular Allergy Overview

Leonard Bielory, MD

*Division of Allergy, Immunology and Rheumatology, University of Medicine and Dentistry,
New Jersey, New Jersey Medical School, 90 Bergen Street, DOC Suite 4700,
Newark, NJ 07103, USA*

Physicians in all specialties frequently encounter various forms of allergic diseases of the eye that present as "red eyes" in their general practice. However, the allergist or clinical immunologist is trained uniquely to understand and manage atopic disorders, because the eye is rarely the only target for an immediate allergic-type response. Typically, many patients have other atopic manifestations, such as rhinoconjunctivitis, rhinosinusitis, asthma, urticaria, or eczema. However, ocular signs and symptoms may be the initial and most prominent features of the entire allergic response that patients present to their physician.

The prevalence of allergies has been increasing during the past several decades, and ranges have been reported as up to 30%–50% of the United States population [1–4]. Industrialized countries report higher allergy prevalence, correlating to the original reports of "vernal catarrh" in Great Britain after the industrial revolution. Many theories abound regarding the increasing prevalence of allergies in the United States, such as the increased industrialization, pollution, urbanization, and the "hygiene theory." The combination of allergic nasal and ocular symptoms (rhinoconjunctivitis) is extremely common (double that of allergic rhinitis symptoms alone), but it is not clear if they are equal (ie, if rhinitis is more common than conjunctivitis or if conjunctivitis is more common than rhinitis). In studies of allergic rhinitis, allergic conjunctivitis is reported in over 75% of patients, while asthma was reported in the range of 10%–20% [5]. However, in some studies that report a high prevalence of seasonal allergic rhinitis in the United States, the ratio of ocular to nasal symptoms appears to double throughout all sections of the United States [6]. Thus, the eye is probably the most common site for the development of allergic inflammatory disorders, because allergens can directly impact on the eye's surface. Ocular allergy commonly is found in conjunction with allergic rhinitis, which is considered the

---

E-mail address: bielory@umdnj.edu

0889-8561/08/$ - see front matter © 2008 Elsevier Inc. All rights reserved.
doi:10.1016/j.iac.2007.12.011   *immunology.theclinics.com*

most common allergic disorder. Although the nasal and ocular symptoms (more appropriately called "conjunctivorhinitis") are perceived as a mere nuisance, their consequences can profoundly affect the patient's quality of life. Seasonal allergic rhinitis and conjunctivitis has been associated with headache and fatigue, impaired concentration and learning, loss of sleep, and reduced productivity [7,8]. Patients also may suffer from somnolence, functional impairment, and increased occupational risks for accidents or injuries secondary to sedating oral antihistamine therapy. In 70% of seasonal allergy patients, conjunctivitis symptoms are at least as severe as rhinitis symptoms [9].

The ocular surface

Allergens and other ocular irritants are deposited easily directly on the surface of the eye. Many agents that are systemically absorbed also can be concentrated and secreted in tears, causing allergic conjunctivitis or an irritant form of conjunctivitis [10]. The overuse of vasoconstrictive agents may lead to a form of conjunctivitis medicamentosa in some patients [11,12]. Other causes of the red eye also may include intraocular conditions associated with systemic autoimmune disorders such as uveitis or scleritis [13]. In addition, allergic inflammatory disorders, such as those that may affect surrounding skin, mucosa or even sinuses and release various mediators of inflammation, including histamine, leukotrienes, and neuropeptides, can have effects on the local ocular tissue [14].

Clinical examination

The clinical examination of the eyes for signs of ocular allergy requires an evaluation of the periorbital tissue and the eye itself. The eyelids and eyelashes are examined for the presence of erythema on the lid margin, telangiectasias, scaling, thickening, swelling, collarettes of debris at the base of the eyelashes, periorbital discoloration, blepharospasm, or ptosis, which are seen in blepharoconjunctivitis and dermatoconjunctivitis. Next, the conjunctivae are examined for hyperemia (injection), cicatrization (scarring), and chemosis (clear swelling). The presence or absence of discharge from the eye is noted for amount, duration, location, and color. The differentiation between scleral injection (scleritis) and conjunctival injection is that scleritis tends to develop over several days and is associated with moderate or severe ocular pain on motion, whereas conjunctivitis is associated with discomfort, but not pain. Scleritis commonly develops in patients who have autoimmune disorders such as systemic lupus erythematosus, rheumatoid arthritis, and Wegener's granulomatosis, but it has been known to occur alone without any other obvious clinical disorders [15–17]. Another form of ocular injection is described as a ring of erythema around the limbal junction of the cornea (ciliary flush), which is a clinical sign for intraocular inflammation such as uveitis. The conjunctival surface also should be examined closely for the presence of inflammatory follicles or papillae involving the bulbar and tarsal conjunctivae. Follicles can be distinguished as grayish, clear, or yellow bumps varying in size from pinpoint to 2 mm in diameter with conjunctival vessels on their surface, whereas papillae contain a centrally located tuft of blood vessels [18]. The cornea is involved rarely in acute forms of allergic conjunctivitis, whereas in the chronic forms of ocular allergy such as vernal keratoconjunctivitis and atopic Keratoconjunctivitis, the "kerato" reflects that the cornea is involved.

Optimal examination of the cornea is completed with the slit-lamp biomiocroscope, although many important clinical features can be seen with the naked eye or with the use of a hand-held direct ophthalmoscope. The direct ophthalmoscope can provide the desired magnification by "plus" (convex) and "minus" (concave) lenses. The cobalt blue filter on the new hand-held ophthalmoscopic heads assists in highlighting anatomic anomalies affecting the cornea or the conjunctiva that have been stained with fluorescein. The cornea should be perfectly smooth and transparent. Mucus adhering to the corneal or conjunctival surfaces is considered pathologic. Dusting of the cornea may indicate punctate epithelial keratitis (a condition commonly seen in chronic eosinophilic conditions of conjunctiva). A localized corneal defect may develop into erosion or a larger ulcer. A corneal plaque may be present if the surface appears dry and white or yellow. The limbus is the zone immediately surrounding the cornea and is normally invisible to the naked eye, but when inflamed, this area becomes visible as a pale or pink swelling. There have been some case reports of limbal allergy [19]. Discrete swellings with small white dots (Trantas-Horner's dots) are indicative of degenerating cellular debris that is seen commonly in chronic forms of conjunctivitis. In addition, since the eye has thin layers of tissue surrounding it, there is an increased tendency to develop secondary infections that can complicate further the clinical presentation [20,21].

Immunopathophysiology of ocular allergy

Allergic diseases affecting the eyes constitute a heterogeneous group of clinicopathologic conditions with a vast array of clinical manifestations that range from simple intermittent symptoms of itching, tearing, or redness, to severe sight-threatening corneal impairment. These conditions may be considered as part of an immunologic spectrum that affects the anterior surface of the eye with a variety of disorders that may overlap and may include seasonal allergic conjunctivitis (SAC) and perennial allergic conjunctivitis (PAC), vernal keratoconjunctivitis (VKC) and atopic keratoconjunctivitis (AKC), and giant papillary conjunctivitis (GPC) [22]. In addition, tear film dysfunction (otherwise known as dry eye syndrome [DES]), commonly complicates ocular allergy and its treatments, especially as the age of the patient increases and is included to reflect the spectrum of hypersensitivity responses from immunoglobulin E (IgE) mast cell hypersensitivity conditions to a mixture of mast cell and cell mediated disorders that involve different mechanisms, cytokines, and cellular populations [23–25]. For example, mast cell degranulation [26–28] and histamine release [29–33] play key roles with limited eosinophil involvement [34–36] in the common forms of SAC and PAC, whereas AKC and VKC are characterized by more chronic inflammatory cellular infiltrates primarily composed of Th2 lymphocytes with an interplay with activated mast cells and eosinophils, and tear film dysfunction, a Th1 mediated disorder, commonly can overlap ocular allergy syndromes (Table 1) [37–39].

Mast cell mediators such as histamine, tryptase, leukotrienes, and prostaglandins in the tear fluid have diverse and overlapping biologic effects [40–42], all of which contribute to the characteristic itching, redness, watering, and mucous discharge associated with both acute and chronic allergic eye disease. Histamine alone has been shown to be involved in the regulation of vascular permeability, smooth muscle contraction, mucus secretion, inflammatory cell migration, cellular activation, and modulation of T-cell function. Histamine is a principal mediator involved in ocular allergy and inflammation [29,32]. In fact, it is estimated that human conjunctival tissue contains approximately 10,000 mast cells per mm^3 [23,39]. Large amounts of histamine are present in several mammalian ocular structures, including the retina, choroid, and optic nerve. Histamine receptors have been found on the conjunctiva, cornea, and ophthalmic arteries. Two separate histamine receptors, H1 and H2, have been identified in the conjunctiva [43–46]. Most ocular allergic reactions are mediated through the effects of histamine on H1 receptors. Histamine concentration in tears of allergic conjunctivitis patients can reach values greater than 100 ng/mL as compared with values of 5–15 ng/mL in controlled patients. Histamine can induce changes in the eye similar to those seen in other parts of the body. These changes include capillary dilatation leading to conjunctival redness, increased vascular permeability leading to chemosis, and smooth-muscle contraction.

In the more severe chronic allergy-related conditions, T cells are the key cellular players in ocular surface impairment, with two predominant inflammatory pathways differentiated by the TH1 and TH2 cell markers, which involve different cytokines and are crudely considered as antagonistic of each other when activated. In previous reports based on conjunctival biopsies in allergic patients, cytokine profiling displayed that TH2 activation occurred in VKC, whereas both TH1 and TH2 activation were found in AKC [39,47–50]. In addition, it is not rare that a patient who is treated for typical SAC also may develop dry eye, tear film disturbance, meibomian dysfunction, adverse effects from the repeated use of toxic preservative-containing topical drugs, or contact cell-mediated conjunctival or eyelid hypersensitivity, all of which are conditions linked to the TH1 cascade [37,51–53].

Table 1
Differential diagnosis of conjunctival inflammatory disorders

	AC	VKC	AKC	GPC	DCS	Bacterial	Viral	CHLMD	DES	BC
Signs										
Predominant cell types	Mast cell eosinophils	Lymphocyte eosinophils	Lymphocyte eosinophils	Lymphocyte eosinophils	Lymphocyte eosinophils	PMN	PMN mono cyte lymphocytes	Monocyte lymphocytes	Lymphocyte monocytes	Monocyte lymphocytes
Chemosis	+	±	±	±	−	±	±	±	−	±
Lymph node	−	−	−	−	−	+	++	±	−	−
Cobblestoning	−	++	++	++	−	−	±	+	−	−
Discharge	Clear mucoid	Stringy mucoid	Stringy mucoid	Clear white mucoid	±	++ Muco-purulent	Clear mucoid	++ Muco-purulent	± Mucoid	++ Muco-purulent
Lid involvement	−	+	+	−	++	+ Glue lids	−	−	−	++
Symptoms										
Pruritus	+	++	++	++	+	−	−	−	−	+
Burning	−	−	−	−	−	−	++	+	+	−
Gritty sensation	±	±	±	+	−	+	+	+	+++	++
Seasonal variation	+	+	±	±	−	±	±	±	−	−

The differential diagnosis of the red eye includes various inflammatory conditions that involves the outside and the inside of the eye. Table 1 focuses on the signs and symptoms of external causes of the red eye that include the predominant cell type found in the conjunctival scraping and the presence or absence of chemosis, lymph node involvement, cobblestoning of the conjunctival surface, discharge, lid involvement, pruritus, gritty sensation, and seasonal variation.
Abbreviations: AC, allergic conjunctivitis; VKC, vernal keratoconjunctivitis; AKC, atopic keratoconjunctivitis; GPC, giant papillary conjunctivitis; DCS, dermatoconjunctivitis; DES, dry eye syndrome; GPC, giant papillary conjunctivitis; PMN, polymorphonuclear cell.
From Bielory L. Allergic diseases of the eye. Med Clin North Am 2006;90(1):129–48; with permission.

Acute allergic conjunctivitis

The eye actually may be the most common target organ of IgE mast cell hypersensitivity mediated reactions [54]. Allergic conjunctivitis is caused by the direct exposure of the ocular mucosal surfaces to environmental allergens (such as pollens from trees, grasses, and weeds) interacting with the pollen-specific IgE found on the mast cells of the eye. Of all the various pollens, ragweed has been identified as the most common cause of conjunctivo-rhinitis in the United States, approaching 75% of all cases of "hay fever" with variations of prevalence in different age groups in various regions of the world [6,55–57]. In the earliest studies on allergy testing, Timothy grass has been identified as one of the most potent ocular allergy inducing allergens [58]. Common conjunctival symptoms include itching, tearing, and perhaps burning. Involvement of the cornea is rare, with blurring of vision being the most common corneal symptom [18,59]. Clinical signs include a milky or pale pink conjunctiva with vascular congestion that may progress to conjunctival swelling (chemosis). A white exudate may form during the acute state and becomes stringy in the chronic form. While ocular signs are typically mild, the conjunctiva frequently takes on a pale, boggy appearance that often evolves into diffuse areas of papillae (small vascularized nodules). These papillae tend to be most prominent on the superior palpebral conjunctiva. Occasionally, dark circles beneath the eyes (allergic shiners) are present as a result of localized venous congestion [60]. PAC, like perennial allergic rhinitis, also exhibits the classic IgE mast cell-mediated hypersensitivity to airborne allergens, which is more commonly sensitive to common perennial household allergens, such as dust mites, molds, and animal dander instead of grass or weed pollens, as with patients who have SAC [61–65]. The ocular reaction seen in both SAC and PAC often resolves quickly once the offending allergen is removed. Obtaining a detailed history from the patient can make the diagnosis of these disorders. Both eyes typically are affected simultaneously, and quite often, a family history of hay fever or atopy is elicited.

Vernal keratoconjunctivitis

VKC is a chronic mast cell/lymphocyte-mediated allergic disorder of the conjunctiva that appears more in males before pubescence, after which it is equally distributed among the sexes and then commonly "burns out" approximately 10 years later (ie, in the third decade of life). As the name implies VKC is recurrent seasonally in the spring (vernal) with symptoms that include intense pruritus induced by nonspecific stimuli, such as exposure to wind, dust, bright light, hot weather, or physical exertion associated with sweating [38]. Although considered a form of ocular allergy, over 50% of patients have a negative skin test or a radioallergosorbent test to allergens [66]. As in other chronic ocular allergy conditions, conjunctival biopsies reveal increased numbers of eosinophils, basophils, and mast cells, and increased numbers of plasma cells and lymphocytes that result with increased corneal involvement with photophobia, foreign body sensation, and lacrimation [39,67]. The most remarkable physical finding is "giant" papillae on the tarsal conjunctiva reaching 7–8 mm in diameter of the upper tarsal plate, which can result in the "cobblestone" appearance on examination [68]. In addition, patients may develop a thin copious milk-white fibrinous secretion, limbal or conjunctival "yellowish-white points" (Horner's points and Trantas' dots), an extra lower eyelid crease (Dennie's line), corneal ulcers, or pseudomembrane formation of the upper lid when everted and exposed to heat (Maxwell-Lyons' sign) [60]. The effects of VKC can be so severe that blindness may result, affecting one eye more than the other in approximately 5% of patients [67,69]. Diffuse areas of punctate corneal epithelial defects can occur in some cases. These defects are best appreciated with a cobalt blue light after the instillation of topical fluorescein dye [70]. In severe cases, these superficial punctate defects may progress to "shield ulcers", which are areas of desquamation of epithelial cells caused by the release of major basic protein from infiltrating eosinophils [71,72].

Atopic keratoconjunctivitis

AK is a chronic inflammatory process and a chronic mast cell/lymphocyte-mediated allergic disorder of the conjunctiva of the eye periorbital tissue that is associated with a familial history for atopy, such as eczema and asthma [73,74]. Allergists or clinical immunologists should expect to see approximately 25% of their elderly patients who have eczema develop some components of AKC. Although AKC commonly is seen in individuals older than 50 years of age, onset can be in selected individuals as early as the late teens. AKC is an eye disorder with disabling symptoms; when it involves the cornea, it can lead to blindness [67]. Ocular symptoms of AKC are similar to the cutaneous symptoms of eczema and include intense pruritus and edematous, coarse, and thickened eyelids. Severe AKC is associated with complications such as blepharoconjunctivitis, cataract, corneal disease, and ocular herpes simplex [75,76]. The symptoms of AKC commonly include itching, burning, and tearing, which are much more severe than in acute conjunctivitis or PAC and tend to be present throughout the year. Seasonal exacerbations are reported by many patients, especially in the winter or summer months, and include exposure to animal dander, dust, and certain foods [38,70,77]. Ocular disease activity has been shown to correlate with exacerbations and remissions of the dermatitis. AKC associated cataracts occur in approximately 10% of patients who have the severe forms of atopic dermatitis, but they occur especially in young adults approximately 10 years after the onset of the atopic dermatitis. A unique feature of AKC cataracts is that they predominantly involve the anterior portion of the lens and may evolve rapidly into complete opacification within 6 months, whereas AKC patients may develop posterior polar type cataracts caused by the prolonged use of topical or oral corticosteroid therapy [78–82]. Keratoconus occurs in a small percentage of patients who have atopic dermatitis. Retinal detachment appears to be increased in patients who have AKC, although it also is increased in patients who have atopic dermatitis in general. The association with specific microorganisms, such as *S aureus* is under investigation presently [20,83,84]. Treatment involves corticosteroids, antihistamines, mast cell stabilizers, and treatment of systemic features of atopic dermatitis. There is a heightened concern regarding the use of antihistamines in older patients who have this condition, because antihistamines may increase dryness of the conjunctival surface.

Giant papillary conjunctivitis

GPC is not truly an "ocular allergy," but many of its features mimic those of the other ocular hypersensitivity syndromes (ie, an increase of symptoms during the spring pollen season and pruritus); thus, it is important to include GPC in the differential diagnosis of ocular allergy [54,85,86]. GPC is becoming more common with the advent of extended-wear soft contact lenses and other foreign bodies, such as suture materials and ocular prosthetics. Symptoms include a white or clear exudate upon awakening, which chronically becomes thick and stringy, and the patient may develop papillary hypertrophy ("cobblestoning") especially in the tarsal conjunctiva of the upper lid, which is more common in soft ($\sim$5%–10%) versus hard contact ($\sim$4%) lens wearers. The contact lens polymer and preservatives such as thimerosal and proteinaceous deposits on the surface of the lens have been implicated as causing GPC, but this concept remains controversial [87–90]. Common symptoms include intense itching, decreased tolerance to contact lens wear, blurred vision, conjunctival injection, and increased mucous production. Treatment involves use of corticosteroids, antihistamines, and mast cell stabilizers and frequent enzymatic cleaning of the lenses, or changing of the lens polymers. Disposable contact lenses have been proposed as an alternative treatment for GPC. It will usually resolve when the patient stops wearing contact lenses or when the foreign body is removed.

Dry eye syndrome (tear film dysfunction)

DES, also know as tear film dysfunction, develops from decreased tear production, increased tear evaporation, or an abnormality in specific components of the aqueous, lipid, or mucin layers that comprise the tear film [91–94]. Symptoms of DES are typically vague and include foreign body sensation, easily fatigued eyes, dryness, burning, ocular pain, photophobia, and blurry vision. Patients initially complain of a mildly injected eye with excessive mucous production and symptoms of gritty sensation as compared with the itching and burning feeling many patients complain of with histamine release onto conjunctiva. Symptoms tend to be worse late in the day after prolonged use of the eyes or exposure to environmental conditions.

Whereas DES may occur as a distinct disorder resulting from intrinsic tear pathology, it is associated more frequently with other ocular and systemic disorders, including ocular allergy, chronic blepharitis, fifth or seventh nerve palsies, vitamin A deficiency, pemphigoid, and trauma [95]. DES is a frequent confounding disorder that may complicate ocular allergic disease with several overlapping signs and symptoms, such as tearing, injection, and exacerbations [96,97]. As the cornea becomes involved, a more scratchy and painful sensation and photophobia may appear. DES and ocular allergy conditions are not exclusive, and as patients age, the likelihood that tear film dysfunction complicating ocular allergies increases [98]. A more systemic form of DES associated with systemic immune diseases (such as Sjögren's syndrome, rheumatoid arthritis or HIV infection [99]) is known commonly as keratoconjunctivitis sicca or hormonal dysregulation that is commonly found in postmenopausal women [100]. The most common cause of DES is not associated with an autoimmune disorder, but rather, the use of medications with anticholinergic properties that decrease lacrimation. Many drugs with antimuscarinic properties include the first-generation antihistamines and even newer agents, such as loratadine and cetirizine [101], phenothiazines, tricyclic antidepressants, atropine, and scopolamine. Other agents that are associated with a sicca syndrome include the retinoids, beta blockers, and chemotherapeutic agents. Tear film dysfunction also is associated with several pharmacologic agents, including antihistamines, anticholinergics, and some psychotropic agents [102]. Exacerbation of symptoms also occurs in the winter months when heating systems decrease the relative humidity in the household to less than 25%. Diagnostic evaluation includes use of the Schirmer test, which typically demonstrates decreased tearing (0–1 mm of wetting at 1 minute and 2–3 mm at 5 minutes). Normal values for the Schirmer test are more than 4 mm at 1 min and 10 mm at 5 min. Treatment includes addressing the underlying pathology, discontinuing the offending drug if possible, and generous use of artificial tears or ocular lubricants. The use of topical cyclosporine has been approved by the FDA for the treatment of DES [37,103]. For severe symptoms, insertion of punctal plugs may be indicated [104].

Contact dermatitis of the eyelids

In contradistinction to ocular allergy, with its predominant activation of the IgE mast cell, contact dermatoconjunctivitis is predominantly a delayed type of lymphocytic hypersensitivity reaction involving the eyelids and the conjunctiva [54,105–107]. The eyelid skin is extremely thin, soft, and pliable and is capable of developing significant swelling and redness with minor degrees of inflammation. This frequently causes the patient to seek medical attention for a cutaneous reaction that, had it appeared elsewhere on the skin, normally would be less of concern. Two principal forms of contact dermatitis attributable to eye area cosmetics are recognized: contact dermatoconjunctivitis and irritant (toxic) contact dermatitis. Contact dermatoconjunctivitis commonly is associated with either cosmetics applied to the hair, face, or fingernails (eg, hair dye and nail polish) or topical ocular medications (eg, neomycin) [108,109]. Preservatives such as thimerosal, found in contact lens cleaning solutions, and benzalkonium chloride, found in many topical ocular therapeutic agents, have been shown by patch tests to be major culprits like the active drugs themselves [110–118]. Stinging and burning of the eyes and itching of the lids are the most common complaints. These subjective symptoms are usually transitory and unaccompanied by objective signs of irritation. The patch test can assist in pinpointing the causative antigen, but interpretation of patch-test results consequently may be difficult, and the likelihood of irritant false-positive reactions must be kept in mind [119–121].

Blepharoconjunctivitis

Blepharitis is a primary inflammation of the eyelid margins that is most often misdiagnosed as an ocular allergy, because it commonly causes conjunctivitis in a secondary fashion [54,110,122–124]. The primary etiologies are various infections or seborrhea. In general, as is also found in patients who have atopic dermatitis, the most common organism isolated from the lid margin is *Staphylococcus aureus*. It has been suggested that antigenic products play the primary role in the induction of chronic eczema of the eyelid margins [20,125–128]. The symptoms include persistent burning, itching, tearing and "a feeling of dryness." Patients commonly complain of more symptoms in the morning than in the evening. This is in contradistinction to patients who have DES and who complain of more symptoms in the evening than in the morning, because the tear film dries out during the day. The crusted exudate that develops in these patients may cause the eye to be "glued shut" when the patient awakens in the morning. The signs of staphylococcal blepharitis include dilated blood vessels, erythema, scales, collarettes of exudative material around the eyelash bases, and foamy exudates in the tear film. Blepharitis can be controlled with improved eyelid hygiene with detergents (eg, nonstinging baby shampoos) and with steroid ointments applied to the lid margin with a cotton tip applicator that loosens the exudate and scales.

Bacterial conjunctivitis

Ocular irritation, conjunctival redness, and a mucopurulent discharge that is worse in the morning characterize acute bacterial conjunctivitis. The absence of itching should indicate an infectious cause of conjunctivitis, such as bacterial or viral [129]. In bacterial conjunctivitis, the eyelids usually become matted to each other; this is noted primarily in the morning when the patient awakens. There is a large accumulation of polymorphonuclear cells on the surface of the eye that causes the discharge to become discolored (yellowish green). Scraping and culturing of the palpebral conjunctiva can assist with the diagnosis and treatment with the appropriate topical antibiotic regimens.

Some forms of bacterial infection, such as inclusion conjunctivitis, that have been associated with chlamydial infections are associated with a preauricular node. Common findings of inclusion conjunctivitis include a mucopurulent discharge and follicular conjunctivitis lasting for more than 2 weeks [130]. A Giemsa stain of a conjunctival scraping may reveal intracytoplasmic inclusion bodies and will assist in confirming the diagnosis. In addition, such prolonged ocular infections commonly are associated with a conjunctival response that reveals grayish follicles on the upper palpebra. The condition can be chronic, and treatment consists of lid margin scrubs, warm compresses, and antibiotics. In general, a topical, broad-spectrum antibiotic (such as sulfacetamide, erythromycin, or a combination of polymyxin B, bacitracin and Neosporin) is appropriate. Cultures are necessary only if the conjunctivitis is severe; it would be best if cultures were examined carefully by an ophthalmologist. The condition should be followed carefully to ensure that the eye improves [131].

Topical gentamicin and tobramycin are indicated if Gram-negative organisms are suspected or seen on Gram stain. All of these antibiotics have the potential to elicit an allergic reaction. A careful history of drug allergies and a time limit for therapy and re-evaluation will minimize complications. Topical ciprofloxacin or ofloxacin offer coverage for a wide spectrum of infecting agents, but they should be used only when there is a likelihood for therapeutic failure or if the conjunctivitis is thought to be caused by multiple infecting organisms or *Pseudomonas* sp [132]. Treatment of inclusion conjunctivitis should be aggressive, because there is the potential for the cornea to perforate in a short time. Both topical and systemic antibiotics should be used. The patient should be observed for other sexually transmitted diseases.

Viral conjunctivitis

Viral conjunctivitis usually has an acute onset, is unilateral, and lasts for approximately one week, but it frequently becomes bilateral [129]. A major clinical symptom that differentiates viral conjunctivitis from allergic conjunctivitis is burning and absence of itching. Adenoviral infections are among the most common viral ocular infections and are extremely contagious. The viral infection produces an inferior follicular response and a serous discharge. It also may involve the cornea as a punctate keratopathy or superficial ulcerations (herpes simplex or herpes zoster infections) [133].

Common findings of viral conjunctivitis include a watery discharge, conjunctival injection, chemosis, and enlargement of the preauricular (pretragal) lymph nodes [129]. Patient history also assists in the diagnosis. Viral conjunctivitis usually is transmitted between family members or among school children. As in chronic bacterial infections, gray elevated vascular areas, known as lymphoid follicles, also may be present. A more serious form of viral conjunctivitis is that caused by herpes simplex, which is one of the leading infectious causes of blindness in Western countries. The viral infection produces an inferior follicular response and a serous discharge, and it can occur without any other sign of a herpetic infection. The pain associated with herpetic infections is excruciating. The pain can occur days before the lesions appear. The absence of pruritus should guide the clinician away from a diagnosis of allergic eye disease and toward an infectious complication. Viral conjunctivitis also may involve the cornea in the form of punctate keratopathy or the classic "dendritic" superficial ulcerations. The possibility of herpes keratitis is one of the most compelling reasons for a primary care physician to examine the cornea with fluorescein staining. Treatment of nonspecific viral conjunctivitis is largely supportive and requires no drug therapy. Topical vasoconstrictors may provide symptomatic relief, and they may decrease conjunctival injection. If the corneal epithelium becomes compromised and there is a risk for secondary infection, prophylactic antibiotics may be indicated [134,135].

Vasomotor conjunctivitis

Mismatches between history and IgE sensitization have been recognized since the use of conjunctival and cutaneous tests in the 1930s. Interestingly, asymptomatic skin cutaneous reactivity appears to be associated with evolution to allergic diathesis, especially when it is paralleled with late phase response that is also associated with the development of a positive conjunctival provocation and increased IL-5 expression and eosinophil proliferation [136,137].

The first use of the term "vasomotor conjunctivitis" can be found in Russian literature from 1971 [138,139]. The possibility of a link between vasomotor rhinitis and conjunctivitis interestingly was reported with bulbar vessel enlargement, diameter nonuniformity, pathologic convolution, and red blood cell aggregation. However, this was noted in a pediatric population, aged 6 to 15 years, that is not known to have a high prevalence of vasomotor [140]. The existence of a nonspecific hyper-reactivity of the conjunctiva to a number of physical agents (ie, temperature [hot and cold air], light, water, dust, and particulate matter [smoke and odors]) chemical agents (eg, volatile organic chemicals) and pharmacologic agents in a common characteristics of allergic subjects, which is strictly related to the inflammatory events consequent to an allergic reaction [139]. The existence of nonallergic hyper-reactivity of the conjunctival surface resurfaced in the literature [49] and subsequently evaluated using a 40% glucose hyperosmolar solution in a conjunctival provocation model that clearly demarcated between normal, allergic conjunctivitis, and nonspecific conjunctival hyperactivity [141]. Such nonallergic stimuli also have been reported to be associated with mast cell mediator release and have been seen in other allergic target organs such as the nose and lung.

Nonallergic ocular hypersensitivity may overlap ocular allergy, as suggested in various studies noted above and in studies of airline crewmembers during the time when smoking had been permitted; the prior history of atopy in the airline crew members was a factor in the development of ocular symptoms (11%) and other symptoms such as fatigue (21%), nasal symptoms (15%), dry or flushed facial skin (12%), and dermal hand symptoms (12%). The aircrew that had a history of atopy had an increase of most symptoms (OR = 1.5–3.8) [142]. In addition, in studies of various large corporate buildings without previously recognized indoor air problems, frequent symptoms included a feeling of eye irritation, fatigue, or heavy-headedness and dry facial skin. Women reported symptoms more frequently than men. Employees who had allergies had a 1.8–2.5 higher risk of reporting a high score for general, skin, or mucosal symptoms.

As with other analyses on ocular allergy, the epidemiologic evidence is cloaked in nasal allergy literature. As one examines the literature regarding nonallergic rhinitis, there is a range of reports from 25 up to 52% in a pediatric population [143–145]. However, many health care observers recognize that patients may have coexisting allergic and nonallergic disease, and in a retrospective analysis of a broader set of patients attending an allergy clinic, 43% of patients had allergic rhinitis, 23% nonallergic rhinitis, and 34% mixed rhinitis. Importantly, 44% of the patients who had been diagnosed with allergic rhinitis also had a nonallergic element. Regarding the nonallergic element, some doctors have tried to explain it as an immune response to viral or bacterial infections of the conjunctiva, an irritant response to a chemical, or a defect in the physiologic homeostasis of the conjunctival surface. An examination of the possible triggers of the nonallergic element creating mucosal hypersensitivity reactions at the conjunctival surface have been reported in several epidemiologic studies focusing on traffic pollution [146–156]. In vitro laboratory findings indicate that diesel exhaust particles can act as an adjuvant and actually enhance IgE production and sensitivity to allergens [146–156]. In other studies of ocular allergy patients who had positive clinical histories that were confirmed by skin testing and then nasal or ocular provocation, there was a constant percentage of patients (24%) who had positive histories but negative serologic or provocation [157].

Ocular examination

The ocular examination begins with the eyelids and lashes. One should look for evidence of lid margin erythema, telangiectasia, thickening, scaling, and lash collars. Then the sclera and conjunctiva are examined for the presence of redness (injection). Certain characteristics that assist in pinpointing the diagnosis are characterized below.

Subconjunctival hemorrhages spontaneously occur after coughing, sneezing, or straining as a result of spontaneous rupture of a conjunctival or episcleral capillary. It is characterized by a painless focal area of solid redness surrounded by normal white sclera on all sides. It commonly resolves without any intervention.

A fundamental principle of the ocular examination is determining whether conjunctival inflammation is nonspecific or punctuated by the presence of follicles or papillae involving the bulbar and tarsal conjunctiva. Follicles appear as grayish, clear, or yellow bumps varying in size from pinpoint to 2mm in diameter, with conjunctival vessels on their surface that generally are distinguishable from papillae that contain a centrally located tuft of vessels that can be seen in the center of papilla as a "red spot." Although a fine papillary reaction is nonspecific, giant papillae (greater than 1mm) on the upper tarsal conjunctiva indicate an allergy and are not seen in active viral or bacterial conjunctivitis. Follicles, a lymphocytic response in the conjunctiva, are a specific finding that occurs primarily in viral and chlamydial infections. Follicle formation is normal in childhood, but in adults, it may indicate significant conjunctival inflammation in the form of viral conjunctivitis (such as adenoviral or primary herpetic conjunctivitis) or chlamydial infection. For a clinician to determine an acceptable (nonpathologic) level of follicular and papillary reactivity, it is advised that they examine the upper and lower tarsal plates and bulbar conjunctiva on a routine basis. Reactive lymphoid hyperplasia is indicated by firm to rubbery nodules under the conjunctiva and without acute inflammatory signs such as erythema, chemosis, or pain.

Conjunctival injection is more intense on the palbebral conjunctiva than the bulbar conjunctiva. The intensity of the injection decreases as one approaches the cornea. In contrast to ciliary injection, the erythema increases as one approaches the cornea. Ciliary injection engorges the ciliary vessels that run one layer deeper than the conjunctiva. It usually appears as a violaceous (purplish) red ring of injection around the cornea when viewed with a handlight. In patients who have ciliary injection, the eversion of the lower eyelids usually reveals normal appearing conjunctiva. If one touches the conjunctiva with a cotton-tipped applicator, the conjunctiva moves freely and the dilated conjunctival vessels move with it. Deeper dilated vessels, such as the ciliary blood vessels, do not move freely with the conjunctiva. In addition, the placement of dilating drops (ie, vasoconstricting agents) constrict the conjunctival blood vessels, making the eye appear less red, while the deeper episcleral vessels remain dilated and engorged.

Episcleritis is the most common and important form of inflammatory disorder that affects the tunic surrounding the ocular globe. The sclera is continuous with the cornea and the lamina cribosa of the optic nerve. The sclera is composed of collagen and elastic fibers and is subject to involvement with systemic autoimmune disorders (eg, systemic lupus erythematosus and rheumatoid arthritis). The episclera, unlike the sclera, is highly vascularized. Episcleritis is a benign self-limiting, sometimes bilateral, inflammatory process in young adults that presents as a red, somewhat painful eye with occasional watering. The inflammatory reaction is located below the conjunctiva and only over the globe of the eye. Severe pain and photophobia are not characteristic features of episcleritis.

Scleritis is much more painful than episcleritis and results in a reddish purple color. Major signs and symptoms of scleritis include moderate to severe ocular pain, tender and inflamed conjunctiva, and thickened and injected sclera. This form of inflammation may extend into the deeper portions of the eye, such as the choroid. In various forms of advanced scleritis, scleral thinning may occur in a painless variety known as scleromalacia. Scleritis tends to develop progressively over the course of several days. The presence of scleritis should prompt a search for other systemic immune mediated disorders, particularly rheumatoid arthritis and Wegener's granulomatosis.

Uveitis is a significant ocular condition that requires immediate ophthalmologic evaluation. One of the signs of this disorder is circumcorneal injection (ciliary flush), which is often described as a ring of redness that completely encircles the edge (limbus) of the cornea. Pupil size also is helpful when forming the diagnosis of a red eye. In iritis, the affected pupil is usually smaller and sluggish. In acute-angle closure glaucoma attacks, the pupil usually is mid-dilated and sluggish or fixed.

The cornea is examined next. A corneal opacity, seen as a whitish infiltrate, is often a sign of a bacterial corneal ulcer. A corneal ulcer is an ophthalmologic emergency. Fluorescein stains help to differentiate among punctate epithelial defects (diffuse punctate staining), herpes simplex keratitis (dendrite-like shaped staining), and abrasion (large solid area of staining seen after trauma).

Ophthalmic procedures and testing

Allergists and clinical immunologists also should be familiar with some ophthalmic procedures and tests to assist in completing a detailed and thorough history and physical examination, which will assist in confirming a diagnosis of ocular allergy [18,70]. More importantly, these various tests help to differentiate between the many disorders that mimic allergic disorders of the eye.

The Schirmer tear test is the most used and easily performed test for the evaluation of DES. Tear production is assessed by the amount of wetting seen on a folded strip of sterile filter paper after it is placed into the conjunctival sac. The patient is seated and the room lights are dimmed, and the patient is asked to "look up" as the lower eyelid is pulled gently downward. Excess moisture and tears are dried along the eyelid margin and conjunctiva with a sterile cotton-tipped applicator. The rounded end of the test strip is bent at the notch approximately 90°–120° and is hooked into the conjunctival sac at the junction of the middle and lateral one third of the lower eyelid margin. The patient's eyes remain closed throughout the examination. The test strips are removed after 5 minutes. The length of the moistened area from the notch to the flat end of the sterile strip is measured using a millimeter ruler or the scale imprinted on the test strip package. Some of the test strips have a leading edge of tear film that changes color, thus improving the reading of the results. The Schirmer I test (without anesthesia) measures both basal and reflex tearing, and the Schirmer II test (with anesthesia) measures only the basal secretion of tearing and is performed as outlined above, but with topical anesthesia instilled.

Fluorescein is a water-soluble dye used to examine the cornea and conjunctival surfaces. It stains the denuded epithelium. It is placed into the eye either with a sterile fluorescein sodium ophthalmic strip or with a dropper in liquid form. A cobalt blue filter is needed to appreciate the fluorescein-staining pattern of the conjunctiva and cornea. This filter produces a blue hue against the intense green color of the fluorescein dye. The patient is asked to blink several times to spread the fluorescein uniformly and evenly over the entire corneal and conjunctival surface. Soft contact lenses must be removed before fluorescein instillation to prevent their permanent staining. At least 1 hour must pass after completion of the examination before the soft contact lenses can be replaced in the eyes.

Conjunctival scraping also can assist in differentiating various forms of red eye. After the administration of a topical local anesthetic, the palpebral conjunctiva (under the upper lid) is scraped gently several times with a spatula for cytologic examination. The sample is spread on a slide and stained with May-Grunwald, Giemsa or another orthochromatic stain to identify eosinophils or neutrophils. The absence of inflammatory cells does not rule out the diagnosis of allergic conjunctivitis, but the presence of eosinophils strongly suggests it.

Conjunctival and eyelid cultures are obtained using a sterile cotton-tipped applicator moistened in thioglycolate broth. The lower palpebral conjunctiva is wiped lightly with the applicator stick for 5 seconds as the patient is asked to look up. Moistened swabs are preferred, because they pick up and release bacteria better than do dry swabs. Then the sample is placed into the transport medium.

Ocular provocation testing can be likened to "skin testing" of the eye. Known quantities of specific allergen are instilled onto the ocular surface, and the resulting allergic response is measured. This technique is performed commonly by allergists in a research study, especially in the assessment of new drugs against ocular allergies.

Summary

The prevalence of ocular allergy clearly is underappreciated and has been under diagnosed and undertreated. The ocular symptoms associated with the most common ocular allergy conditions, such as SAC and PAC, are twice as likely to affect the allergy sufferer rather than nasal symptoms alone. The differential diagnosis of conjunctivitis is quite broad, with the most common forms associated with allergies, infections, and hormones. There are common features and some discerning features that, with a good history and examination, may provide a more focused and appropriate management.

References

[1] Singh K, Bielory L, Kavosh E. Allergens associated with ocular and nasal symptoms: an epidemiologic study. J Allergy Clin Immunol 2007;119(1 Suppl 1):S223.
[2] Singh K, Bielory L. Ocular allergy: a national epidemiologic study. J Allergy Clin Immunol 2007;119(1 Suppl 1):S154.
[3] Singh K, Bielory L. Epidemiology of ocular allergy symptoms in United States adults (1988–1994). Ann Allergy 2007;(1).
[4] Singh K, Bielory L. Epidemiology of ocular allergy symptoms in regional parts of the United States in the adult population (1988–1994). Ann Allergy 2007;(1).
[5] Bousquet J, Knani J, Hejjaoui A, et al. Heterogeneity of atopy. I. Clinical and immunologic characteristics of patients allergic to cypress pollen. Allergy 1993;48(3):183–8.
[6] Nathan H, Meltzer EO, Selner JC, et al. Prevalence of allergic rhinitis in the United States. J Allergy Clin Immunol 1999;99(6):s808–14.
[7] Juniper EF, Howland WC, Roberts NB, et al. Measuring quality of life in children with rhinoconjunctivitis. J Allergy Clin Immunol 1998;101(2 Pt 1):163–70.
[8] Juniper EF, Thompson AK, Ferrie PJ, et al. Validation of the standardized version of the Rhinoconjunctivitis Quality of Life Questionnaire. J Allergy Clin Immunol 1999;104(2 Pt 1):364–9.
[9] Wuthrich B, Brignoli R, Canevascini M, et al. Epidemiological survey in hay fever patients: symptom prevalence and severity and influence on patient management. Schweiz Med Wochenschr 1998;128(5):139–43.
[10] Palmer RM, Kaufman HE. Tear film, pharmacology of eye drops, and toxicity. Curr Opin Ophthalmol 1995;6(4):11–6.
[11] Spector SL, Raizman MB. Conjunctivitis medicamentosa. J Allergy Clin Immunol 1994; 94(1):134–6.
[12] Soparkar CN, Wilhelmus KR, Koch DD, et al. Acute and chronic conjunctivitis due to over-the-counter ophthalmic decongestants. Arch Ophthalmol 1997;115(1):34–8.
[13] Zierhut M, Schlote T, Tomida II, et al. Immunology of uveitis and ocular allergy. Acta Ophthalmol Scand 2000;78(Suppl 230):22–5.
[14] Udell IJ, Abelson MB. Chemical mediators of inflammation. Int Ophthalmol Clin 1983; 23(1):15–26.
[15] Dinowitz K, Aldave AJ, Lisse JR, et al. Ocular manifestations of immunologic and rheumatologic inflammatory disorders. Curr Opin Ophthalmol 1994;5(6):91–8.
[16] Haynes BF, Fishman ML, Fauci AS, et al. The ocular manifestations of Wegener's granulomatosis. Fifteen years experience and review of the literature. Am J Med 1977;63(1): 131–41.
[17] Bistner S. Allergic- and immunologic-mediated diseases of the eye and adnexae. Vet Clin North Am Small Anim Pract 1994;24(4):711–34.
[18] Dinowitz M, Rescigno R, Bielory L. Ocular allergic diseases: differential diagnosis, examination techniques, and testing. Clin Allergy Immunol 2000;15:127–50.
[19] Butrus SI, Abelson MB. Importance of limbal examination in ocular allergic disease. Ann Ophthalmol 1988;20(3):101–4.
[20] Tuft SJ, Ramakrishnan M, Seal DV, et al. Role of Staphylococcus aureus in chronic allergic conjunctivitis. Ophthalmology 1992;99(2):180–4.

[21] Cvenkel B, Globocnik M. Conjunctival scrapings and impression cytology in chronic conjunctivitis. Correlation with microbiology. Eur J Ophthalmol 1997;7(1):19–23.

[22] Hodges MG, Keane-Myers AM. Classification of ocular allergy. Curr Opin Allergy Clin Immunol 2007;7(5):424–8.

[23] Allansmith MR, Ross RN. Ocular allergy. Clin Allergy 1988;18(1):1–13.

[24] Rothenberg ME, Owen WF Jr, Stevens RL. Ocular allergy. Mast cells and eosinophils. Int Ophthalmol Clin 1988;28(4):267–74.

[25] Leonardi A. The central role of conjunctival mast cells in the pathogenesis of ocular allergy. Curr Allergy Asthma Rep 2002;2(4):325–31.

[26] Udell IJ, Kenyon KR, Hanninen LA, et al. Time course of human conjunctival mast cell degranulation in response to compound 48/80. Acta Ophthalmol Suppl 1989;192:154–61.

[27] Li Q, Luyo D, Hikita N, et al. Compound 48/80-induced conjunctivitis in the mouse: kinetics, susceptibility, and mechanism. Int Arch Allergy Immunol 1996;109(3):277–85.

[28] Woodward DF, Ledgard SE, Nieves AL. Conjunctival immediate hypersensitivity: re-evaluation of histamine involvement in the vasopermeability response. Invest Ophthalmol Vis Sci 1986;27(1):57–63.

[29] Bachert C. Histamine–a major role in allergy? Clin Exp Allergy 1998;28(Suppl 6):15–9.

[30] Leonardi AA, Smith LM, Fregona IA, et al. Tear histamine and histaminase during the early (EPR) and late (LPR) phases of the allergic reaction and the effects of lodoxamide. Eur J Ophthalmol 1996;6(2):106–12.

[31] Lightman S. Therapeutic considerations: symptoms, cells and mediators. Allergy 1995; 50(Suppl 21):10–3 [discussion: 34–8].

[32] Struck HG, Wicht A, Ponicke K, et al. [Histamine in tears in allergic rhinoconjunctivitis]. Ophthalmologe 1998;95(4):241–6.

[33] Kari O, Salo OP, Halmepuro L, et al. Tear histamine during allergic conjunctivitis challenge. Graefes Arch Clin Exp Ophthalmol 1985;223(2):60–2.

[34] Trocme SD, Aldave AJ. The eye and the eosinophil. Surv Ophthalmol 1994;39(3):241–52.

[35] Hingorani M, Calder V, Jolly G, et al. Eosinophil surface antigen expression and cytokine production vary in different ocular allergic diseases. J Allergy Clin Immunol 1998;102(5): 821–30.

[36] Leonardi A, Borghesan F, Avarello A, et al. Effect of lodoxamide and disodium cromoglycate on tear eosinophil cationic protein in vernal keratoconjunctivitis. Br J Ophthalmol 1997;81(1):23–6.

[37] Bielory L. Ocular allergy and dry eye syndrome. Curr Opin Allergy Clin Immunol 2004; 4(5):421–4.

[38] Bielory L. Allergic and immunologic disorders of the eye. Part II: ocular allergy. J Allergy Clin Immunol 2000;106(6):1019–32.

[39] Bielory L. Allergic and immunologic disorders of the eye. Part I: immunology of the eye. J Allergy Clin Immunol 2000;106(5):805–16.

[40] Gary RK Jr, Woodward DF, Nieves AL, et al. Characterization of the conjunctival vasopermeability response to leukotrienes and their involvement in immediate hypersensitivity. Invest Ophthalmol Vis Sci 1988;29(1):119–26.

[41] Woodward DF, Nieves AL, Williams LS, et al. Interactive effects of peptidoleukotrienes and histamine on microvascular permeability and their involvement in experimental cutaneous and conjunctival immediate hypersensitivity. Eur J Pharmacol 1989;164(2): 323–33.

[42] Simons FE. H1-receptor antagonists: does a dose-response relationship exist? Ann Allergy 1993;71(6):592–7.

[43] Umemoto M, Tanaka H, Miichi H, et al. Histamine receptors on rat ocular surface. Ophthalmic Res 1987;19(4):200–4.

[44] Cook EB, Stahl JL, Barney NP, et al. Mechanisms of antihistamines and mast cell stabilizers in ocular allergic inflammation. Curr Drug Targets Inflamm Allergy 2002;1(2): 167–80.

[45] Bielory L, Ghafoor S. Histamine receptors and the conjunctiva. Curr Opin Allergy Clin Immunol 2005;5(5):437–40.

[46] Abelson MB, Udell IJ. H2-receptors in the human ocular surface. Arch Ophthalmol 1981; 99(2):302–4.

[47] McGill J. Conjunctival cytokines in ocular allergy. Clin Exp Allergy 2000;30(10):1355–7.

[48] Foster CS. The pathophysiology of ocular allergy: current thinking. Allergy 1995;50(Suppl 21):6–9 [discussion: 34–8].

[49] Bonini S, Bonini S. IgE and non-IgE mechanisms in ocular allergy. Ann Allergy 1993;71(3): 296–9.

[50] Metz DP, Bacon AS, Holgate S, et al. Phenotypic characterization of T cells infiltrating the conjunctiva in chronic allergic eye disease. J Allergy Clin Immunol 1996;98(3):686–96.

[51] Dursun D, Wang M, Monroy D, et al. Experimentally induced dry eye produces ocular surface inflammation and epithelial disease. Adv Exp Med Biol 2002;506(Pt A):647–55.

[52] Stern ME, Gao J, Siemasko KF, et al. The role of the lacrimal functional unit in the pathophysiology of dry eye. Exp Eye Res 2004;78(3):409–16.

[53] Gao J, Morgan G, Tieu D, et al. ICAM-1 expression predisposes ocular tissues to immune-based inflammation in dry eye patients and Sjogrens syndrome-like MRL/lpr mice. Exp Eye Res 2004;78(4):823–35.

[54] Bielory L. Differential diagnoses of conjunctivitis for clinical allergist-immunologists. Ann Allergy Asthma Immunol 2007;98(2):105–14, quiz 114–7, 152.

[55] Nowak D, Wichmann HE, Magnusson H. Asthma and atopy in Western and Eastern communities–current status and open questions. Clin Exp Allergy 1998;28(9):1043–6.

[56] Sly RM. Changing prevalence of allergic rhinitis and asthma. Ann Allergy Asthma Immunol 1999;82(3):233–48, quiz 248–52.

[57] Strachan D, Sibbald B, Weiland S, et al. Worldwide variations in prevalence of symptoms of allergic rhinoconjunctivitis in children: the International Study of Asthma and Allergies in Childhood (ISAAC). Pediatr Allergy Immunol 1997;8(4):161–76.

[58] Noon L, Cantab B. Prophylactic inoculation against hay fever. Lancet 1911;1572–3.

[59] Friedlaender MH. Management of ocular allergy. Ann Allergy Asthma Immunol 1995; 75(3):212–22, quiz 223–4.

[60] Bielory L. Chapter 5: Allergic and immunologic disorders of the eye. In: Adelman DC, Corren J, Casale T, editors. Manual of allergy and immunology. 4th edition. Philadelphia: Lippincott Williams and Wilkins; 2002. p. 75–92.

[61] Dart JK, Buckley RJ, Monnickendan M, et al. Perennial allergic conjunctivitis: definition, clinical characteristics and prevalence. A comparison with seasonal allergic conjunctivitis. Trans Ophthalmol Soc U K 1986;105(Pt 5):513–20.

[62] Boquete M, Carballada F, Armisen M, et al. Factors influencing the clinical picture and the differential sensitization to house dust mites and storage mites. J Investig Allergol Clin Immunol 2000;10(4):229–34.

[63] Valdivieso R, Acosta ME, Estupinan M. Dust mites but not grass pollen are important sensitizers in asthmatic children in the Ecuadorian Andes. J Investig Allergol Clin Immunol 1999;9(5):288–92.

[64] Bertel F, Mortemousque B, Sicard H, et al. [Conjunctival provocation test with Dermatophagoides pteronyssinus in the diagnosis of allergic conjunctivitis from house mites]. J Fr Ophtalmol 2001;24(6):581–9.

[65] van Hage-Hamsten M, Johansson SG, Zetterstrom O. Predominance of mite allergy over allergy to pollens and animal danders in a farming population. Clin Allergy 1987;17(5): 417–23.

[66] Montan PG, Ekstrom K, Hedlin G, et al. Vernal keratoconjunctivitis in a Stockholm ophthalmic centre–epidemiological, functional, and immunologic investigations. Acta Ophthalmol Scand 1999;77(5):559–63.

[67] Tanaka M, Dogru M, Takano Y, et al. The relation of conjunctival and corneal findings in severe ocular allergies. Cornea 2004;23(5):464–7.

[68] Bonini S, Lambiase A, Marchi S, et al. Vernal keratoconjunctivitis revisited: a case series of 195 patients with long-term followup. Ophthalmology 2000;107(6):1157–63.

[69] Rehany U, Rumelt S. Corneal hydrops associated with vernal conjunctivitis as a presenting sign of keratoconus in children. Ophthalmology 1995;102(12):2046–9.

[70] Bielory L, Dinowitz M, Rescigno R. Ocular allergic diseases: differential diagnosis, examination techniques and testing. J Toxicol Cutaneous Ocul Toxicol 2002;21:329–51.

[71] Giuri S. [Corneal ulcerative lesions in type-I immediate hypersensitivity]. Oftalmologia 1998;44(3):20–6.

[72] Tabbara KF. Ocular complications of vernal keratoconjunctivitis. Can J Ophthalmol 1999; 34(2):88–92.

[73] Casey R, Abelson MB. Atopic keratoconjunctivitis. Int Ophthalmol Clin 1997;37(2):111–7.

[74] Tuft SJ, et al. Clinical features of atopic keratoconjunctivitis. Ophthalmology 1991;98(2): 150–8.

[75] Bonini S, Lambiase A, Matricardi P, et al. Atopic and vernal keratoconjunctivitis: a model for studying atopic disease. Curr Probl Dermatol 1999;28:88–94.

[76] Power WJ, Tugal-Tutkun I, Foster CS. Long-term follow-up of patients with atopic keratoconjunctivitis. Ophthalmology 1998;105(4):637–42.

[77] Bielory L, Goodman PE, Fisher EM. Allergic ocular disease. A review of pathophysiology and clinical presentations. Clin Rev Allergy Immunol 2001;20(2):183–200.

[78] Norris PG, Rivers JK. Screening for cataracts in patients with severe atopic eczema. Clin Exp Dermatol 1987;12(1):21–2.

[79] Ibarra-Duran MG, Mena-Cedillos CA, Rodriguez-Almaraz M. [Cataracts and atopic dermatitis in children. A study of 68 patients]. Bol Med Hosp Infant Mex 1992;49(12): 851–5.

[80] Ohmachi N, Sasabe T, Kojima M, et al. [Eye complications in atopic dermatitis]. Arerugi 1994;43(7):796–9.

[81] Hutnik CM, Nichols BD. Cataracts in systemic diseases and syndromes. Curr Opin Ophthalmol 1999;10(1):22–8.

[82] Castrow FF II. Atopic cataracts versus steroid cataracts. J Am Acad Dermatol 1981;5(1): 64–6.

[83] Chan LS, Robinson N, Xu L. Expression of interleukin-4 in the epidermis of transgenic mice results in a pruritic inflammatory skin disease: an experimental animal model to study atopic dermatitis. J Invest Dermatol 2001;117(4):977–83.

[84] Nivenius E, Montan PG, Chryssanthou E, et al. No apparent association between periocular and ocular microcolonization and the degree of inflammation in patients with atopic keratoconjunctivitis. Clin Exp Allergy 2004;34(5):725–30.

[85] Katelaris CH. Giant papillary conjunctivitis–a review. Acta Ophthalmol Scand Suppl 1999;(228):17–20.

[86] Calonge M. Classification of ocular atopic/allergic disorders and conditions: an unsolved problem. Acta Ophthalmol Scand Suppl 1999;(228):10–3.

[87] Palmisano PC, Ehlers WH, Donshik PC. Causative factors in unilateral giant papillary conjunctivitis. CLAO J 1993;19(2):103–7.

[88] Mondino BJ, Salamon SM, Zaidman GW. Allergic and toxic reactions of soft contact lens wearers. Surv Ophthalmol 1982;26(6):337–44.

[89] Meisler DM, Krachmer JH, Goeken JA. An immunopathologic study of giant papillary conjunctivitis associated with an ocular prosthesis. Am J Ophthalmol 1981;92(3):368–71.

[90] Ballow M, Donshik PC, Rapacz P, et al. Immune responses in monkeys to lenses from patients with contact lens induced giant papillary conjunctivitis. CLAO J 1989;15(1): 64–70.

[91] Berdy GJ, Hedqvist B. Ocular allergic disorders and dry eye disease: associations, diagnostic dilemmas, and management. Acta Ophthalmol Scand Suppl 2000;(230):32–7.

[92] Stern ME, Beuerman RW, Fox RI, et al. The pathology of dry eye: the interaction between the ocular surface and lacrimal glands. Cornea 1998;17(6):584–9.

[93] The definition and classification of dry eye disease: report of the Definition and Classification Subcommittee of the International Dry Eye WorkShop (2007). Ocul Surf 2007;5(2): 75–92.

[94] The epidemiology of dry eye disease: report of the Epidemiology Subcommittee of the International Dry Eye WorkShop (2007). Ocul Surf 2007;5(2):93–107.

[95] Pflugfelder SC. Differential diagnosis of dry eye conditions. Adv Dent Res 1996;10(1):9–12.

[96] Michelson PE. Red eye unresponsive to treatment. West J Med 1997;166(2):145–7.

[97] Fujishima H, Toda I, Shimazaki J, et al. Allergic conjunctivitis and dry eye. Br J Ophthalmol 1996;80(11):994–7.

[98] Moss SE, Klein R, Klein BE. Incidence of dry eye in an older population. Arch Ophthalmol 2004;122(3):369–73.

[99] Chronister CL. Review of external ocular disease associated with aids and HIV infection. Optom Vis Sci 1996;73(4):225–30.

[100] Pflugfelder SC. Hormonal deficiencies and dry eye. Arch Ophthalmol 2004;122(2):273–4.

[101] Ousler GW, Wilcox KA, Gupta G, et al. An evaluation of the ocular drying effects of 2 systemic antihistamines: loratadine and cetirizine hydrochloride. Ann Allergy Asthma Immunol 2004;93(5):460–4.

[102] Burstein NL. The effects of topical drugs and preservatives on the tears and corneal epithelium in dry eye. Trans Ophthalmol Soc U K 1985;104(Pt 4):402–9.

[103] Pflugfelder SC. Antiinflammatory therapy for dry eye. Am J Ophthalmol 2004;137(2): 337–42.

[104] Calonge M. The treatment of dry eye. Surv Ophthalmol 2001;45(Suppl 2):S227–39.

[105] Calonge M. Ocular allergies: association with immune dermatitis. Acta Ophthalmol Scand Suppl 2000;(230):69–75.

[106] Zug KA, Palay DA, Rock B. Dermatologic diagnosis and treatment of itchy red eyelids. Surv Ophthalmol 1996;40(4):293–306.

[107] Bielory L, Wagner RS. Allergic and immunologic pediatric disorders of the eye. J Investig Allergol Clin Immunol 1995;5(6):309–17.

[108] Gurwood AS, Altenderfer DS. Contact dermatitis. Optometry 2001;72(1):36–44.

[109] Anibarro B, Barranco P, Ojeda JA. Allergic contact blepharoconjunctivitis caused by phenylephrine eyedrops. Contact Dermatitis 1991;25(5):323–4.

[110] Rafael M, Pereira F, Faria MA. Allergic contact blepharoconjunctivitis caused by phenylephrine, associated with persistent patch test reaction. Contact Dermatitis 1998;39(3): 143–4.

[111] Wilson FM II. Adverse external ocular effects of topical ophthalmic medications. Surv Ophthalmol 1979;24(2):57–88.

[112] de Groot AC, Beverdam EG, Ayong CT, et al. The role of contact allergy in the spectrum of adverse effects caused by cosmetics and toiletries. Contact Dermatitis 1988;19(3):195–201.

[113] Estlander T, Kari O, Jolanki R, et al. Occupational conjunctivitis associated with type IV allergy to methacrylates. Allergy 1996;51(1):56–9.

[114] Estlander T, Kari O, Jolanki R, et al. Occupational allergic contact dermatitis and blepharoconjunctivitis caused by gold. Contact Dermatitis 1998;38(1):40–1.

[115] Fisher AA. Allergic contact dermatitis and conjunctivitis from benzalkonium chloride. Cutis 1987;39(5):381–3.

[116] Fuchs T, Meinert A, Aberer W, et al. [Benzalkonium chloride–a relevant contact allergen or irritant? Results of a multicenter study of the German Contact Allergy Group]. Hautarzt 1993;44(11):699–702.

[117] Stern GA, Killingsworth DW. Complications of topical antimicrobial agents. Int Ophthalmol Clin 1989;29(3):137–42.

[118] Tosti A, Tosti G. Thimerosal: a hidden allergen in ophthalmology. Contact Dermatitis 1988;18(5):268–73.

[119] Gaspari AA. Contact allergy to ophthalmic dipivalyl epinephrine hydrochloride: demonstration by patch testing. Contact Dermatitis 1993;28(1):35–7.

[120] Marsh RJ, Towns S, Evans KF. Patch testing in ocular drug allergies. Trans Ophthalmol Soc U K 1978;98(2):278–80.

[121] Villarreal O. Reliability of diagnostic tests for contact allergy to mydriatic eyedrops. Contact Dermatitis 1998;38(3):150–4.

[122] Mannis MJ. Allergic blepharoconjunctivitis. Avoiding misdiagnosis and mismanagement. Postgrad Med 1989;86(4):123–9.

[123] Resano A, Esteve C, Fernandez Benitez M. Allergic contact blepharoconjunctivitis due to phenylephrine eye drops. J Investig Allergol Clin Immunol 1999;9(1):55–7.

[124] Kaiserman I. Severe allergic blepharoconjunctivitis induced by a dye for eyelashes and eyebrows. Ocul Immunol Inflamm 2003;11(2):149–51.

[125] O'Callaghan RJ. Role of exoproteins in bacterial keratitis: the Fourth Annual Thygeson Lecture, presented at the Ocular Microbiology and Immunology Group Meeting, November 7, 1998. Cornea 1999;18(5):532–7.

[126] Leung DY, Meissner HC, Fulton DR, et al. Toxic shock syndrome toxin-secreting Staphylococcus aureus in Kawasaki syndrome. Lancet 1993;342(8884):1385–8.

[127] Marrack P, Kappler J. The staphylococcal enterotoxins and their relatives. Science 1990; 248(4959):1066.

[128] Seal DV, McGill JI, Jacobs P, et al. Microbial and immunological investigations of chronic non-ulcerative blepharitis and meibomianitis. Br J Ophthalmol 1985;69(8):604–11.

[129] Weber CM, Eichenbaum JW. Acute red eye. Differentiating viral conjunctivitis from other, less common causes. Postgrad Med 1997;101(5):185–6, 189–92, 195–6.

[130] Rao SK, Madhavan HN, Padmanabhan P, et al. Ocular chlamydial infections. Clinicomicrobiological correlation. Cornea 1996;15(1):62–5.

[131] Chung CW, Cohen EJ. Eye disorders: bacterial conjunctivitis. West J Med 2000;173(3): 202–5.

[132] Chisari G, Reibaldi M. Ciprofloxacin as treatment for conjunctivitis. J Chemother 2004; 16(2):156–9.

[133] Rietveld RP, van Weert HC, ter Riet G, et al. Diagnostic impact of signs and symptoms in acute infectious conjunctivitis: systematic literature search. BMJ 2003;327(7418): 789.

[134] Weinstock FJ, Weinstock MB. Common eye disorders: six patients to treat, pitfalls to avoid. Postgrad Med 1996;99(4):119–23.

[135] Ruppert SD. Differential diagnosis of pediatric conjunctivitis (red eye). Nurse Pract 1996; 21(7):12, 15–8, 24 Passim.

[136] Bodtger U. Prognostic value of asymptomatic skin sensitization to aeroallergens. Curr Opin Allergy Clin Immunol 2004;4(1):5–10.

[137] Bodtger U, Poulsen LK, Malling HJ. Asymptomatic skin sensitization to birch predicts later development of birch pollen allergy in adults: a 3-year follow-up study. J Allergy Clin Immunol 2003;111(1):149–54.

[138] Sivko MT. [Vasomotor conjunctivitis]. Oftalmol Zh 1971;26(4):306–7.

[139] Bielory L. Vasomotor (perennial chronic) conjunctivitis. Curr Opin Allergy Clin Immunol 2006;6(5):355–60.

[140] Feniksova LV, Rybalkin SV, Pekli FF. [Study of the changes in microcirculatory bed in children with vasomotor rhinitis based on biomicroscopy of conjunctival blood vessels]. Vestn Otorinolaringol 1990;(4):42–4.

[141] Sacchetti M, Lambiase A, Aronni S, et al. Hyperosmolar conjunctival provocation for the evaluation of nonspecific hyperreactivity in healthy patients and patients with allergy. J Allergy Clin Immunol 2006;118(4):872–7.

[142] Lindgren T, Andersson K, Dammstrom BG, et al. Ocular, nasal, dermal and general symptoms among commercial airline crews. Int Arch Occup Environ Health 2002;75(7): 475–83.

[143] Enberg RN. Perennial nonallergic rhinitis: a retrospective review. Ann Allergy 1989;63 (6 Pt 1):513–6.

[144] Leynaert B, Bousquet J, Neukirch C, et al. Perennial rhinitis: an independent risk factor for asthma in nonatopic subjects: results from the European Community Respiratory Health Survey. J Allergy Clin Immunol 1999;104(2 Pt 1):301–4.

[145] Mullarkey MF, Hill JS, Webb DR. Allergic and nonallergic rhinitis: their characterization with attention to the meaning of nasal eosinophilia. J Allergy Clin Immunol 1980;65(2):122–6.

[146] Davies RJ, Rusznak C, Devalia JL. Why is allergy increasing?–environmental factors. Clin Exp Allergy 1998;28(Suppl 6):8–14.

[147] Rusznak C, Devalia JL, Davies RJ. The impact of pollution on allergic disease. Allergy 1994;49(Suppl 18):21–7.

[148] Riedl MA, Landaw EM, Saxon A, et al. Initial high-dose nasal allergen exposure prevents allergic sensitization to a neoantigen. J Immunol 2005;174(11):7440–5.

[149] Devouassoux G, Landaw EM, Saxon A, et al. Chemical constituents of diesel exhaust particles induce IL-4 production and histamine release by human basophils. J Allergy Clin Immunol 2002;109(5):847–53.

[150] Diaz-Sanchez D, Penichet-Garcia M, Saxon A. Diesel exhaust particles directly induce activated mast cells to degranulate and increase histamine levels and symptom severity. J Allergy Clin Immunol 2000;106(6):1140–6.

[151] Saxon A, Diaz-Sanchez D. Diesel exhaust as a model xenobiotic in allergic inflammation. Immunopharmacology 2000;48(3):325–7.

[152] Diaz-Sanchez D, Garcia MP, Wang M, et al. Nasal challenge with diesel exhaust particles can induce sensitization to a neoallergen in the human mucosa. J Allergy Clin Immunol 1999;104(6):1183–8.

[153] Nel AE, Diaz-Sanchez D, Ng D, et al. Enhancement of allergic inflammation by the interaction between diesel exhaust particles and the immune system. J Allergy Clin Immunol 1998;102(4 Pt 1):539–54.

[154] Diaz-Sanchez D, Tsien A, Fleming J, et al. Combined diesel exhaust particulate and ragweed allergen challenge markedly enhances human in vivo nasal ragweed-specific IgE and skews cytokine production to a T helper cell 2-type pattern. J Immunol 1997;158(5):2406–13.

[155] Peterson B, Saxon A. Global increases in allergic respiratory disease: the possible role of diesel exhaust particles. Ann Allergy Asthma Immunol 1996;77(4):263–8, quiz 269–70.

[156] Takenaka H, Zhang K, Diaz-Sanchez D, et al. Enhanced human IgE production results from exposure to the aromatic hydrocarbons from diesel exhaust: direct effects on B-cell IgE production. J Allergy Clin Immunol 1995;95(1 Pt 1):103–15.

[157] Pastorello EA, Codecasa LR, Pravettoni V, et al. Clinical reliability of diagnostic tests in allergic rhinoconjunctivitis. Boll Ist Sieroter Milan 1988;67(5–6):377–85.

ELSEVIER
SAUNDERS

Immunol Allergy Clin N Am
28 (2008) 25–42

IMMUNOLOGY
AND ALLERGY
CLINICS
OF NORTH AMERICA

Ocular Mast Cells and Mediators

Anne-Marie A. Irani, MD*

*Division of Pediatric Allergy, Immunology, and Rheumatology, Virginia Commonwealth
University Health System, 1112 East Clay Street, Mc Guire Hall Annex Room 4-421,
Richmond, VA 23229, USA*

Mast cells have long been recognized for their role in immediate hypersensitivity reactions, by virtue of the presence of high affinity receptors for IgE (FcεRI) on their surface. More recently, mast cells have been postulated to be involved in a variety of chronic inflammatory disorders as numerous mediators released by activated mast cells are characterized. This article summarizes current information on mast cell mediators, heterogeneity, and differentiation, and it reviews studies of mast cells in the normal eye and various ocular disorders.

Mast cell mediators

The humoral and cellular inflammatory responses occurring during immediate hypersensitivity reactions are initiated by numerous mediators of mast cells and possibly by basophils. Some mediators are stored preformed inside the secretory granules of mast cells and are released rapidly upon mast cell activation by a process of regulated secretion or degranulation. Other mediators are synthesized de novo upon mast cell activation and are released without a prolonged intracellular storage phase after variable time intervals. In humans, the principal preformed mediators of mast cells include histamine, proteoglycans, neutral proteases, and possibly, basic fibroblast growth factor. Newly generated mediators include the arachidonic acid metabolites prostaglandin (PG) D_2, and leukotriene (LT) C_4, and TH2-like cytokines such as interleukins (IL) 4, 5, 6, and 13, and tumor necrosis factor-α (TNF-α).

Portions of this article previously appeared in Irani A. Ocular mast cells and mediators. Immunol Allergy Clin North Am 1997;17(1):1–18.

* Virginia Commonwealth University, Box 980225, Richmond, VA 23298-0225, USA.
E-mail address: airani@vcu.edu

doi:10.1016/j.iac.2007.12.006
immunology.theclinics.com

Preformed granule-associated mediators

Biogenic amines

Histamine is stored in secretory granules of mast cells, is bound to carboxyl and sulfate groups on proteins and proteoglycans, and is the sole biogenic amine in human mast cells and basophils. Human mast cells contain 1 to 5 pg of histamine per cell [1], which is equivalent to a concentration of 0.1 M inside the secretory granules. In contrast, plasma histamine concentration averages 2 nM. Intermediate concentrations in various biologic fluids, such as nasal lavage fluid, reflect local rates of production and diffusion or metabolism. After mast cell degranulation, released histamine is metabolized within minutes. Elevated levels of histamine in plasma or urine are found following anaphylactic reactions and indicate mast cell or basophil involvement. Histamine exerts potent biologic effects through its interaction with cell-specific receptors designated H1, H2, and H3 receptors [2–4]. Stimulation of H1 receptors results in vasodilation and increased capillary permeability, contraction of bronchial and gastrointestinal smooth muscle, and increased mucous secretion at mucosal sites. H2 receptor agonists stimulate gastric acid secretion and exert numerous effects on cells of the immune system, including augmentation of suppression by T lymphocytes [2], inhibition of mediator secretion by cytotoxic lymphocytes and granulocytes, and suppression of eosinophil chemotaxis [5]. Additional effects include activation of endothelial cells to release prostacyclin, a potent inhibitor of platelet aggregation. Stimulation of H3 receptors affects neurotransmitter release and histamine production in the central and peripheral nervous system [6]. H3 receptors are postulated to mediate interactions between mast cells and peripheral nerves, and they may be involved in histamine-mediated neurogenic hyperexcitability.

Proteoglycans

The presence of highly sulfated proteoglycans in secretory granules of mast cells confers the metachromatic staining properties of these cells when stained with basic dyes, such as toluidine blue or alcian blue. In human mast cells, heparin and chondroitin sulfate E are the major intracellular proteoglycans [7,8]. Heparin is found in all mature mast cells [9], but not in other cell types. The biologic functions of endogenous mast cell proteoglycans await further clarification. These proteoglycans bind to histamine, neutral proteases, and acid hydrolases at the acidic pH found inside the mast cell secretory granules, and may play an important role in intracellular packaging. Heparin facilitates processing of chymase and tryptase forms to their active forms. The stabilizing effect of heparin and (to a lesser degree) chondroitin sulfate E on tryptase activity may be critical for mast cell physiology [10,11]. Heparin and (to a lesser extent) chondroitin sulfate E express anticoagulant, anticomplement, and antikallikrein activities.

Heparin facilitates fibroblast growth factor activity in cutaneous mast cells [12,13] and modulates the cell adhesion properties of matrix proteins, such as vitronectin, fibronectin, and laminin.

Neutral proteases

Neutral proteases cleave peptide bonds near neutral pH and are the dominant protein components of secretory granules in rodent and human mast cells [14]. These enzymes also serve as selective markers that distinguish mast cells from other cell types and distinguish different types of mast cells from one another. Tryptase is a serine class protease with tryptic-like activity [15,16]. It is stored in secretory granules bound to heparin, which is essential for tryptase to retain its enzymatic activity [10], and it is not inhibited by biologic inhibitors of serine proteases present in plasma and urine. Tryptase is present in all mast cells at concentrations that vary from 10 pg per mast cell derived from the lung to 35 pg per mast cell derived from the skin [1]. Negligible amounts have been detected in human basophils (0.04 pg/cell) [17], but not in any other cell type. Tryptase is released together with histamine during degranulation [18] and serves as a specific marker of human mast cells. At least two homologous tryptase genes, termed α and β, have been identified on human chromosome 16, and the corresponding recombinant proteins have been synthesized [19–21]. A mutation in the leader sequence of α-tryptase prevents it from processing to a mature form and packaging in secretory granules. Thus, α-protryptase is thought to be constitutively secreted, is enzymatically inactive, and is the principal form of tryptase detected in the peripheral circulation in normal controls. Mature β-tryptase is the principal form of tryptase stored in secretory granules, is enzymatically active, is usually undetectable in normal controls, and is released during mast cell degranulation. Therefore, elevated serum levels of α/β-protryptases reflect mast cell hyperplasia such as what occurs in systemic mastocytosis, whereas elevated serum levels of mature β-tryptase reflect mast cell activation such as what occurs in systemic anaphylaxis [22]. Because β-tryptase accounts for all of the tryptase enzymatic activity, it is the principal form measured by enzymatic assays, whereas the currently commercially available tryptase immunoreactive assay (Pharmacia, Uppsala, Sweden) measures a combination of α and β tryptases. Potential biologic activities of tryptase include inactivation of fibrinogen, with subsequent anticoagulant effect, which explains the lack of fibrin deposition in reactions involving urticaria and angioedema, and consequently, their rapid resolution [23]. Tryptase augments histamine constriction effects on airway smooth muscles [24] and degrades vasoactive intestinal peptide (an intrinsic neuropeptide with bronchodilating properties), effects that may result in increased bronchospasm. In synovial cells derived from subjects who have rheumatoid arthritis, tryptase activates latent collagenase [25]. Tryptase stimulates growth of smooth muscle cells and fibroblasts in vitro [26,27].

The recent development of tryptase inhibitors as potential therapeutics should help better identify the physiologic role of this enzyme in vivo.

Chymase is a serine protease with chymotryptic-like activity that was purified from human skin [28], and the corresponding gene was cloned and localized to human chromosome 14 [29]. Like tryptase, chymase is bound to heparin but remains stable after dissociation from heparin [30]. Chymase activity is inhibited by the classical biologic inhibitors of serine proteases, such as α_1-antichymotrypsin, α_1-proteinase inhibitor, and α_2-macroglobulin [31]. Dispersed skin mast cells contain 4.5 pg of chymase per cell, whereas neither chymotrypsin enzymatic activity nor chymase mRNA are detected in lung mast cells, thus localizing chymase to a subpopulation of human mast cells [17,32]. Potential biologic activity of chymase includes potent activation of angiotensin I [33] and procollagenase [34] and inactivation of bradykinin [35]. Chymase digests the lamina lucida of the basement membrane at the dermal-epidermal junction of human skin [36] and degrades substance P, vasoactive intestinal peptide, and probably other neuropeptides [37,38]. Dog chymase stimulates mucus production from glandular cells in vitro [39], suggesting a similar role in allergic disorders at various organ sites, such as mucous hypersecretion in asthma and allergic rhinitis and mucous hypersecretion in allergic ocular disorders.

Cathepsin G is a serine neutral protease with chymotryptic activity that colocalizes with chymase in human mast cells [28]. It also is found in neutrophils and monocytes and therefore cannot be used as a specific marker of mast cells. Human mast cell carboxypeptidase also resides with chymase and cathepsin G in a subpopulation of human mast cells [40]. It cleaves the carboxyterminal His^9/Leu^{10} bond of angiotensin I and behaves like a zinc metalloexopeptidase; it is inhibited by o-phenanthroline [41]. Dispersed human skin mast cells contain 5 to 16 pg of carboxypeptidase per cell.

Newly generated mediators

Lipid mediators

Unstimulated human mast cells incorporate exogenous arachidonic acid into membrane and cytoplasmic lipid [42]. Upon activation of mast cells, arachidonate released by hydrolysis of these lipids is metabolized along the cyclooxygenase pathway, giving rise to PGs and thromboxanes, or (along the lipoxygenase pathway) LTs. Dispersed preparations of human mast cells obtained from lung, skin, or small intestine and subjected to activation produce PGD_2, in excess over LTC_4, and smaller amounts of LTB_4 [43]. In contrast, activated basophils produce LTC_4, but no PGD_2. The production of arachidonic acid metabolites begins within minutes of cell activation and lasts up to about 30 minutes. These mediators also are produced by many other cell types, and their detection in biologic fluids cannot be used as a specific marker of mast cell or basophil activation. Relative production of these lipid mediators cannot be used to distinguish various types of mast cells. The biologic activity of arachidonic acid metabolites has been underscored by the favorable clinical effects of 5-lipoxygenase inhibitors in atopic and aspirin-induced asthma, where mast cell activation occurs [44]. PGD_2 production may be involved in the pathogenesis of recurrent hypotensive episodes in a subgroup of subjects who have systemic mastocytosis, as evidenced by clinical improvement following inhibition of cyclooxygenase with aspirin [45].

Cytokines

Upon activation, human mast cells produce an array of cytokines, including up-regulation of the IL-4 gene cluster on human chromosome 5 (IL-4, IL-5, IL-6, IL-9, IL-13, and granulocyte macrophage-colony-stimulating factor), and of TNF-α on human chromosome 6 [46–48]. Mast cells preferentially produce IL-13 over IL-4 as opposed to basophils, which produce more IL-4. Cytokine production occurs minutes to hours following mast cell activation. Cytokines derived from activated mast cells serve to activate endothelial cells to recruit eosinophils and other inflammatory cell types at the site of immediate hypersensitivity reactions, thus giving rise to the late phase of allergic response and sustained inflammation. These cytokines also may be involved in modulating the local distribution of the Th1 and Th2 types of T lymphocytes, thereby expanding the biologic role of mast cells far beyond type I hypersensitivity reactions only.

In conjunctival biopsy specimens obtained from normal subjects, and those with seasonal allergic conjunctivitis during and outside the pollen season, mast cells comprised greater than 90% of IL-4$^+$ immunoreactive cells and the majority of IL-5$^+$, IL-6$^+$, and IL-13$^+$ cells [49].

Mast cell heterogeneity

Phenotypic heterogeneity

Mast cell heterogeneity was recognized first in the rodent system with the early work of Enerback and colleagues [14], who demonstrated variations in the metachromatic staining properties of rat mast cells based on the type of fixative. Thus, mast cells in the gastrointestinal mucosa required fixation in Carnoys fluid or in isotonic formaldehyde acetic acid to be visualized with metachromatic stains and were referred to as "mucosal mast cells" or "formalin-sensitive mast cells". Mast cells in the skin and the peritoneal cavity were seen easily with metachromatic stains after fixation in formalin and the previously mentioned fixatives, and they were termed "connective-tissue mast cells" or "formalin-resistant mast cells".

A similar differentiation was difficult to reproduce in the human system. Instead, differentiation of human mast cells based on their neutral protease content was demonstrated first in 1986 [32]. At least two types of mast cells were defined in humans. MC_T cells were found to contain tryptase, but none of the other mast cell proteases, whereas MC_{TC} cells contained tryptase and chymase, cathepsin G, and human mast cell carboxypeptidase [50,51]. These proteases appear to reflect qualitative differences, as evidenced by a lack of chymase mRNA and the enzyme in morphologically mature MC_T cells [17]. Furthermore, cultured MC_T cells from lungs remained deficient in chymase protein and chymase mRNA [52]. MC_T cells were found to predominate in the gastrointestinal mucosa of the small intestine and in the alveolar lining and epithelium of the lung, whereas MC_{TC} cells predominated in the skin and in gastrointestinal submucosa of the small intestine [32]. The subepithelium of the nasal mucosa and the bronchial walls contained a mixture of both types of mast cells. More recently, mature MC_{TC} cells obtained from human lung and skin preparations were shown to express surface CD88 (C5aR) and could be separated from MC_T cells by cell sorting [52]. The relative abundance of MC_T and MC_{TC} cells varies with tissue inflammation or fibrosis [53,54], and the protease phenotype cannot be deduced based on location alone. Therefore, the nomenclature of mucosal mast cells and connective tissue mast cells appeared inadequate in this system. Mast cell heterogeneity based on differential expression of various neutral proteases was characterized later in the mouse system by the elegant experiments of Stevens and colleagues [55,56]. Variations in expressions of mouse mast cell proteases 1 through 7 were demonstrated initially at the message level and were demonstrated later at the protein level as well; variations depended on stages of maturation of the mast cells and tissue localization, suggesting that local environmental factors were involved in directing mast cell differentiation.

Mast cell heterogeneity based on differential expression of various cytokines was demonstrated first by Bradding and colleagues [57]. Skin mast cells were found to express IL-4, but little if any IL-5 and IL-6, whereas lung and nasal mast cells expressed predominantly IL-5 and IL-6 and lesser amounts of IL-4. At this time, it is unclear if the differential expression of cytokines corresponds to the different protease phenotypes, but it suggests that MC_{TC} mast cells, which are almost the exclusive type of mast cell found in the skin, express predominantly IL-4, whereas MC_T cells, which predominate in the lung, express predominantly IL-5 and IL-6. This concept was supported further by studies of conjunctival biopsies with sequential in situ hybridization and double immunohistochemistry; these studies demonstrated that MC_{TC} cells comprised 89.2%–93.3% of IL-4$^+$ cells and 77.8% of IL-4$^+$ cells in seasonal allergic conjunctivitis and normal subjects, respectively [49]. Similarly, IL-13 appeared to colocalize preferentially to the MC_{TC} cells, while IL-5 and IL-6 were more commonly expressed in the MC_T cells. Functional differences between these two types of mast cells could be postulated based on differential expression of cytokines.

Functional heterogeneity

Mast cell heterogeneity also can be defined on the basis of functional differences. Stimulation by way of the FcɛRI receptor and calcium ionophores activates all tissue-derived mast cells. Nonimmunologic agonists, however, show selectivity for mast cells isolated from various tissue sites. Agents, such as morphine sulfate, substance P, vasoactive intestinal peptide, somatostatin, calcitonin gene-related protein, and the anaphylatoxins C5a and C3a, cause histamine release from skin mast cells but not from mast cells derived from the lung, the tonsils, the adenoids, and the colon, regardless of protease phenotype [58–62]. Heart mast cells respond to C5a but not to substance P [63,64]. Dispersed conjunctival mast cells are activated by morphine, but not substance P, to release low levels of histamine, tryptase, leukotrienes, and PGD_2. Conjunctival mast cells also respond to compound 48/80 [65]. Such tissue-specific differences in the mast cell secretory response may be caused by microenvironmental influences rather than to lineage. For example, the rat basophil leukemia cell line (which represents rat mucosal mast cell) is unresponsive to substance P at baseline, but responds well when cocultured with murine 3T3 fibroblasts without otherwise changing its phenotype [66]. Such microenvironmental influences may result from intrinsic changes in the mast cell brought about by accessory cells or by way of acquisition of new membrane components from accessory cells. A further level of functional heterogeneity occurs in MC_{TC} cells derived from lungs versus skin. Thus, although lung-derived MC_{TC} cells produce LTC_4 upon activation, skin-derived MC_{TC} cells do not [52].

Pharmacologic heterogeneity

Pharmacologic responsiveness of mast cells also varies depending on the tissue source. Sodium cromoglycate and nedocromil, when used at high concentrations, are weak inhibitors of activation of lung-derived mast cells, but they have no effect on mast cells from the skin and intestines [67–69]. Adrenoceptor agonists, cyclosporine A, and FK-506 produce inhibition of IgE-dependent histamine release in vitro from skin- and lung-derived mast cells [70–72]. Lodoxamide reduces the allergic response in rat conjunctiva in vivo following allergen challenge, and inhibits histamine release in vitro from rat conjunctival mast cells in a dose-dependent manner [73]. Dexamethasone in vitro does not inhibit activation-secretion by human lung-derived mast cells [74]. In vivo, topical nasal glucocorticosteroids result in diminished mediator release in response to nasal allergen challenge [75], perhaps caused by decreased mast cell concentration after prolonged topical administration as demonstrated in the skin and in the synovium [54,76]. Recent studies using IL-10 knockout mice have demonstrated a protective effect of IL-10 on degranulation of conjunctival mast cells in response to compound 48/80 [77].

Mast cell differentiation

Mast cells originate from hematopoietic stem cells and differentiate under the influence of stem cell factor (SCF), the ligand for Kit, a product of the c-kit proto-oncogene [78–80]. Unlike most other hematopoietic cells, mast cell progenitors circulate in the peripheral blood and complete their differentiation in peripheral tissues along a distinct myeloid lineage, which is different from that of basophils, monocytes, or other leukocytes [81,82]. Whereas other myelocytes stop expressing surface Kit as they complete their differentiation, mast cells express increasing amounts of Kit as they mature and require the persistent presence of SCF for their continued survival [79,80,83]. The critical effects of SCF in mast cell development and survival are evident particularly in certain strains of mice, with genetic defects in either Kit expression or SCF production, in which a profound mast cell deficiency occurs [84]. Although IL-3 serves as an important growth and differentiation factor for rodent mast cells [85], it appears to have little influence on human mast cells, which lack a surface receptor for IL-3 [86]. Although SCF appears to be an essential growth factor, other factors or accessory cells may be involved in regulation of mast cell development. For example, IL-4 down-regulates the expression of Kit in mast cells [87], including conjunctival mast cells [88], and results in inhibition of SCF-dependent development of mast cells from progenitors in vitro, but IL-4 has little effect on mature mast cells [89,90]. This effect may be responsible, in part, for the absence of mast cells in normal bone marrow despite the presence of large amounts of SCF. Glucocorticosteroids have a similar inhibitory effect on SCF-dependent mast cell development, whereas mature mast cells are relatively resistant to the effect of glucocorticoids. Furthermore, mast cells developing in cultures of fetal liver cells in the presence of SCF appear immature by morphologic criteria and lack the high affinity receptor for IgE, whereas mast cells developing from cord blood mononuclear cells cocultured with murine 3T3 fibroblasts (which produce SCF) appear mature and possess surface FcεRI. Thus, cell-associated SCF found on the surface of fibroblasts or other factors produced by fibroblasts may contribute to the maturational effect on mast cell development.

Conditions that influence the selective development of MC_T, or MC_{TC}, cells are not understood yet; however, commitment to a particular mast cell phenotype appears to occur by the time granule formation begins, so the compositional differences between MC_T and MC_{TC} cells can be appreciated at the electron microscopy level in morphologically immature cells [91], which suggests parallel rather than sequential development. However, studies of cord-blood-derived or bone-marrow-derived human mast cell cultures have demonstrated the acquisition of chymase staining over time in previously tryptase-positive, chymase-negative mast cells, implying sequential development [92–95]. Another possibility is that immature MC_{TC} cells may produce little, if any, chymase protein, and would thus resemble MC_T cells until they mature and start expressing chymase protein. Alternatively, MC_{TC} cells may have a survival advantage over MC_T cells in the culture conditions tested, because the latter undergo apoptosis in the presence of IL-4 [96], while skin-derived MC_{TC} cells proliferate better in serum-free medium than do lung-derived MC_T cells [97]. For individuals who have congenital combined immunodeficiency syndromes and patients who have AIDS, marked and selective decreases in MC_T cells occur in the bowel, whereas the concentration and distribution of MC_{TC} cells are unaffected, which suggests that T lymphocyte factors are involved in the normal growth and differentiation of MC_T but not MC_{TC} cells [98].

Ocular mast cells

The normal eye

Several studies have attempted to characterize the number, distribution, and phenotypes of mast cells in the normal eye of various species. As early as 1937, Jorpes and colleagues [99] noted mast cells in the limbal area of normal human eyes. Later, Feeney and Hogan [100] described the presence of mast cells among the nonpigmented cells of the normal human choroid stroma. Using flat whole mounts of the entire uvea stained with toluidine blue at pH 1.6, large numbers of mast cells could be detected in the posterior choroid of the eyes of guinea pigs, rabbits, and rats [101]. The mast cells often were seen lining the external walls of branching arterial vessels. In guinea pigs, concentration of mast cells in the posterior choroid averaged $250/mm^2$ compared with 2 to 12 mast cells/mm^2 in the intestinal mesentery and the kidney capsule, respectively. In contrast, the iris and ciliary body contained very few, if any, mast cells. Similarly, very few mast cells were identified in the sclera, retina, and cornea. A different pattern of distribution was noted in ferrets and dogs, where few mast cells were seen in the choroid, and most intraocular mast cells were found in the anterior uvea of dogs and in the deep part of the ciliary body in ferrets [102]. Rat choroidal mast cells released histamine when exposed to compound 48/80, indicating properties similar to those of connective tissue mast cells [103]. In humans, most studies of ocular mast cells have been concentrated on the conjunctival tissue. In normal subjects, few, if any, mast cells were found in the conjunctival epithelium, and they appeared to be of the MC_T type. The substantia propria of the normal conjunctiva contained large numbers of mast cells with a concentration of $11,054/mm^3$; 95% of which were of the MC_{TC} type (Fig. 1A) [104]. Allansmith [105] estimated the number of mast cells in the ocular and adnexal tissues of one human eye at 50 million, and confirmed the virtual absence of mast cells from the normal conjunctival epithelium, cornea, iris, retina, and optic nerve. Mast cells were found scattered in the meninges of optic nerves, usually in perivascular locations.

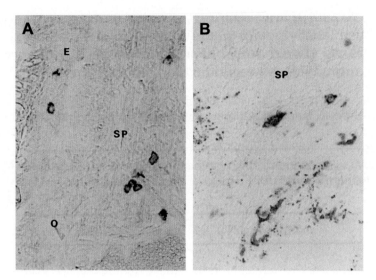

Fig. 1. Sections of human conjunctiva stained by double irnrnunohistochernistry with anti-tryptase and anti-chymase antibodies. MC_T cells are visualized in blue. MC_{TC} cells are visual-ized in brown. (A) Section of normal conjunctiva showing two MC_T cells in the epithelium and several MC_{TC} cells in the substantia propria (original magnification ×1100). (B) Section of vernal conjunctivitis showing one intact MC_T cell, one intact MC_{TC} cell, and numerous free MC_{TC} granules in the substantia propria (original magnification ×1700). E, epithelium; SP, substantia propria.

Mast cells in diseases of the eye

The eye is a target organ for many pathologic reactions involving im-mune reactions. Mast cell involvement has been postulated in a variety of ocular disorders, including those involving IgE-mediated reactions and chronic inflammatory disorders of the conjunctiva or the uveal tract.

Allergic conjunctivitis

Direct exposure of the ocular mucosal surface to environmental allergens (and with the large number of conjunctival mast cells), results in the frequent occurrence of immediate hypersensitivity reactions affecting the conjunctiva in atopic subjects. Mast cell activation in allergic conjunctivitis is evidenced by an increase in tryptase levels in unstimulated tear fluid of subjects who have symptomatic allergic conjunctivitis [6]. Similarly, conjunctival provo-cation of atopic individuals who have relevant allergens results in the release of histamine, kinins, PGD, and TAME-esterase activity in tears [106]. The total number of conjunctival mast cells found in the substantia propria in subjects who have allergic conjunctivitis has been reported to increase mildly $(15,389/mm^3)$ compared with normal control subjects [104]. The number of epithelial conjunctival mast cells is increased, which is similar to findings in the nasal mucosa of subjects who have allergic rhinitis [107,108]. A marked increase in subepithelial mast cell numbers and epithelial invasion with mast cells has been reported in atopic keratoconjunctivitis as well [109,110]. Whether the epithelial mast cells seen in these conditions represent an increase in precursor mast cells differentiating locally or a migration of subepithelial mast cells into the epithelial layer is not known. However, the characterization of epithelial mast cells as tryptase-positive only (MC_T cells) would argue toward the former theory, because subepithelial mast cells are mostly of the MC_{TC} type. The increase in lymphocytic infiltrate seen in the epithelium of subjects who have atopic keratoconjunctivitis may provide the necessary local environmental factors for differentiation of mast cells toward the MC_T type. Sodium cromoglycate had been reported to cause partial inhibition of degranulation of lung mast cells (mostly MC_T cells), whereas skin mast cells (MC_{TC} cells) appeared resistant to its effects. Therefore, the clinical response seen in subjects who had allergic conjunctivitis treated with topical sodium cromoglycate may result from inhibition of degranulation of conjunctival MC_T cells found in the epithelium.

Vernal conjunctivitis

Increased concentration of mast cells in the conjunctival substantia propria of subjects with vernal conjunctivitis has been reported at the electron microscopy level as well as by immunohistochemistry [111]. Mast cell concentrations averaged $24,689/mm^3$ and reached an upper limit of $60,632/mm^3$ in one subject, similar to mast cell concentrations in cutaneous mastocytosis. Furthermore, a significant number of MC_T cells are seen in the epithelium and subepithelium of the bulbar conjunctiva, although MC_{TC} remains the predominant type [104]. The presence of MC_T cells in the inflamed conjunctiva of subjects who have vernal conjunctivitis may reflect permissive local environmental factors, because large numbers of CD4-positive T lymphocytes are known to infiltrate this tissue. Extensive degranulation of mast cells is apparent at the electron microscopy level and by light microscopy, where large numbers of free granules scattered around the substantia propria were observed (Fig. 1B). These findings are consistent with previous results showing elevated histamine and tryptase levels in tears [110,112]. It is unclear if mast degranulation is a primary event in vernal conjunctivitis or if it is a result of the severe eye rubbing associated with this condition, because eye rubbing has been demonstrated to lead to an increase in tryptase level in tear fluid. Treatment of vernal conjunctivitis with cyclosporine eye drops does not alter the numbers, phenotype, or fragmented appearance of mast cells in the conjunctiva (K. Tabbara and Anne-Marie Irani, MD, personal communication, 1995).

Giant papillary conjunctivitis

Contrary to findings in vernal conjunctivitis, mast cell hyperplasia appears to be minimal in giant papillary conjunctivitis, with concentrations of mast cells averaging 17,313/mm^3 [104]. Epithelial mast cells were seen in four out of six subjects studied and were exclusively MC_{TC} cells. A recent report in prosthesis-associated giant papillary conjunctivitis also demonstrated epithelial mast cells in 5 of 17 specimens, but none were demonstrated in normal conjunctiva [113]. In asymptomatic soft contact lens wearers, the concentration and protease phenotype of conjunctival mast cells were similar to normal controls, and no epithelial mast cells were found. Thus, the distribution of MC_T and MC_{TC} cells may contribute to the distinct clinical presentations and have important implications regarding the pathogenesis and treatment of these ocular disorders.

Experimental autoimmune uveitis

In this animal model of human autoimmune ocular diseases, an intense bilateral panophthalmic inflammation develops 10 to 18 days after inoculation with the retinal S-antigen emulsified in an appropriate adjuvant, or 3 days after adoptive transfer with a uveitogenic T-lymphocyte line. Several studies have documented an association between baseline mast cell numbers in the anterior uvea and choroid, and the susceptibility to experimental autoimmune uveitis (EAU) [111,114,115]. Two inbred rat strains, CAR and Lewis, are high responders to the induction of EAU, and essentially all animals develop the disorders postimmunization with retinal antigens. On the other hand, only one fourth of Brown Norway (BN) rats and one half of F_1 hybrids of Lewis and BN rats (LBNF) developed EAU. The corresponding mast cell measurement revealed significant numbers of mast cells in the iris, ciliary body, and choroid of Lewis rats and CAR rats, revealed almost absent mast cells in these locations in the BN strain of rats, and revealed intermediate numbers in the LBNF hybrids. These patterns of susceptibility to EAU are identical to the patterns of susceptibility to experimental autoimmune encephalitis (EAE) in the same animal strains. Mice with a genetic mutation in the c-kit tyrosine kinase receptor resulting in mast cell deficiency are resistant to induction of EAU and exhibit delayed onset and decreased severity of the disease as compared with wild-type littermates [116]. Furthermore, reconstitution of mast cell development following bone marrow transplant from syngeneic wild-type animals restores susceptibility to EAE, indicating an important role for mast cells in the disease pathogenesis.

The evidence pointing to mast cell degranulation in EAU is weaker and consists of demonstrating a variable degree of decreasing mast cell numbers in the anterior uvea and choroid following immunization with the retinal antigen, and before or immediately following the development of clinical disease. Mediator levels were measured in tissue homogenates in only one study, and they showed a decrease from control values in the anterior portion of the eye, concomitant with the decrease in mast cell numbers. Histamine level in aliquots of aqueous fluid from the eyes of EAU rats did not vary significantly from those of saline controls [111]. These results would argue against the occurrence of mast cell degranulation and in favor of apoptosis of mast cells or inhibition of mast cell differentiation. Histamine levels were reported to be increased in the choroid and the retina.

Summary

Mast cells are resident cells in the ocular and adnexal tissues of the normal eye and are concentrated in the conjunctival subepithelium, posterior choroid, and along limbal vessels. In normal conjunctiva, the majority of mast cells are of the MC_{TC} type. The cornea, iris, retina, and optic nerve are devoid of mast cells in humans. Species difference in the distribution of ocular mast cells may account for differing disease susceptibility to autoimmune phenomenon. The role of mast cells in ocular allergy is well established, as it is in allergic disorders involving other organs, such as the nose, lungs, and skin. In addition, involvement of mast cells in chronic inflammatory disorders of the eye, such as vernal conjunctivitis, giant papillary conjunctivitis, and atopic keratoconjunctivitis, is suggested by epithelial invasion of the conjunctiva with mast cells by an altered mast cell phenotype and by the release of mast cell mediators in tear fluid. Advances in the understanding of mast cell biology in general, and of mast cell involvement in ocular disorders in particular, should lead to the development of new therapeutic approaches based on the specific immunopathology and the selective participation of different types of mast cells.

References

[1] Schwartz LB, Irani AMA, Roller K, et al. Quantitation of histamine, tryptase and chymase in dispersed human T and TC mast cells. J Immunol 1987;138:2611–5.

[2] Arrang JM, Garbarg M, Lancelot JC, et al. Highly potent and selective ligands for histamine H3-receptors. Nature 1987;327:117–23.

[3] Black JW, Duncan WA, Durant CJ, et al. Definition and antagonism of histamine H2-receptors. Nature 1972;236:385–90.

[4] Polk RE, Healy DP, Schwartz LB, et al. Vancomycin and the red-man syndrome: pharmacodynamics of histamine release. J Infect Dis 1988;157:502–7.

[5] Clark RA, Gallin JI, Kaplan AP. The selective eosinophil chemotactic activity of histamine. J Exp Med 1975;142:1462–76.

[6] Arrang JM, Devaux B, Chodkiewicz JP, et al. H3-receptors control histamine release in human brain. J Neurochem 1988;51:105–8.

[7] Stevens RL, Fox CC, Lichtenstein LM, et al. Identification of chondroitin sulfate E proteoglycans and heparin proteoglycans in the secretory granules of human lung mast cells. Proc Natl Acad Sci U S A 1988;85:2284–7.

[8] Thompson HL, Schulman ES, Metcalfe DD. Identification of chondroitin sulfate E in human lung mast cells. J Immunol 1988;140:2708–13.

[9] Craig SS, Irani AMA, Metcalfe DD, et al. Ultrastructural localization of heparin to human mast cells of the MC_{TC} and MC_T types by labeling with antithrombin III-gold. Lab Invest 1993;69:552–61.

[10] Schwartz LB, Bradford TR. Regulation of tryptase from human lung mast cells by heparin. Stabilization of the active tetramer. J Biol Chem 1986;261:7372–9.

[11] Alter SC, Metcalfe DD, Bradford TR, et al. Regulation of human mast cell tryptase. Effects of enzyme concentration, ionic strength and the structure and negative charge density of polysaccharides. Biochem J 1987;248:821–7.

[12] Reed JA, Albino AP, McNutt NS. Human cutaneous mast cells express basic fibroblast growth factor. Lab Invest 1995;72:215–22.

[13] Spivak-Kroizman T, Lemmon MA, Dikic I, et al. Heparin-induced oligomerization of FGF molecules is responsible for FGF receptor dimerization, activation, and cell proliferation. Cell 1994;79:1015–24.

[14] Schwartz LB. Neutral proteases of mast cells. Monograph in Allergy, Volume 27. 2nd edition. Basel (Germany): Karger; 1990.

[15] Hopsu VK, Glenner GG. A histochemical enzyme kinetic system applied to the trypsin-like amidase and esterase activity in human mast cells. J Cell Biol 1963;17:503–10.

[16] Schwartz LB, Lewis RA, Austen KF. Tryptase from human pulmonary mast cells. Purification and characterization. J Biol Chem 1981;256:11939–43.

[17] Xia H-Z, Kepley CL, Sakai K, et al. Quantitation of tryptase, chymase, FceRIa, and FceRIgamma mRNAs in human mast cells and basophils by competitive reverse transcription-polymerase chain reaction. J Immunol 1995;154:5472–80.

[18] Schwartz LB, Lewis RA, Seldin D, et al. Acid hydrolases and tryptase from secretory granules of dispersed human lung mast cells. J Immunol 1981;126:1290–4.

[19] Miller JS, Westin EH, Schwartz LB. Cloning and characterization of complementary DNA for human tryptase. J Clin Invest 1989;84:1188–95.

[20] Miller JS, Moxley G, Schwartz LB. Cloning and characterization of a second complementary DNA for human tryptase. J Clin Invest 1990;86:864–70.

[21] Vanderslice P, Ballinger SM, Tam EK, et al. Human mast cell tryptase: multiple cDNAs and genes reveal a multigene serine protease family. Proc Natl Acad Sci U S A 1990;87: 3811–5.

[22] Schwartz LB. Diagnostic value of tryptase in anaphylaxis and mastocytosis. Immunol Allergy Clin North Am 2006;26(3):451–63.

[23] Schwartz LB, Bradford TR, Littman BH, et al. The fibrinogenolytic activity of purified tryptase from human lung mast cells. J Immunol 1985;135:2762–7.

[24] Sekizawa K, Caughey GH, Lazarus SC, et al. Mast cell tryptase causes airway smooth muscle hyperresponsiveness in dogs. J Clin Invest 1989;83:175–9.

[25] Gruber BL, Marchese MJ, Suzuki K, et al. Synovial procollagenase activation by human mast cell tryptase dependence upon matrix metalloproteinase 3 activation. J Clin Invest 1989;84:1657–62.

[26] Brown JK, Jones CA, Tyler CL, et al. Tryptase-induced mitogenesis in airway smooth muscle cells: potency, mechanisms, and interactions with other mast cell mediators. Chest 1995;107(Suppl):95S–6S.

[27] Hartmann T, Ruoss SJ, Raymond WW, et al. Human tryptase as a potent, cell-specific mitogen: role of signaling pathways in synergistic responses. Am J Phys 1992;262:L528–34.

[28] Schechter NM, Fraki JE, Geesin JC, et al. Human skin chymotryptic protease. Isolation and relation to cathepsin G and rat mast cell proteinase. J Biol Chem 1983;258:2973–8.

[29] Caughey GH, Zerweck EH, Vanderslice P. Structure, chromosomal assignment, and deduced amino acid sequence of a human gene for mast cell chymase. J Biol Chem 1991; 266:12956–63.

[30] Sayama S, Iozzo RV, Lazarus GS, et al. Human skin chymotrypsin-like proteinase chymase. Subcellular localization to mast cell granules and interaction with heparin and other glycosaminoglycans. J Biol Chem 1987;262:6808–15.

[31] Schechter NM, Sprows JL, Schoenberger OL, et al. Reaction of human skin chymotrypsin-like proteinase chymase with plasma proteinase inhibitors. J Biol Chem 1989;264:21308–15.

[32] Irani AA, Schechter NM, Craig SS, et al. Two types of human mast cells that have distinct neutral protease compositions. Proc Natl Acad Sci U S A 1986;83:4464–8.

[33] Wintroub BU, Schechter NB, Lazarus GS, et al. Angiotensin I conversion by human and rat chymotryptic proteinases. J Invest Dermatol 1984;83:336–9.

[34] Saarinen J, Kalkkinen N, Welgus HG, et al. Activation of human interstitial procollagenase through direct cleavage of the Leu^{83}-Thr^{84} bond by mast cell chymase. J Biol Chem 1994; 269:18134–40.

[35] Reilly CF, Tewksbury DA, Schechter NM, et al. Rapid conversion of angiotensin I to angiotensin II by neutrophil and mast cell proteinases. J Biol Chem 1982;257:8619–22.

[36] Briggaman RA, Schechter NM, Fraki J, et al. Degradation of the epidermal-dermal junction by a proteolytic enzyme from human skin and human polymorphonuclear leukocytes. J Exp Med 1984;160:1027–42.

[37] Caughey GH. Roles of mast cell tryptase and chymase in airway function. Am J Phys 1989; 257:L39–46.

[38] Church MK, Lowman MA, Robinson C, et al. Interaction of neuropeptides with human mast cells. Int Arch Allergy Appl Immunol 1989;88:70–8.

[39] Sommerhoff CP, Caughey GH, Finkbeiner WE, et al. Mast cell chymase. A potent secretagogue for airway gland serous cells. J Immunol 1989;142:2450–6.

[40] Irani AMA, Goldstein SM, Wintroub BU, et al. Human mast cell carboxypeptidase: selective localization to MC_{TC} cells. J Immunol 1991;147:247–53.

[41] Goldstein SM, Kaempfer CE, Proud D, et al. Detection and partial characterization of a human mast cell carboxypeptidase. J Immunol 1987;139:2724–9.

[42] Peters SP, MacGlashan DW, Schulman ES, et al. Arachidonic acid metabolism in purified human lung mast cells. J Immunol 1984;132:1972–9.

[43] Robinson C. Mast cells and newly-generated lipid mediators. In: Holgate ST, editor. Immunology and medicine: mast cells, mediators and disease. London: Kluwer Academic Publishers; 1988. p. 149–74.

[44] Israel E, Rubin P, Kemp JP, et al. The effect of inhibition of 5-lipoxygenase by zileuton in mild-to-moderate asthma. Ann Intern Med 1993;119:1059–66.

[45] Roberts LJ II, Sweetman BJ, Lewis RA, et al. Increased production of prostaglandin D2 in patients with systemic mastocytosis. N Engl J Med 1980;303:1400–4.

[46] Walsh LJ, Trinchieri G, Waldorf HA, et al. Human dermal mast cells contain and release tumor necrosis factor a, which induces endothelial leukocyte adhesion molecule 1. Proc Natl Acad Sci U S A 1991;88:4220–4.

[47] Bradding P, Feather IH, Wilson S, et al. Immunolocalization of cytokines in the nasal mucosa of normal and perennial rhinitic subjects. The mast cell as a source of IL-4, IL-5, and IL-6 in human allergic mucosal inflammation. J Immunol 1993;151:3853–65.

[48] Burd PR, Thompson WC, Max EE, et al. Activated mast cells produce interleukin 13. J Exp Med 1995;181:1373–80.

[49] Anderson DF, Zhang SL, Bradding P, et al. The relative contribution of mast cell subsets to conjunctival T(H)2-like cytokines. Invest Ophthalmol Vis Sci 2001;42(5):995–1001.

[50] Irani AA. Tissue and developmental variation of protease expression in human mast cells. In: Caughey GH, editor. Mast cell proteases in immunology and biology, vol. 6. New York: Marcel Dekker; 1995. p. 127–44.

[51] Irani A-MA, Bradford TR, Kepley CL, et al. Detection of MC_T and MC_{TC} types of human mast cells by immunohistochemistry using new monoclonal anti-tryptase and anti-chymase antibodies. J Histochem Cytochem 1989;37:1509–15.

[52] Oskeritzian CA, Zhao W, Min HK, et al. Surface CD88 functionally distinguishes the MCTC from the MCT type of human lung mast cell. J Allergy Clin Immunol 2005; 115(6):1162–8.

[53] Hawkins RA, Claman HN, Clark RA, et al. Increased dermal mast cell populations in progressive systemic sclerosis: a link in chronic fibrosis. Ann Intern Med 1985;102:182–6.

[54] Malone DG, Wilder RL, Saavedra-Delgado AM, et al. Mast cell numbers in rheumatoid synovial tissues. Correlations with quantitative measures of lymphotic infiltration and modulation by anti-inflammatory therapy. Arthritis Rheum 1987;30:130–7.

[55] Stevens RL. Gene expression in different populations of mouse mast cells. Ann N Y Acad Sci 1991;629:31–7.

[56] Stevens RL, Friend DS, McNeil HP, et al. Strain-specific and tissue-specific expression of mouse mast cell secretory granule proteases. Proc Natl Acad Sci U S A 1994;91: 128–32.

[57] Bradding P, Okayama Y, Howarth PH, et al. Heterogeneity of human mast cells based on cytokine content. J Immunol 1995;155:297–307.

[58] Bloch JG, Asch L, Landry Y, et al. Effects of different secretagogues on synovial fluid mast cells from patients with rheumatoid arthritis. Agents Actions 1992;36(Suppl):CC290–3.

[59] Church MK, Pao GJ, Holgate ST. Characterization of histamine secretion from mechanically dispersed human lung mast cells: effects of anti-IgE, calcium ionophore A 23187, compound 48/80, and basic polypeptides. J Immunol 1982;129:2116–21.

[60] El-Lati SG, Dahinden CA, Church MK. Complement peptides C3a- and C5a-induced mediator release from dissociated human skin mast cells. J Invest Dermatol 1994;102(5): 803–6.

[61] Fox CC, Dvorak AM, Peters SP, et al. Isolation and characterization of human intestinal mucosal mast cells. J Immunol 1985;135:483–91.

[62] Schmutzler W, Delmich K, Eichelberg D, et al. The human adenoidal mast cell. Susceptibility to different secretagogues and secretion inhibitors. Int Arch Allergy Appl Immunol 1985;77:177–8.

[63] Patella V, Marinò I, Lampärter B, et al. Human heart mast cells: isolation, purification, ultrastructure, and immunologic characterization. J Immunol 1995;154:2855–65.

[64] Sperr WR, Bankl HC, Mundigler G, et al. The human cardiac mast cell: localization, isolation, phenotype, and functional characterization. Blood 1994;84:3876–84.

[65] Miller S, Cook E, Graziano F, et al. Human conjunctival mast cell responses in vitro to various secretagogues. Ocul Immunol Inflamm 1996;4:39–49.

[66] Swieter M, Midura RJ, Nishikata H, et al. Mouse 3T3 fibroblasts induce rat basophilic leukemia (RBL- 2H3) cells to acquire responsiveness to compound 48/80. J Immunol 1993;150:617–24.

[67] Ting S, Zweiman B, Lavker RM. Cromolyn does not modulate human allergic skin reactions in vivo. J Allergy Clin Immunol 1983;71:12–7.

[68] Schulman ES, Post TJ, Vigderman RJ. Density heterogeneity of human lung mast cells. J Allergy Clin Immunol 1988;82:78–86.

[69] Sommerhoff CP, Osborne ML, Lazarus SC. Effect of inhibitors on histamine release from mast cells recovered by bronchoalveolar lavage in basenji-greyhound and mongrel dogs. Agents Actions 1990;31:183–9.

[70] Sperr WR, Agis H, Czerwenka K, et al. Effects of cyclosporin A and FK-506 on stem cell factor-induced histamine secretion and growth of human mast cells. J Allergy Clin Immunol 1996;98(2):389–99.

[71] Marone G, Triggiani M, Cirillo R, et al. Cyclosporin A inhibits the release of histamine and peptide leukotriene C4 from human lung mast cells. Ric Clin Lab 1988;18:53–9.

[72] Dráberová L. Cyclosporin A inhibits rat mast cell activation. Eur J Immunol 1990;20: 1469–73.

[73] Yanni JM, Weimer LK, Glaser RL, et al. Effect of lodoxamide on in vitro and in vivo conjunctival immediate hypersensitivity responses in rats. Int Arch Allergy Immunol 1993;101:102–6.

[74] Schleimer RP, Schulman ES, MacGlash DW, et al. Effects of dexamethasone on mediator release from human lung fragments and purified human lung mast cells. J Clin Invest 1983; 71:1830–5.

[75] Pipkorn U, Proud D, Lichtenstein LM, et al. Inhibition of mediator release in allergic rhinitis by pretreatment with topical glucocorticosteroids. N Engl J Med 1987;316:1506–10.

[76] Lavker RM, Schechter NM. Cutaneous mast cell depletion results from topical corticosteroid usage. J Immunol 1985;135(4):2368–73.

[77] Bundoc VG, Keane-Myers A. IL-10 confers protection from mast cell degranulation in a mouse model of allergic conjunctivitis. Exp Eye Res 2007;85(4):575–9.

[78] Irani AA, Nilsson G, Miettinen U, et al. Recombinant human stem cell factor stimulates differentiation of mast cells from dispersed human fetal liver cells. Blood 1992;80:3009–21.

[79] Valent P, Spanblöchl E, Sperr WR, et al. Induction of differentiation of human mast cells from bone marrow and peripheral blood mononuclear cells by recombinant human stem cell factor/kit-ligand in long-term culture. Blood 1992;80:2237–45.

[80] Mitsui H, Furitsu T, Dvorak AM, et al. Development of human mast cells from umbilical cord blood cells by recombinant human and murine c-kit ligand. Proc Natl Acad Sci U S A 1993;90:735–9.

[81] Agis H, Willheim M, Sperr WR, et al. Monocytes do not make mast cells when cultured in the presence of SCF: characterization of the circulating mast cell progenitor as a c-kit^+, $CD34^+$, Ly^-, $CD14^-$, $CD17^-$, colony- forming cell. J Immunol 1993;151:4221–7.

[82] Valent P. The phenotype of human eosinophils, basophils, and mast cells. J Allergy Clin Immunol 1994;94(Suppl):1177–83.

[83] Iemura A, Tsai M, Ando A, et al. The c-kit ligand, stem cell factor, promotes mast cell survival by suppressing apoptosis. Am J Pathol 1994;144:321–8.

[84] Kitamura Y, Tsujimura T, Jippo T, et al. Regulation of mast cell development by c-kit receptor and its ligand. Acta Histochem Cytochem 1994;27:17–22.

[85] Ihle JN, Keller JR, Oroszlan S, et al. Biologic properties of homogeneous interleukin 3. I. Demonstration of WEHI-3 growth factor activity, mast cell growth factor activity, p cell-stimulating factor activity, colony- stimulating factor activity, and histamine-producing cell- stimulating factor activity. J Immunol 1983;131:282–7.

[86] Valent P, Besemer J, Sillaber C, et al. Failure to detect IL-3-binding sites on human mast cells. J Immunol 1990;145:3432–7.

[87] Sillaber C, Strobl H, Bevec D, et al. IL-4 regulates c-kit proto-oncogene product expression in human mast and myeloid progenitor cells. J Immunol 1991;147:4224–8.

[88] Stahl JL, Cook EB, Graziano FM, et al. Human conjunctival mast cells–expression of FceRI, c-kit, ICAM-1, and IgE. Arch Ophthalmol 1999;117(4):493–7.

[89] Nilsson G, Miettinen U, Ishizaka T, et al. Interleukin-4 inhibits the expression of Kit and tryptase during stem cell factor-dependent development of human mast cells from fetal liver cells. Blood 1994;84(5):1519–27.

[90] Sillaber C, Sperr WR, Agis H, et al. Inhibition of stem cell factor dependent formation of human mast cells by interleukin-3 and interleukin-4. Int Arch Allergy Immunol 1994;105: 264–8.

[91] Craig SS, Schechter NM, Schwartz LB. Ultrastructural analysis of maturing human T and TC mast cells in situ. Lab Invest 1989;60:147–57.

[92] Ahn K, Takai S, Pawankar R, et al. Regulation of chymase production in human mast cell progenitors. J Allergy Clin Immunol 2000;106(2):321–8.

[93] Dvorak AM, Furitsu T, Kissell-Rainville S, et al. Ultrastructural identification of human mast cells resembling skin mast cells stimulated to develop in long-term human cord blood mononuclear cells cultured with 3T3 murine skin fibroblasts. J Leukoc Biol 1992;51: 557–69.

[94] Shimizu Y, Sakai K, Miura T, et al. Characterization of 'adult-type' mast cells derived from human bone marrow CD34(+) cells cultured in the presence of stem cell factor and interleukin-6. Interleukin-4 is not required for constitutive expression of CD54, Fc epsilon RI alpha and chymase, and CD13 expression is reduced during differentiation. Clin Exp Allergy 2002;32(6):872–80.

[95] Toru H, Eguchi M, Matsumoto R, et al. Interleukin-4 promotes the development of tryptase and chymase double-positive human mast cells accompanied by cell maturation. Blood 1998;91(1):187–95.

[96] Oskeritzian CA, Wang Z, Kochan JP, et al. Recombinant human (rh)IL-4-mediated apoptosis and recombinant human IL- 6-mediated protection of recombinant human stem cell factor-dependent human mast cells derived from cord blood mononuclear cell progenitors. J Immunol 1999;163(9):5105–15.

[97] Kambe N, Kambe M, Kochan JP, et al. Human skin-derived mast cells can proliferate while retaining their characteristic functional and protease phenotypes. Blood 2001; 97(7):2045–52.

[98] Irani AM, Craig SS, DeBlois G, et al. Deficiency of the tryptase-positive, chymase-negative mast cell type in gastrointestinal mucosa of patients with defective T lymphocyte function. J Immunol 1987;138:4381–6.

[99] Jorpes JE, Holmgren H, Wilander O. Uber das vorkommen von heparin in den gefässwänden und in den augen. Z Mikrosk Anat Forsch 1937;42:279–300.

[100] Feeney L, Hogan MJ. Electron microscopy of the human choroid. I. Cells and supporting structures. Am J Ophthalmol 1961;51:1057–72.

[101] Smelser GK, Silver S. The distribution of mast cells in the normal eye. A method of study. Exp Eye Res 1963;2:134–40.

[102] Louden C, Render JA, Carlton WW. Mast cell numbers in normal and glaucomatous canine eyes. Am J Vet Res 1990;51:818–9.

[103] Godfrey WA. Characterization of the choroidal mast cell. Trans Am Ophthalmol Soc 1987; 85:557–99.

[104] Irani A-MA, Butrus SI, Tabbara KF, et al. Human conjunctival mast cells: distribution of MC_T and MC_{TC} in vernal conjunctivitis and giant papillary conjunctivitis. J Allergy Clin Immunol 1990;86:34–40.

[105] Allansmith MR. Immunology of the external ocular tissues. J Am Optom Assoc 1990;61(6): S16–22.

[106] Proud D, Sweet J, Stein P, et al. Inflammatory mediator release on conjunctival provocation of allergic subjects with allergen. J Allergy Clin Immunol 1990;85:896–905.

[107] Baddeley SM, Bacon AS, McGill JI, et al. Mast cell distribution and neutral protease expression in acute and chronic allergic conjunctivitis. Clin Exp Allergy 1995;25:41–50.

[108] Morgan SJ, Williams JH, Walls AF, et al. Mast cell numbers and staining characteristics in the normal and allergic human conjunctiva. J Allergy Clin Immunol 1991;87:111–6.

[109] Foster CS, Rice BA, Dutt JE. Immunopathology of atopic keratoconjunctivitis. Ophthalmology 1991;98:1190–6.

[110] Morgan SJ, Williams JH, Walls AF, et al. Mast cell hyperplasia in atopic keratoconjunctivitis. An immunohistochemical study. Eye 1991;5:729–35.

[111] Lee CH, Lang LS, Orr EL. Changes in ocular mast cell numbers and histamine distribution during experimental autoimmune uveitis. Reg Immunol 1993;5:106–13.

[112] Butrus SI, Ochsner KI, Abelson MB, et al. The level of tryptase in human tears: an indicator of activation of conjunctival mast cells. Ophthalmology 1990;97:1678–83.

[113] Bozkurt B, Akyurek N, Irkec M, et al. Immunohistochemical findings in prosthesis-associated giant papillary conjunctivitis. Clin Experiment Ophthalmol 2007;35(6):535–40.

[114] Li Q, Fujino Y, Caspi RR, et al. Association between mast cells and the development of experimental autoimmune uveitis in different rat strains. Clin Immunol Immunopathol 1992;65:294–9.

[115] Mochizuki M, Kuwabara T, Chan CC, et al. An association between susceptibility to experimental autoimmune uveitis and choroidal mast cell numbers. J Immunol 1984;133: 1699–701.

[116] Brown MA, Tanzola MB, Robbie-Ryan M. Mechanisms underlying mast cell influence on EAE disease course. Mol Immunol 2002;38(16–18):1373–8.

ELSEVIER
SAUNDERS

Immunol Allergy Clin N Am
28 (2008) 43–58

IMMUNOLOGY
AND ALLERGY
CLINICS
OF NORTH AMERICA

Allergic Conjunctivitis

Leonard Bielory, MD[a],
Mitchell H. Friedlaender, MD[b],*

[a]*Division of Allergy, Immunology, and Rheumatology, UMDNJ–New Jersey Medical School,
90 Bergen Street, DOC Suite 4700, Newark, NJ 07103, USA*
[b]*Division of Ophthalmology, Scripps Clinic, 10666 North Torrey Pines Road,
La Jolla, CA 92037, USA*

Allergic conjunctivitis affects up to 40% of the general population [1–3] and is a common clinical problem for ophthalmic and allergic practices [4]. In one study of 5000 allergic children, 32% had ocular symptoms as the single manifestation of their allergies [5]. Although many cases are seasonal, a large number of patients have year-round symptoms.

The conjunctiva can be affected by allergies to airborne pollens, animal dander, and other environmental antigens. The conjunctiva, like the nasal mucosa, is an active immunologic tissue that undergoes lymphoid hyperplasia in response to a stimulant [6]. The conjunctiva represents a thin mucous membrane that extends from the limbus of the eye to the lid margin of the eyelid. The conjunctiva is divided into three portions: the bulbar conjunctiva, which covers the anterior portion of the sclera; the palpebral conjunctiva, which lines the inner surface of the eyelids; and the space bounded by the bulbar and palpebral conjunctiva, which is the fornix or the conjunctival sac. The conjunctiva is histologically divided into two layers: epithelial and substantia propria. The epithelial layer is composed of two to five cells of stratified columnar cells, whereas the substantia propria is composed of loose connective tissue.

As in other forms of allergic inflammation, the mast cell plays a key role. Mast cells are widely distributed, especially in connective tissue and mucosal surfaces. In the eye, they are classically found in the conjunctiva, choroid, ciliary body, iris, and optic nerve. Mast cells ($6000/mm^3$) and other inflammatory cells are normally found in the substantia propria, just below the epithelial junction [7]. Initial reports of conjunctival mast cell populations were

---

* Corresponding author.
E-mail address: friedlaender.mitch@scrippshealth.org (M.H. Friedlaender).

0889-8561/08/$ - see front matter © 2008 Elsevier Inc. All rights reserved.
doi:10.1016/j.iac.2007.12.005
immunology.theclinics.com

based on the differential physiologic response to compound 48/80, which causes connective tissue mast cells (but not mucosal mast cells) to degranulate. In the rat animal model, the response to a single application of 48/80 suggested that the conjunctival mast cells primarily belong to the connective tissue type of mast cells [8–10]. Mononuclear cell populations of the normal human conjunctiva are primarily located in the epithelium and include Langerhans cells (CD1$^+$; 85 $\pm$ 16 cells/mm^2) and CD3$^+$ lymphocytes (189 $\pm$ 27 cells/mm^2), with a CD4$^+$:CD8$^+$ ratio of 0.75 [11]. The Langerhans cells are known to facilitate immune reactions in the skin by functioning as an antigen-presenting cell, but their function in the cornea has yet to be clarified [12]. Of interest, the Langerhans cells of the eye are recognized by the CD1$^+$ marker, not the CD6$^+$ thymocyte marker, which is commonly found on Langerhans cells of the skin or in histiocytes from patients who have histiocytosis X [13]. Normal ocular epithelium does not contain any mast cells, eosinophils, or basophils, although in ocular inflammatory disorders such as vernal and giant papillary conjunctivitis, such cells are seen, as evidenced by the conjunctival deposition of eosinophil major basic protein deposition [14]. Conjunctival epithelial cells, however, may also play an active role in allergic inflammation because they have been shown to express RANTES in large amounts when stimulated in vitro with tumor necrosis factor α or interferon-γ [15].

Histamine concentration in tears can reach values greater than 100 ng/mL compared with normal values of 5 to 15 ng/mL [16–19]. Histamine can cause changes in the eye similar to changes in other parts of the human body, such as capillary dilatation, increased vascular permeability, and smooth muscle contraction. A histamine concentration of 240 nmol/L (10 μL of a 50-ng/mL histamine phosphate concentration) can cause conjunctival redness and increased vascular permeability in 50% of the subjects studied. Tear histamine levels in nonatopic control subjects were not found to be different from those in allergic patients during their symptom-free periods [17].

History

A detailed history may reveal recent exposure to individuals who have conjunctivitis or upper respiratory tract infection within the family, school, or workplace. Such a history may help confirm an adenovirus infection in an endemic area. Knowledge of the patient's sexual activities and any associated discharge may suggest chlamydial disease or *Neisseria* infection. Frequently, the patient does not mention the use of over-the-counter topical medications such as vasoconstrictors or artificial tears, cosmetics, or contact lens wear. Direct questioning often reveals the use of these products or other topical and systemic medications, which are capable of producing inflammation that can mimic seasonal allergic conjunctivitis (SAC) or perennial allergic conjunctivitis (PAC). Knowledge of any systemic disease such as rheumatoid arthritis or other collagen vascular diseases raises the clinician's suspicion for keratoconjunctivitis sicca, although a patient referred for irritated eyes who has thyroid dysfunction suggests superior limbic keratoconjunctivitis.

The offending allergens vary from one location to another, but the symptoms appear to be similar throughout the world. Often, symptoms are not severe enough to precipitate a visit to the allergist or the ophthalmologist. Among patients who seek help, some may not require treatment and others may simply be able to avoid the allergens responsible for their disease.

Symptoms usually consist of low-grade ocular and periocular itching (pruritus), tearing (epiphora), burning, stinging, photophobia, and watery discharge. Redness and itching seem to be the most consistent symptoms. Although symptoms persist throughout the allergy season, they are subject to exacerbations and remission, depending on the weather and the patient's activities. Symptoms are generally worse when the weather is warm and dry; cooler temperatures and rain tend to alleviate symptoms. Although itching is generally mild, occasionally it can be severe, and rarely patients may be incapacitated by their symptoms. Many of the symptoms of ocular allergy are nonspecific, such as tearing, irritation, stinging, burning, and photophobia.

The symptom of itching is strikingly characteristic of allergic conjunctivitis. It is often said that ocular itching implies allergy until proven otherwise. Furthermore, ocular itching is rare in other conditions, although it is not unknown. Patients who have blepharitis, dry eye, and other types of conjunctivitis may experience itching. It is worthwhile to pinpoint the location of itching. For example, patients who complain of ocular itching may be presumed to be describing conjunctival itching; however, some patients who have ocular itching describe symptoms related to the skin of their eyelids. Careful questioning can distinguish itching of the conjunctiva from itching of the eyelid skin. Although the former is usually associated with allergic rhinoconjunctivitis, which affects the conjunctiva, the latter may indicate contact allergy, which affects the skin and the conjunctiva. The discharge is usually watery and may be described as tearing. Sometimes there is a scan mucus component. The discharge may range from serous (watery) to mucopurulent and grossly purulent. A stringy or ropy discharge is characteristic of allergy. In severe forms of allergic conjunctivitis, such as vernal conjunctivitis, tenacious strands of mucus can be removed from the eye by the patient or the doctor. Environmental allergens are ubiquitous and nonselective, most commonly affecting both eyes at the same time. Conjunctival injection is commonly associated with discomfort, and when the patient complains of ocular pain, the physician must search for other causes.

In allergic patients, it is unusual to have conjunctival symptoms without nasal symptoms [20]. The nasal mucosa is expected to react in the same fashion as the conjunctival mucosa; however, at times the physician encounters allergic patients whose symptoms appear to be ocular. These patients may indicate that they do not have systemic allergies because they have not experienced typical allergic rhinitis. It is not known why the conjunctiva should be the main target in certain patients who have allergies. There may be emotional or psychologic factors that make ocular symptoms more disturbing than nasal symptoms. Often, when patients deny nasal or respiratory symptoms, careful questioning can sometimes elicit such symptoms, even though they may be mild.

Examination

The eye should be carefully examined for evidence of eyelid involvement (ie, blepharitis, dermatitis, swelling, discoloration, ptosis, blepharospasm), conjunctival involvement (ie, chemosis), hyperemia, palpebral and bulbar papillae, cicatrization, and presence of increased or abnormal-appearing secretions. In addition, a funduscopic examination should be performed for uveitis associated with autoimmune disorders and chronic steroid use.

The bulbar conjunctiva is examined by looking directly at the eye and asking the patient to look up and then down while gently retracting the opposite lid (ie, looking down while holding up the upper eyelid). Examination of the palpebral (tarsal) conjunctiva is performed by asking the patient to look down, grasping the upper lid at its base with a cotton swab on the upper portion of the lid, and then pulling out and up. The patient should be looking down during the examination. To return the lid to its normal position, the patient should look up. The lower tarsal conjunctiva is examined by everting the lower eyelid while placing a finger near the lid margins and drawing downward. Conjunctivitis can be differentiated from inflammation involving the anterior portion of the eye by the involvement of the fornix and the palpebral conjunctiva. A velvety, beef-red conjunctiva suggests a bacterial cause. A "milky" appearance, the result of obscuration of blood vessels by conjunctival edema (Fig. 1), is characteristic of allergy. The combination of these two features gives the conjunctiva a pinkish or milky appearance. Because the conjunctival blood vessels are partially obscured, they are best evaluated with a slit-lamp microscope. Often, chemosis is so marked that it is obvious without magnification. If edema is severe, patients exhibit periorbital edema (Fig. 2), which is more prominent around the lower lids because of gravity. Ecchymosis, or the "allergic shiner," has also been described in allergic patients and is thought to be the result of impaired venous return from the skin and subcutaneous tissues, although proof of this is lacking [21].

The signs of allergic conjunctivitis may not be striking. One expects the allergic eye to show mild to moderate redness. Severe redness would suggest a different diagnosis. It seems, however, that swelling or chemosis is

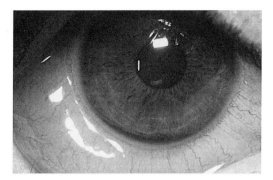

Fig. 1. Chemosis and injection of allergic conjunctivitis.

somewhat out of proportion to the amount of redness that is present. No doubt, some of the mediators released during allergic inflammation promote extravasation of serum out of the blood vessels and into the surrounding tissues. If chemosis is subtle, it can sometimes be detected at the medial aspect of the bulbar conjunctiva in the small fold of bulbar conjunctiva on the inner corner of the eye known as the plica semilunaris. This looser conjunctival tissue may appear more elevated and boggy than expected.

It is worthwhile to examine the superior limbus and the superior tarsal conjunctiva. In more severe allergies, these tissues are the site of Trantas' dots and giant papillae, respectively. They appear to be peculiar, anatomic targets for allergic inflammation and sometimes provide a subtle indication of the activity of ocular allergic disease. The direct (handheld) ophthalmoscope provides approximately 14× magnification. The physician may need to adjust the ophthalmoscope power setting to accommodate the patient's or the physician's refractive errors; the minus (red-numbered) lenses correct for nearsightedness, whereas the positive (green-numbered) lenses correct for farsighted errors. While using the lens, settings of +8 with the

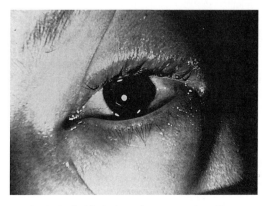

Fig. 2. Periorbital edema in acute ocular allergy.

ophthalmoscope held close to the patient's eye assist the physician in focusing on the anterior segment to reveal corneal opacities or changes in the iris or lens. Decreasing the power of the lens from +8 to −8 increases the depth of focus so that the examiner may move from the anterior segment progressively through the vitreous and reach the retina. The red-free (green) light filter is employed to sharply delineate small aneurysms and hemorrhages as black in patients who have autoimmune disorders (eg, systemic lupus erythematosus, vasculitis). Recently, attempts to measure the ocular allergic reaction objectively have been published [22]. The aim of objective measurements is greater accuracy and reproducibility, especially for clinical trials with antiallergic medications.

Seasonal and perennial allergic conjunctivitis

Because SAC and PAC are linked to allergic rhinitis (more commonly known as allergic rhinoconjunctivitis), they are the most prevalent forms of ocular allergy [7,23–25]. Of the two, SAC is more common. The importance of this condition is due more to its frequency than its severity [21].

Seasonal allergic conjunctivitis

SAC is the most common form of allergic conjunctivitis, representing more than half of all cases of allergic conjunctivitis [26,27]. The onset of symptoms is seasonally related to specific circulating aeroallergens. Grass pollens have been noted to be associated with increased ocular symptoms during the spring and, in some areas, during the fall (Indian summer). The ocular symptoms are frequently associated with nasal or pharyngeal complaints. Patients present with complaints of itchy eyes or a burning sensation with a watery discharge. A white exudate may form during the acute state, which becomes stringy in the chronic form. Rarely, SAC may also include corneal symptoms of photophobia and blurring of vision. The conjunctival surfaces are mildly injected with various levels of chemosis (conjunctival edema). Lid edema and papillary hypertrophy along the tarsal conjunctival surface may sometimes occur. Symptoms are usually bilateral, although the degree of involvement may not be symmetric. Affected individuals usually have a history of atopy. Allergic conjunctivitis, unlike several other ocular diseases, is seldom followed by permanent visual impairment.

Conjunctival cytology has revealed eosinophil infiltration in 25% of patients who have SAC. Elevated serum immunoglobulin (Ig)E levels have been noted in 78% of patients who have SAC, whereas tear fluid IgE is present in almost all (96%) tear fluid samples.

Perennial allergic conjunctivitis

PAC is considered to be a variant of SAC that persists throughout the year, although 79% of patients who have PAC experience a seasonal exacerbation. Dust mites, animal dander, and feathers are the most common airborne allergens implicated in PAC, and PAC is more likely than SAC to be associated with perennial rhinitis. Patients who have PAC and SAC are similar in age and sex, and both patient groups have the same prevalence of associated symptoms of asthma or eczema. In the older literature, the prevalence appears to be much lower than SAC (3/5 per 10,000 population) [28], but recent epidemiologic studies have reflected this prevalence to be as high as 40%. PAC is similar to SAC in affected age range and length of history, although SAC is subjectively more severe. When patients who had PAC were compared with patients who had SAC, a history to exposure to house dust was more common (42% versus 0%), as was the association of perennial rhinitis (75% versus 12%).

SAC and PAC are typical mast cell–mediated hypersensitivity reactions affecting the eye, in which the allergens react with specific IgE antibodies bound to the surface of conjunctival mast cells. The activation of mast cells leads to the release of powerful vasoactive amines, which is responsible for the itching, vasodilatation, and edema encountered in allergic conjunctivitis.

Patients who have SAC and PAC have been noted to have aeroallergen sensitivity and elevated IgE in tears and in serum. Differences between PAC and SAC include the findings that 89% of patients who had PAC had specific serum IgE for house dust compared with only 43% of patients who had SAC. Similarly, 78% of patients who had PAC had tear-specific IgE for house dust, whereas no patients who had SAC had measurable IgE specific for house dust in tears [29]. Mediators released by the degranulation of mast cells include preformed mediators such as histamine and prostaglandins. Tear samplings have also been shown to contain elevated levels of eosinophil major basic protein. Eosinophils have been demonstrated in conjunctival scrapings from 25% to 84% of patients who have PAC and from 43% of patients who have SAC.

Procedures

Scraping the conjunctival surface to look for eosinophils is a helpful diagnostic test. The procedure is done by placing a drop of topical anesthetic such as tetracaine hydrochloride 0.5% in the lower conjunctival sac. The anesthetic takes effect within 10 seconds. Using a platinum spatula, the inner surface of the lower lid is gently scraped several times. The material is then spread on a microscope slide. The slide is stained with Hansel stain, Giemsa stain, or another common reagent. Slides are examined for the presence of eosinophils or eosinophil granules. Eosinophils are not ordinarily found in the conjunctival scrapings from nonallergic individuals. The presence of even one eosinophil or eosinophil granule is considerable evidence in favor of a diagnosis of allergic conjunctivitis [30]. The absence of eosinophils should not rule out a diagnosis of allergy. Eosinophils are often present in the deeper layers of the conjunctiva and may be absent or undetectable in the upper layers. The frequency of eosinophils in the conjunctival scrapings from patients who have allergic conjunctivitis may vary from 20% to 80% [31] depending on the patient population, the chronicity of the allergic condition, and the persistence of the examiner [31]. Corneal infiltrates may occasionally be seen in severe allergic patients and tend to be nummular, subepithelial, and peripheral.

Conjunctival provocation tests (CPTs), which consist of instilling an offending pollen into the conjunctival sac, also produce the typical symptoms of hay fever conjunctivitis [32,33] and were the original method for evaluating allergic responses. Ocular challenge is used as a pharmacologic model for the evaluation of new antiallergic medications and immunotherapy [34]. The positivity of the challenge may be assessed by a sign and symptom scoring system that includes subjective and objective signs such as conjunctival erythema, chemosis, tearing, and pruritus. CPTs have also been shown to have a relatively good reproducibility in both eyes [32,35]. A CPT of ocular mast cells by way of opioid receptors has shown that 80% of normal patients reflect mast cell activation by detection of the release of histamine (7 versus 18 nm/L) and prostaglandin D_2 (0 versus 273 ng/L). The release of these mediators can be blocked by pretreating patients with cromolyn [36]. In assessing the potential usefulness of CPTs as a diagnostic tool, it was found that CPTs directly correlated to the radioallergosorbent test (RAST) in 71% (n = 130/183) of allergic patients. Of the 29% of uncorrelated cases, 23% (43/183) were positive by RAST but not by CPT, whereas 6% (10/183) were positive by CPT but not by RAST [37]. This finding suggests that there may be local sensitization of the target organ without evidence for systemic sensitization to the same antigen that clinically may reflect allergens causing ocular symptoms without any evidence of pulmonary or nasal allergic symptoms.

Late-phase reaction

A conjunctival late-phase reaction (LPR) has been described [38–41]. In the guinea pig model used by Leonardi and colleagues [42], the LPR manifested in several forms, including a classic biphasic response (33%), a multiphasic response (25%), and a single prolonged response (41%). The histologic evaluation of the conjunctiva revealed the typical influx of nonspecific cells of the inflammatory response, including neutrophils, basophils, and eosinophils. Tears collected from timed periods over the course of 6 hours after allergen challenge or CPT reflected the ability of mediators released during the LPR to reproduce the influx of cells commonly seen after ocular allergen testing [43]; however, clinical symptoms were not reproduced in this single patient. Direct application of leukotriene B_4 has been found to increase the number of eosinophils and neutrophils in rat conjunctiva [41].

Ocular challenge with platelet-activating factor also resulted in an inflammatory response. The substantia propria was the primary site of the vascular changes that included endothelial cell swelling, capillary dilatation, and edema. In one study, 7 of 10 patients revealed a resurgence of ocular symptoms 6 hours after the initial challenge. Scrapings of the conjunctiva revealed an influx of eosinophils, neutrophils, and lymphocytes; however, the study did not evaluate the total time sequence for the arrival of the cells in the conjunctiva, and some researchers have questioned whether this may be part of the initial immediate hypersensitivity reaction. Ocular challenge with histamine revealed vascular permeability but not an inflammatory response, as measured by the epithelial expression of intracellular adhesion molecule (ICAM; CD54) [44]. In another study evaluating the efficacy of a new antihistamine, 14 of 22 patients (64%) developed signs and symptoms of an ocular LPR 2 to 9 hours after the ocular challenge dose [45]. In that study, the three most severe ocular LPRs occurred in patients who had previously been treated with a topical antihistamine, although the itching score of the LPR was less than the immediate reaction. Because the investigators were searching for an increased tolerance of allergen for an "immediate" reaction, this observation raises the possibility that the topical H_1 antagonist used in that study blocked the immediate ocular response but permitted the administration of a higher dose of allergen in the ocular conjunctival challenge. In another study, loratadine was thought to have a protective effect on the LPR induced in the CPT [46]. Various mediators have been detected in the tears of allergic patients and may help guide future drug development [47,48].

Treatment

Antihistamines

Antihistamines may be given systemically to relieve allergic symptoms. These drugs may only partially relieve ocular symptoms, and patients often complain of side effects such as drowsiness and dryness of the eyes, nose, and mouth. Antihistamines such as antazoline and pheniramine are available as eye drops and are usually combined with a topical vasoconstrictor such as naphazoline hydrochloride. These antihistamine-vasoconstrictor eye drops are now available over-the-counter and are useful in treating mild allergic conjunctivitis [49]. Most are used four times a day, and the side effects are minimal. They whiten the eyes by constricting the conjunctival blood vessels. They also relieve itching in most patients [30,50].

Mast cell stabilizers

Mast cell stabilizers have been a useful addition to the other drugs available for treating allergic conjunctivitis. Several studies have confirmed their therapeutic value in allergic conjunctivitis [51,52]. Often, patients notice improvement within 24 to 48 hours. Mast cell stabilizers are most useful for relief of mild and moderate symptoms of allergic conjunctivitis. More severe cases may require the addition of topical corticosteroids. Unlike corticosteroids, mast cell stabilizers have minimal ocular side effects. An acute chemotic reaction to cromolyn was reported in two patients [53–55], but as in the treatment of asthma, cromolyn side effects are rare. An extra benefit of mast cell stabilizers is the relief of nasal symptoms caused by the drainage of tear fluid into the nasal passages. Nedocromil sodium is available in the United States and in Europe.

Lodoxamide tromethamine 0.1% (Alomide)

Lodoxamide tromethamine 0.1% (Alomide) is a mast cell stabilizer that prevents the release of histamine and leukotrienes [56]. Lodoxamide inhibits mediator release from mast cells, presumably by inhibiting calcium influx, thereby indirectly inhibiting increased vascular permeability. It is 2500 times more potent than cromolyn in inhibiting mediator release from mast cells; however, it appears to be roughly equivalent to cromolyn in controlling the symptoms of allergic conjunctivitis, vernal conjunctivitis, and giant papillary conjunctivitis. It is preserved in benzalkonium chloride.

Ketorolac tromethamine (Acular)

This nonsteroidal anti-inflammatory drug (NSAID) is preserved in benzalkonium chloride. It has been shown to relieve itching associated with allergic conjunctivitis. It also reduces levels of prostaglandin $(PG)E_2$ in tears. There may be some burning on instillation. It is unexpected that an NSAID would relieve itching, but research by Woodward and colleagues [57] suggested that some of the prostaglandins, particularly PGE_2 and PGI_2, may be pruritogenic.

Olopatadine (Patanol, Pataday)

Olopatadine inhibits mast cell degranulation and antagonizes histamine receptors to manage the itching, redness, chemosis, tearing, and lid swelling of the ocular allergic reaction [58,59]. Its mast cell stabilizing ability has been demonstrated in vitro (using human conjunctival mast cells) and in vivo (human clinical experience). A new formulation has recently been approved for once-a-day administration [60].

Ketotifen (Zaditor)

This benzocycloheptathiopen derivative is approved for the temporary prevention of itching due to allergic conjunctivitis [61]. It is a selective, non-competitive blocker of the H_1 histamine receptor. It inhibits inflammatory mediator release from mast cells, basophils, and eosinophils. It inhibits chemotaxis and degranulation of eosinophils, type 1 hypersensitivity reactions, and leukotriene activity. It is also an inhibitor of platelet-activating factors. In animal studies, it decreases vascular permeability and extravasation of Evan's blue dye in rat and guinea pig models of anaphylaxis. In human clinical trials using conjunctival allergen challenge, it reduces itching significantly and has a more modest effect on the reduction of conjunctival injection associated with allergy.

Nedocromil (Alocril)

This disodium salt of pyranoquinolone dicarboxylic acid is approved for treatment of itching associated with allergic conjunctivitis. It inhibits histamine, LTC4, and tumor necrosis factor α. It decreases chemotaxis of neutrophils and eosinophils and renders them unresponsive to mediators. It blocks the expression of cell surface adhesion molecules involved in eosinophil chemotaxis and decreases vascular permeability induced by inflammation. It reduces itching and, to a lesser extent, redness associated with allergic conjunctivitis. It has an onset of action 2 minutes after dosing and a duration of about 8 hours.

Pemirolast (Alamast)

Pemirolast is a mast cell stabilizer with antihistamine properties [62]. It is approved for the prevention of itching associated with allergic conjunctivitis. In SAC studies, it decreased itching and, to a lesser extent, redness, throughout the allergy season. It also decreased itching after conjunctival allergen challenge.

Azelastine (Optivar)

This phthalazinone derivative has been approved for the prevention or treatment of itching due to allergic conjunctivitis [63]. It inhibits histamine release from allergen-stimulated mast cells and suppresses inflammation. It decreases expression of ICAM-1, reduces eosinophil chemotaxis, and inhibits platelet-activating factor. It interferes with calcium influx in mast cells and inhibits the H_1 histamine receptor. It reduces itching, and, to a lesser extent, redness in SAC, in PAC, and after conjunctival allergen challenge.

Epinastine (Elestat)

Epinastine is a topically active, direct H_1 receptor antagonist and has affinity for the H_2, α_1, α_2, and 5-HT_2 receptors [64]. It also inhibits histamine release from mast cells. Epinastine has a duration of action of at least 8 hours and it is administered twice a day. It is indicated for the prevention of itching associated with allergic conjunctivitis. It can be used safely in patients older than 3 years.

Corticosteroids (Vexol, Lotemax)

Corticosteroids may be extremely effective in relieving symptoms of allergic rhinitis, but because the disease is a chronic, recurrent, benign condition, these drugs should be used only in extreme situations, commonly as a "burst" treatment for no more than 1 to 2 weeks. Topical steroids are associated with glaucoma, cataract formation, and infections of the cornea and conjunctiva [65]. Any prolonged use (ie, longer than 2 weeks) should therefore be used with the greatest caution, and the patient should preferably be monitored by an ophthalmologist. Under no circumstances should patients be allowed to use corticosteroid eye drops without medical supervision or be given prescriptions for unlimited refills.

Fluorometholone 0.1% eye drops are often selected as a useful treatment of external ocular inflammation. This steroid is highly effective in allergic conjunctivitis. It appears that fluorometholone penetrates the cornea well but is inactivated quickly in the anterior chamber. Thus, the complications of fluorometholone are rare. It may be that fluorometholone is inactivated before it has an opportunity to combine with trabecular meshwork or lens receptors. Thus, the incidence of glaucoma and cataract formation is expected to be lower than with prednisolone or dexamethasone.

Two "modified" steroids have recently been investigated for their efficacy in allergic conjunctivitis. Rimexolone (Vexol) [66] is a derivative of prednisolone that is quickly inactivated in the anterior chamber. During a 4-week treatment period in patients who had uveitis, rimexolone caused an increase in intraocular pressure of 10 mm or more in 5% of patients, whereas prednisolone acetate 1% caused elevation in nearly 14% of patients. In a 6-week steroid-responder study, prednisolone 1% and dexamethasone 0.1% caused mean pressures to rise to 30 mmHg after 3 weeks. Rimexolone and fluorometholone caused mean pressures to rise to only 22 mmHg at 3 weeks and 24 mmHg at 6 weeks. Rimexolone has recently been approved for treatment of postcataract inflammation and for iritis.

Another modified corticosteroid that shows great promise is loteprednol etabonate (Lotemax) [67]. Lotemax also seems to be highly effective in allergic conjunctivitis and is only rarely associated with a significant rise in intraocular pressure. A low-dose loteprednol etabonate (Alrex) has been approved for the relief of allergic conjunctivitis. Alrex is a useful treatment when mast cell stabilizers have been inadequate.

Other antiallergic drugs are being investigated and show promising results in the treatment of allergic conjunctivitis, including emedastine [68], a selective blocker of the H_1 histamine receptor. Cyclosporine, a fungal antimetabolite that can be used as an anti-inflammatory drug [69,70], inhibits interleukin-2 activation of lymphocytes. It is used systemically to prevent rejection of various solid-tissue transplants. It has been used as an eye drop in a variety of conditions including dry eye vernal conjunctivitis and in high-risk corneal transplants patients. Cyclosporine appears to interfere with antigen processing and presentation of antigen to the uncommitted T lymphocytes.

Immunotherapy has been successful in treating allergic conjunctivitis and may alter the progression of other atopic conditions [71].

Summary

Allergic conjunctivitis is common, especially during the allergy season. Ocular symptoms are usually accompanied by nasal symptoms, and there may be other allergic events in the patient's history that support the diagnosis of ocular allergy. Diagnostic tests can be helpful, especially conjunctival scrapings, to look for eosinophils. Consultation with the allergist to perform skin tests or in vitro tests may be useful and confirmatory in the diagnosis of ocular allergy. Symptoms may be mild, and many patients do not require treatment. If treatment is necessary, several antiallergic drugs are available. The selection of an antiallergic drug is based on the patient's need and a determination of which drug is well tolerated and most effective. Various antiallergic drugs are available for the eye. Antihistamines, mast cell stabilizers, and NSAIDs are safe and reasonably effective. Corticosteroids are an order of magnitude more potent than noncorticosteroids; however, they have attendant side effects that are best monitored by the ophthalmologist. The development of modified corticosteroids has been a boon to the treatment of ocular allergy because these drugs may reduce potential side effects without sacrificing potency.

References

[1] Singh K, Bielory L. Ocular allergy: a national epidemiologic study. J Allergy Clin Immunol 2007;119(1 Suppl 1):S154.

[2] Singh K, Bielory L. Epidemiology of ocular allergy symptoms in United States adults (1988–1994). Ann Allergy 2007;98:A22.

[3] Singh K, Bielory L. Epidemiology of ocular allergy symptoms in regional parts of the United States in the adult population (1988–1994). Ann Allergy 2007;98:A22.

[4] Friedlaender MH. Current concepts in ocular allergy. Ann Allergy 1991;67(1):5–10, 13.

[5] Marrache F, Brunet D, Frandeboeuf J, et al. The role of ocular manifestations in childhood allergy syndromes. Rev Fr Allergol Immunol Clin 1978;18.

[6] Isaacson P, Wright DH. Extranodal malignant lymphoma arising from mucosa-associated lymphoid tissue. Cancer 1984;53(11):2515–24.

[7] Bielory L. Allergic and immunologic disorders of the eye. Part I: immunology of the eye. J Allergy Clin Immunol 2000;106(5):805–16.

[8] Allansmith MR, Baird RS, Kashima K, et al. Mass cells in ocular tissues of normal rats and rats infected with Nippostrongylus brasiliensis. Invest Ophthalmol Vis Sci 1979;18:863–7.

[9] Henriquez AS, Bloch KJ, Kenyon KR, et al. Ultrastructure of mast cells in rat ocular tissue undergoing anaphylaxis. Arch Ophthalmol 1983;101:1439–46.

[10] Allansmith MR, Baird RS, Ross RN, et al. Effect of multiple applications of compound 48/80 on mast cells of rat conjunctiva. Acta Ophthalmol (Copenh) 1987;65:406–12.

[11] Soukiasian SH, Rice B, Foster CS, et al. The T cell receptor in normal and inflamed human conjunctiva. Invest Ophthalmol Vis Sci 1992;33(2):453–9.

[12] Gillette TE, Chandler JW, Greiner JV. Langerhans cells of the ocular surface. Ophthalmology 1982;89(6):700–11.

[13] Seto SK, Gillette TE, Chandler JW. HLA-DR+/T6– Langerhans cells of the human cornea. Invest Ophthalmol Vis Sci 1987;28(10):1719–22.

[14] Trocme SD, Kephart GM, Allansmith MR, et al. Conjunctival deposition of eosinophil granule major basic protein in vernal keratoconjunctivitis and contact lens–associated giant papillary conjunctivitis. Am J Ophthalmol 1989;108(1):57–63.

[15] Fukagawa K, Saito H, Tsubota K, et al. RANTES production in a conjunctival epithelial cell line. Cornea 1997;16(5):564–70.

[16] Angi MR, Bettero A, Filippi F, et al. [Quantitative evaluation of conjunctival irritation by simultaneous determination of histamine, serotonin and leukotriene C4 in tears]. Ophtalmologie 1987;1:509–11 [in French].

[17] Kari O, Salo OP, Halempuro L, et al. Tear histamine during allergic conjunctivitis challenge. Graefes Arch Clin Exp Ophthalmol 1985;223(2):60–2.

[18] Angi MR, Bettero A, Benassi CA. Histamine in tears: developments in collection and HPLC-fluorimetric detection. Agents Actions 1985;16:84–6.

[19] Abelson MB, Baird RS, Allansmith MR. Tear histamine levels in vernal conjunctivitis and other ocular inflammations. Ophthalmology 1980;87:812–4.

[20] Singh K, Bielory L, Kavosh E. Allergens associated with ocular and nasal symptoms: an epidemiologic study. J Allergy Clin Immunol 2007;119(1 Suppl 1):S223.

[21] Weeke ER. Epidemiology of hay fever and perennial allergic rhinitis. Monogr Allergy 1987; 21:1–20.

[22] Friedlaender MH. Objective measurement of allergic reactions in the eye. Curr Opin Allergy Clin Immunol 2004;4(5):447–53.

[23] Bielory L. Allergic diseases of the eye. Med Clin North Am 2006;90(1):129–48.

[24] Bielory L, Dinowitz M, Rescigno R. Ocular allergic diseases: differential diagnosis, examination techniques and testing. J Toxicol Cutaneous Ocul Toxicol 2002;21:329–51.

[25] Bielory L. Allergic and immunologic disorders of the eye. Part II: ocular allergy. J Allergy Clin Immunol 2000;106(6):1019–32.

[26] Ono SJ, Abelson MB. Allergic conjunctivitis: update on pathophysiology and prospects for future treatment. J Allergy Clin Immunol 2005;115(1):118–22.

[27] Bielory L. Differential diagnoses of conjunctivitis for clinical allergist-immunologists. Ann Allergy Asthma Immunol 2007;98(2):105–14 [quiz 114–7, 152].

[28] Dart JK, Buckley RJ, Monnickendan M, et al. Perennial allergic conjunctivitis: definition, clinical characteristics and prevalence. A comparison with seasonal allergic conjunctivitis. Trans Ophthalmol Soc U K 1986;105(Pt 5):513–20.

[29] Ballow M, Mendelson L, Donshik P, et al. Pollen-specific IgG antibodies in the tears of patients with allergic-like conjunctivitis. J Allergy Clin Immunol 1984;73(3):376–80.

[30] Friedlaender MH, Okumoto M, Kelley J. Diagnosis of allergic conjunctivitis. Arch Ophthalmol 1984;102(8):1198–9.

[31] Abelson MB, Madiwale N, Weston JH. Conjunctival eosinophils in allergic ocular disease. Arch Ophthalmol 1983;101(4):555–6.

[32] Stegman R, Miller D. A human model of allergic conjunctivitis. Arch Ophthalmol 1975; 93(12):1354–8.

[33] Friedlaender MH. Conjunctival provocation testing: overview of recent clinical trials in ocular allergy. Int Ophthalmol Clin 2003;43(1):95–104.

[34] Abelson MB, Smith LM. Levocabastine. Evaluation in the histamine and compound 48/80 models of ocular allergy in humans. Ophthalmology 1988;95(11):1494–7.

[35] Aichane A, Campbell AM, Chanal I, et al. Precision of conjunctival provocation tests in right and left eyes. J Allergy Clin Immunol 1993;92(1 Pt 1):49–55.

[36] Campbell AM, Demoly P, Michel FB, et al. Conjunctival provocation tests with codeine phosphate. Effect of disodium cromoglycate. Ann Allergy 1993;71(1):51–5.

[37] Leonardi A, Fregona IA, Gismondi M, et al. Correlation between conjunctival provocation test (CPT) and systemic allergometric tests in allergic conjunctivitis. Eye 1990;4(Pt 5):760–4.

[38] Bonini S, Bonini S, Bucci MG, et al. Allergen dose response and late symptoms in a human model of ocular allergy. J Allergy Clin Immunol 1990;86(6 Pt 1):869–76.

[39] Bonini S, Bonini S, Vecchione A, et al. Inflammatory changes in conjunctival scrapings after allergen provocation in humans. J Allergy Clin Immunol 1988;82(3 Pt 1):462–9.

[40] Leonardi A, Bloch KJ, Briggs R, et al. Histology of ocular late-phase reaction in guinea pigs passively sensitized with IgG1 antibodies. Ophthalmic Res 1990;22(4):209–19.

[41] Trocme SD, Bonini S, Barney NP, et al. Late-phase reaction in topically induced ocular anaphylaxis in the rat. Curr Eye Res 1988;7(5):437–43.

[42] Leonardi A, Briggs RM, Bloch KJ, et al. Clinical patterns of ocular anaphylaxis in guinea pigs passively sensitized with IgG1 antibody. Ophthalmic Res 1990;22(2):95–105.

[43] Bonini S, Centofanti M, Schiavone M, et al. Passive transfer of the ocular late phase reaction. Ocular Immunol Inflammat 1993;1:323–5.

[44] Ciprandi G, Buscaglia S, Pesce GP, et al. Ocular challenge and hyperresponsiveness to histamine in patients with allergic conjunctivitis. J Allergy Clin Immunol 1993;91(6):1227–30.

[45] Zuber P, Pecoud A. Effect of levocabastine, a new H1 antagonist, in a conjunctival provocation test with allergens. J Allergy Clin Immunol 1988;82(4):590–4.

[46] Ciprandi G, Buscaglia S, Marchesi E, et al. Protective effect of loratadine on late phase reaction induced by conjunctival provocation test. Int Arch Allergy Immunol 1993;100(2):185–9.

[47] Schultz BL. Pharmacology of ocular allergy. Curr Opin Allergy Clin Immunol 2006;6(5):383–9.

[48] Cook EB. Tear cytokines in acute and chronic ocular allergic inflammation. Curr Opin Allergy Clin Immunol 2004;4(5):441–5.

[49] Greiner JV, Udell IJ. A comparison of the clinical efficacy of pheniramine maleate/naphazoline hydrochloride ophthalmic solution and olopatadine hydrochloride ophthalmic solution in the conjunctival allergen challenge model. Clin Ther 2005;27(5):568–77.

[50] Abelson MB, Allansmith MR, Friedlaender MH. Effects of topically applied ocular decongestant and antihistamine. Am J Ophthalmol 1980;90(2):254–7.

[51] Friday GA, Biglan AW, Hiles DA, et al. Treatment of ragweed allergic conjunctivitis with cromolyn sodium 4% ophthalmic solution. Am J Ophthalmol 1983;95(2):169–74.

[52] Greenbaum J, Cockcroft D, Hargreave FE, et al. Sodium cromoglycate in ragweed-allergic conjunctivitis. J Allergy Clin Immunol 1977;59(6):437–9.

[53] Ostler HB. Acute chemotic reaction to cromolyn. Arch Ophthalmol 1982;100(3):412–3.

[54] Ostler HB. Alpha 1-antitrypsin and ocular sensitivity to cromoglycate. Lancet 1982;2(8310):1287.

[55] Settipane GA, Klein DE, Boyd GK, et al. Adverse reactions to cromolyn. JAMA 1979;241(8):811–3.

[56] Caldwell DR, Verin P, Hartwich-Young R, et al. Efficacy and safety of lodoxamide 0.1% vs cromolyn sodium 4% in patients with vernal keratoconjunctivitis. Am J Ophthalmol 1992;113(6):632–7.

[57] Woodward DF, Nieves AL, Friedlaender MH. Characterization of receptor subtypes involved in prostanoid-induced conjunctival pruritus and their role in mediating allergic conjunctival itching. J Pharmacol Exp Ther 1996;279(1):137–42.

[58] Abelson MB. A review of olopatadine for the treatment of ocular allergy. Expert Opin Pharmacother 2004;5(9):1979–94.

[59] Abelson MB, Gomes PJ, Vogelson CT, et al. Effects of a new formulation of olopatadine ophthalmic solution on nasal symptoms relative to placebo in two studies involving subjects with allergic conjunctivitis or rhinoconjunctivitis. Curr Med Res Opin 2005;21(5):683–91.

[60] Sharif NA, Xu SX, Yanni JM. Olopatadine (AL-4943A): ligand binding and functional studies on a novel, long acting H1-selective histamine antagonist and anti-allergic agent for use in allergic conjunctivitis. J Ocul Pharmacol Ther 1996;12(4):401–7.

[61] Avunduk AM, Tekelioglu Y, Turk A, et al. Comparison of the effects of ketotifen fumarate 0.025% and olopatadine HCI 0.1% ophthalmic solutions in seasonal allergic conjunctivities: a 30-day, randomized, double-masked, artificial tear substitute-controlled trial. Clin Ther 2005;27:1392–402.

[62] Abelson MB, Berdy GJ, Mundorf T, et al. Pemirolast potassium 0.1% ophthalmic solution is an effective treatment for allergic conjunctivitis: a pooled analysis of two prospective, randomized, double-masked, placebo-controlled, phase III studies. J Ocul Pharmacol Ther 2002;18(5):475–88.

[63] Bielory L, Buddiga P, Bigelson S. Ocular allergy treatment comparisons: azelastine and olopatadine. Curr Allergy Asthma Rep 2004;4(4):320–5.

[64] Friedlaender MH. Epinastine in the management of ocular allergic disease. Int Ophthalmol Clin 2006;46(4):85–6.

[65] Friedlaender MH. Corticosteroid therapy of ocular inflammation. Int Ophthalmol Clin 1983;23(1):175–82.

[66] Assil KK, Massry G, Lehmann R, et al. Control of ocular inflammation after cataract extraction with rimexolone 1% ophthalmic suspension. J Cataract Refract Surg 1997;23: 750–7.

[67] Friedlaender MH, Howes J. A double-masked, placebo-controlled evaluation of the efficacy and safety of loteprednol etabonate in the treatment of giant papillary conjunctivitis. The Loteprednol Etabonate Giant Papillary Conjunctivitis Study Group I. Am J Ophthalmol 1997;123:455–64.

[68] Sharif NA, Xu S, Yanni J. Emedastine: Pharmacological profile of a novel antihistamine for use in allergic conjunctivitis. Invest Ophthalmol Vis Sci 1995;36:s135.

[69] Hakin KN, Ham J, Lightman SL. Use of cyclosporin in the management of steroid dependent non-necrotising scleritis. Br J Ophthalmol 1991;75(6):340–1.

[70] Kilicu A, Gurler B. Topical 2% cyclosporine A in preservative-free artificial tears for the treatment of vernal keratoconjunctivitis. Can J Ophthalmol 2006;41(6):693–8.

[71] Bielory L, Mongia A. Current opinion of immunotherapy for ocular allergy. Curr Opin Allergy Clin Immunol 2002;2(5):447–52.

ELSEVIER
SAUNDERS

Immunol Allergy Clin N Am
28 (2008) 59–82

IMMUNOLOGY
AND ALLERGY
CLINICS
OF NORTH AMERICA

Vernal Conjunctivitis

Jason Jun, BA[a], Leonard Bielory, MD[b],
Michael B. Raizman, MD[a,c],*

[a]Tufts University School of Medicine, Boston, MA, USA
[b]Division of Allery, Immunology, and Rheumatology, UMDNJ–New Jersey Medical School,
90 Bergen Street, DOC Suite 4700, Newark, NJ 07103, USA
[c]Cornea and Anterior Segment Service, New England Eye Center, 20 Tremont Street,
Biewend Buidling, 10th Floor, Boston, MA 02111, USA

Vernal conjunctivitis (VC) is a bilateral, seasonal, external ocular inflammatory disease of unknown cause. VC most commonly begins in the spring, hence the name "vernal." Afflicted patients experience intense itching, tearing, photophobia, and mucous discharge, and usually demonstrate large cobblestone papillae on their superior tarsal conjunctiva and limbal conjunctiva. VC primarily affects children, may be related to atopy, and has environmental and racial predilections. Although usually self-limited, VC can result in potentially blinding corneal complications. Treatment of chronic forms of ocular allergies may necessitate collaborative efforts between the ophthalmologist and the allergist or immunologist.

History

The first reported description of VC was in 1846 by Arlt, who reported what would be one of the classic VC presentations of perilimbal swelling, while von Graefe in 1871 reported cobblestone papillae on the upper tarsal conjunctiva. Shortly thereafter, in 1872, Saemisch observed seasonal flares of the disease in 182 VC patients and coined the term "vernal catarrh" or "spring catarrh." Other characteristic features, such as white points at the

Portions of this article originally appeared in Lee Y, Raizman M. Vernal conjunctivitis. Immunology and Allergy Clinics of North America 1997;17(1):33–51.

* Corresponding author. Cornea, External Disease, and Cataract Service, New England Medical Center, 260 Tremont Street, Biewend Building, 10th Floor, Boston, MA 02111.

E-mail address: mraizman@tufts-nemc.org (M.B. Raizman).

0889-8561/08/$ - see front matter © 2008 Elsevier Inc. All rights reserved.
doi:10.1016/j.iac.2007.12.007

limbus, were reported in 1879 by Horner (Horner's points), and further characterized by Trantas (Horner-Trantas dots) in 1899. During this time, in 1888, Emmert categorized VC into three types:

Palpebral, with papillae primarily involving the upper tarsal conjunctiva
Limbal, with papillae located at the limbus
Mixed, with components of both palpebral and limbal types [1]

With the evolution of histology, Herbert, in 1903, observed eosinophils in the peripheral blood of VC patients; in 1908 Pascheff found a prevalence of mast cells in the tarsal conjunctival epithelium of VC patients [1]; and in 1909 Gabrielides reported finding eosinophils in conjunctival secretions in addition to providing a detailed description of the vernal plaque.

Epidemiology

Although VC has a world-wide distribution, it does have racial and regional variations. There is a greater prevalence of VC in hot, dry environments, such as the Middle East, the Mediterranean basin, North and West Africa, parts of India, and Central and South America [2–4]. This disease accounts for 0.1% to 0.5% of the patients presenting with ocular problems and appears to be increasing. A cross-sectional study performed in eastern Africa reported that VC affects as many as 5% of school-aged children [5], 10% of 74,400 outpatient visits to ophthalmic clinics in Israel [6], and up to 15% in Italy [4]. A recent case series from Nigeria identified VC as the most common conjunctival disease seen in a major teaching hospital over a 2-year period [7]. In that same study the association with atopy was noted to be 5%, while in another Nigerian study it was found to be as high as 20%, with approximately 6% connected to asthma, 5% allergic rhinitis, and 4% eczema [8]. The greater prevalence in hotter regions could be because of a higher level of atmospheric pollution by pollens and other allergens [1]. Seasonal variation, association with atopy, and regression of the disease are also less common in these regions. In a Japanese study, the breakdown of patients with ocular allergies included seasonal allergic conjunctivitis (SAC) (81.2%), perennial allergic conjunctivitis (10.6%), atopic keratoconjunctivitis (AKC) (4.4%), and vernal keratoconjunctivitis (VC) (3.8%), with a mean age in each disease of 52.9, 56.1, 25.7, and 16.6 years, respectively. Total clinical score, based on 10 objective ocular clinical findings of conjunctival, limbal, and corneal lesions, resulted in a progressively increasing scores of 1.54, 2.13, 3.72, and 12.68, respectively [9].

The prevalence of VC in temperate areas, such as Northern Europe, has been shown to be affected by the immigration of African and Asian children [10]. While this suggests the contribution of genetic factors to the pathogenesis of this disease, substantive work in this area is still ongoing [11].

VC is primarily a disease of childhood and youth. VC has been reported in patients as young as 1 month old to patients over the age of 70. However, the majority of patients are between 5 and 25 years of age. Approximately 60% are between 11 and 20 years of age, 17% between 21 and 30 years of age, and 6% greater than 30 years of age [12]. The mean age of onset is between 6 and 7 years old, with a slightly earlier onset in boys than in girls [3,13]. Boys are more frequently affected than girls, with a reported ratio of 4:1 to 2:1 until puberty. By age 20 this ratio approaches 1:1 [3,13]. Recurrent episodes usually occur over a 2- to 10-year period and often resolve spontaneously around puberty. In middle-aged patients, the disease may persist and become protracted. Some of these patients develop an ocular condition that is indistinguishable from the typical atopic conjunctivitis of adulthood.

A recent case series of 128 VC subjects from the Padua region of Italy found that the incidence of VC was 1 in 100,000 for all inhabitants, regardless of age and gender. For the population under 15 years of age, the mean incidence was 7.2 in 100,000 (10 in 100,000 in males, 4.2 in 100,000 in females). In the population over 15 years of age, the mean incidence was 0.06 in 100,000 (0.04 in 100,000 in males, 0.08 in 100,000 in females) [3].

Clinical manifestation

VC is an allergic conjunctival inflammation disorder, often with secondary keratopathy. Invariably, patients complain of itching, which can be severe. In a pediatric quality of life study, the most commonly reported symptoms were itching (93%), burning (90%), redness (90%), the need to use eye drops (90%), tearing (83%), and photophobia (80%). The children's greatest concerns were limitations on going to the pool (71%), playing sports (58%), and meeting friends (58%) [14]. Discharge is common: an accumulation of ropy mucus can be found in the conjunctival fornix. Tearing, photophobia, burning or foreign body sensation, and conjunctival injection may also be prominent.

Although typically a bilateral disease, VC can present asymmetrically. Giant papillae, the classic hallmark, form on the superior tarsal or limbal conjunctiva. The papillae in the upper lid may become so severe as to cause a mechanical ptosis from their weight. White dots (Horner's points or Trantas' dots) can occur in the limbus and persist for 2 days to 1 week [15–17]. With continued inflammation, inflammatory mediators, such as eosinophilic major basic protein in the tear film, can cause epithelial toxicity, compounding the mechanical effects of the large upper lid papillae on the cornea. A punctate epithelial keratopathy may develop and, in severe cases, the epithelium can break down to form a shield-like ulcer. These corneal ulcerations are more common in children and may compromise visual acuity if scarring develops. These defects are thought to be trophic and are usually resistant to the standard treatments (lubrication, patching, bandage contact lenses). A secondary infectious keratitis also can develop. The most common corneal degenerative change from the chronic inflammation is a pseudogerontoxon, resembling corneal arcus. Changes in corneal curvature can also result, and keratoconus may develop late in the disease course.

As the disease continues, the symptoms can progress and can become chronic or perennial. Approximately 23% of patients have a perennial form of VC from disease onset and more than 60% have additional recurrences during the winter [13].

Conjunctival signs

VC affects the palpebral and limbal conjunctiva. The cobblestone papillae characteristic of VC are easily visible with eversion of the upper lid (Fig. 1). On slit lamp examination, they are 1 mm to 8 mm in diameter, have a central core of blood vessels, and stain with fluorescein at their apices from erosion during active inflammation. Laced between and on top of the giant papillae is a ropy mucoid discharge that can form a pseudomembrane [1]. Follicles are not a feature of this disease. VC can cause a reticular subepithelial fibrosis but does not cause keratoconjunctivitis sicca and only rarely causes cicatrization of the conjunctiva (Figs. 2 and 3) [1].

Limbal signs

Limbal VC was first described by Arlt in 1846 and is more common in highly pigmented individuals. It consists of large papillae in the limbal conjunctiva. These tend to involve the superior limbus and consist of inflammatory cells rich in eosinophils at their apices. Focal areas of mucinous degeneration of epithelial cells and eosinophils form the white Horner-Trantas dots. In severe forms of limbal VC, accumulation of inflammatory cells may form a frank mound on the peripheral cornea [18]. The limbal conjunctiva also can become thickened and opacified (Fig. 4) [1].

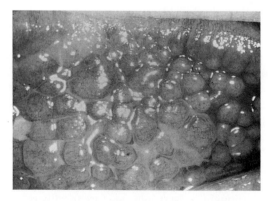

Fig. 1. Palpebral vernal conjunctivitis. The upper tarsal conjunctiva typically has multiple large, cobblestone-like papillae interlaced with a ropy mucus discharge. (*Reprinted from* Lee Y, Raizman M. Vernal conjunctivitis. Immunology and Allergy Clinics of North America 1997;17(1):33–51; with permission.)

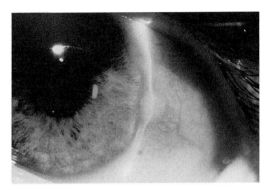

Fig. 2. Limbal vernal conjunctivitis. Large papillae can present at the corneoscleral limbus. They consist of inflammatory cells rich in eosinophils at their apices. (*Reprinted from* Lee Y, Raizman M. Vernal conjunctivitis. Immunology and Allergy Clinics of North America 1997;17(1):33–51; with permission.)

Corneal signs

Corneal involvement is associated with more severe disease. A superficial punctate epithelial keratopathy most commonly involves the superior half of the cornea. These can become confluent to form a shield ulcer: a shallow erosion with raised edges consisting of cellular debris and mucus. Named for their oval or shield-like shape, they tend to occur in the superior cornea and usually only affect very young patients. Mucus and fibrin can accumulate on the base of these trophic ulcers and inhibit re-epithelialization [1]. They can also scar, creating a subepithelial, gray opacity and can become vascularized with chronic corneal inflammation. With a compromised epithelial surface, these erosions are at risk for a secondary bacterial infection [19]. Shield

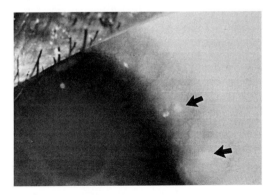

Fig. 3. Limbal vernal conjunctivitis. White Horner-Trantas dots (*arrows*) are often found at the limbus and represent focal areas of mucinous degeneration of epithelial cells and eosinophils. (*Reprinted from* Lee Y, Raizman M. Vernal conjunctivitis. Immunology and Allergy Clinics of North America 1997;17(1):33–51; with permission.)

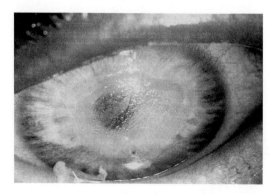

Fig. 4. Vernal shield ulcer. Named for their shield-like shape, they tend to occur in the superior cornea, are slow to re-epithelialize, and can result in visually significant corneal scarring. (*Reprinted from* Lee Y, Raizman M. Vernal conjunctivitis. Immunology and Allergy Clinics of North America 1997;17(1):33–51; with permission.)

ulcers have been reported to occur in 3% to 20% of VC cases [13,20–23]. Shield ulcers may also be complicated by amblyopia, strabismus, microbial keratitis, and corneal perforation [13,19,21,22,24].

A degenerative pseudogerontoxon resembling corneal arcus can develop in the peripheral cornea. Further degeneration can result in a peripheral furrow with steepening of the corneal curvature [25]. A superior pannus can also result from chronic inflammatory changes at the limbus.

Atypical corneal changes also have been reported in the literature. Shuler and colleagues [26] described inferior corneal ulcerations associated with palpebral VC. Cameron and colleagues [27] reported corneal ectasias (keratoconus, keratoglobus, pellucid marginal degeneration, superior marginal corneal thinning) in a series of VC patients. In general, VC rarely results in severe corneal scarring or pannus formation or other visually significant complications except for when the disease transforms into AKC (Fig. 5).

Pathogenesis

VC traditionally has been considered to be an IgE-mast cell lymphocyte-mediated hypersensitivity reaction, as suggested by its seasonal incidence, association with personal or family history of atopy, elevated levels of mast cells, eosinophils, specific IgE, and its response to antiallergic therapy [1, 28–38]. However, a large proportion of VC patients lack one or more of these characteristics. Bonini and colleagues [13] found that 42% and 47% of their cohort of VC subjects had negative skin prick and radio-allergosorbent (RAST) tests, respectively. Other studies indicate that at least 35% of VC patients lack either personal or family history of atopic conditions [39]. There appears to be a significant geographic variation as well. A large case series from Africa indicated associated atopy in as little as 5% of patients [7].

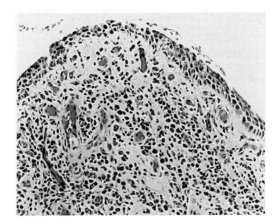

Fig. 5. Papillae from upper tarsal conjunctiva of patient with vernal conjunctivitis. Note the vascular stalks to the surface and the cellular infiltration (hematoxylin-eosin, original magnification ×200). (*Reprinted from* Lee Y, Raizman M. Vernal conjunctivitis. Immunology and Allergy Clinics of North America 1997;17(1):33–51; with permission.)

Histopathologic examination of affected conjunctiva shows an increased number of mast cells, eosinophils (cells associated with allergic reactions), and lymphocytes, both in the subepithelium and epithelium [11], as well as mononuclear cells, fibroblasts, and newly secreted collagen. As the disease progresses, cellular infiltration and new collagen deposition form the giant papillae. These findings have led many to conclude that the pathogenesis of VC represents a complex interaction between the IgE-mast cell hypersensitivity and the predominantly lymphocytic type hypersensitivity, and nonspecific mechanisms [28–31,40,41].

Activation and degranulation of mast cells, whether by the classic IgE-mediated pathway or from other specific or nonspecific stimuli, play a critical role in the pathogenesis of VC and other ocular allergies. Mast cells appear to be heavily concentrated in the epithelium and subepithelial stroma [39] of VC patients. Total mast cell concentrations are also significantly greater in the substantia propria, suggesting that active recruitment of mast cells into inflamed conjuctiva plays a key role in pathogenesis [35,37].

Preformed mast cell derivatives, such as histamine and tryptase, have repeatedly been found to be elevated in VC patients [32,42–44]. Histamine is responsible for the itching and redness experienced in ocular allergy. VC patients have also been shown to respond to a histamine conjunctival challenge at a lower threshold than normal controls, which suggests a non-specific conjunctival hyperreactivity in these patients [33]. Further work has demonstrated that this hyperreactivity may be caused in part by a deficiency of histaminase, the main histamine-metabolizing enzyme, in VC patients [45]. Histamine may also play a role in the remodeling of tissues seen in VC through its stimulation of conjunctival fibroblasts, which increase production of procollagen I and other proinflammatory cytokines, such as interleukin (IL)-1, IL-6, and IL-8 [46,47].

Tryptase, a neutral protease present only in mast cells, is considered a better marker for mast cell activation than histamine. Tryptase is held at a higher concentration in mast cells and is detectable for longer periods after release [43,48]. Tabbara [49] observed that tear tryptase levels were significantly decreased after medical therapy and were correlated with improvement in the clinical signs and symptoms of VC. Tabbara goes on to suggest that tear tryptase levels may serve as a good diagnostic tool for ocular allergy and for monitoring of activity of the disease. Tryptase may play its own role in VC pathogenesis through the further activation of proteases, such as metalloproteinase-2. The expression of metalloproteinases have been demonstrated in various chronic atopic disease states, such VKC, nasal polyps, and asthma, and play a role in the remodeling [50].

The release of IL-4, IL-13, and tumor necrosis factor (TNF)-α by activated mast cells has also been shown to induce production of chemokines and expression of adhesion molecules, such as vascular cell adhesion molecule (VCAM)-1 and intercellular adhesion molecule (ICAM)-1 by corneal fibroblasts [51–54]. These findings highlight the importance of mast cell-fibroblast interactions in ocular allergy.

Eosinophils are found in all stages of VC and have been shown to comprise 90% of the cytologic picture in the active phase of the disease [39]. Up-regulation of eosinophils by IL-5 and fibroblast-derived chemokines, such as eotaxin [53], likely plays an important role in the corneal findings associated with VC.

Large amounts of eosinophil major basic protein (MBP) and eosinophil cationic protein have been found in conjunctiva [55] and tears [56], and significantly higher levels of eosinophil cationic protein (ECP) have been found in tears [57] and serum [58] of VC patients over controls. The levels of both mediators correlate with the severity of disease. MBP has been implicated in the pathogenesis of corneal shield ulcers [59–61]. ECP also has demonstrated epithelial toxicity [57,58]. A histopathologic study revealed granular, deeply-eosinophilic, laminar material, firmly attached to the Bowman layer that was confirmed via immunohistochemistry to be eosinophil-derived major basic protein, suggesting that MBP plaques precipitate on the denuded stromal bed, thereby playing a pathogenic role in nonhealing shield ulcers [62]. Although the corneal manifestations of VC are often described as "frictional," from the enlarged upper lid papillae and from eye rubbing, the chemical toxicity from degranulated mast cells and eosinophils is probably a more important cause [63].

Recent attention has turned to the role of Th2 lymphocytes in the pathogenesis of VC. Bonini [41] has suggested that VC shares similarities to asthma, another Th2-driven disease. Several studies have demonstrated the abundance of Th2 cells and Th2-derived cytokines in both the conjunctiva and tears of VC patients [11,42,64–66]. Leonardi and colleagues [46] have shown that over two-thirds of VC patients have CD4+/IL-4+ lymphocytes (Th2 cells) in tears, versus only 8% of patients displaying CD4+/INF-γ+ (Th1) cells. Th2-derived cytokines (IL-3, IL-4, IL-5, IL-10, IL-13, and granulocyte-macrophage colony-stimulating factor or GM-CSF) fuel local hyperproduction of IgE (IL-4) and lead to increased levels of eosinophils (IL-5) and mast cells (IL-3). Th2 cells and their derivatives have been found in VC patients regardless of IgE allergy test results [46]. The overabundance of Th2 cells and resulting local hyperproduction of IgE may also explain an increased reactivity to nonspecific environmental factors, such as wind, sunlight, and heat [46].

Bonini and colleagues [11] have hypothesized that VC may result from an up-regulation of a "cytokine gene cluster" located on chromosome 5q, including genes for IL-3, IL-4, IL-5, IL-13 (an IL-4-like cytokine), and GM-CSF, which would further suggest that VC is a Th2 cell-driven disease. Unique genetic loci, such as the eotaxin 1 locus, have been associated with SAC [67,68], and similar genome-wide analyses for VC are now nearing completion.

Other inflammatory cells, such as neutrophils, basophils, macrophages, natural killer, and dendritic cells have also been implicated in VC through the release of proinflammatory mediators, enzymes, and cytokines [11,13,39,41,46,69–71]. In particular, leukotrienes, produced from the metabolism of arachadonic acid in mast cells, neutrophils, and macrophages, are potent mediators of hypersensitivity and inflammatory reactions [40,72,73]. Leukotriene concentrations in tear fluid have been shown to increase in allergic patients upon allergen challenge [74,75]. Leukotrienes act on the conjunctiva to produce venodilation, edema, hyperemia, and the infiltration of leukocytes and eosinophils [76–78], leading some to suggest that these compounds play a critical role in eliciting some of the common features of VC [79].

Additional areas that are currently under investigation and have demonstrated promise in animal models include immunomodulation of IL-1, IL-10, and local dendritic cells within the conjunctiva [80]. Allam and colleagues [81] have shown that early dendritic cell activation by allergens is a very early step in disease pathogenesis, with dermal allergy as the prototype.

Differences have also been noted in tear film abnormalities between VC and AKC patients. The mean tear breakup time, corneal sensitivity, and conjunctival goblet cell density values in VC patients and controls were significantly higher when compared with AKC patients. The squamous metaplasia grades in eyes with AKC were significantly higher when compared with eyes with VC and controls. The inflammatory cell response in brush cytology specimens was different between patients with AKC and VC. Eyes with AKC showed significantly higher MUC1, -2, and –4, and lower MUC5AC mRNA expression when compared with eyes with VC [82].

Other investigators have looked beyond the immune system for clues into the pathogenetic origins of VC. Substance P and nerve growth factor (NGF) receptors have been found in the tears and conjunctiva of VC patients [83–85]. Serum assays have detected high levels of both Substance P and NGF during the acute phase of the disease. In a study evaluating tear fluid Substance P levels in SAC, atopic dermatitis without keratoconjunctivitis, VC, and normal controls, found subjects with atopic dermatitis and normal controls had low levels, whereas subjects with SAC and VC showed significant elevation of Substance P [83]. Furthermore, the differential prevalence by gender and the commonly observed resolution of the disease after puberty suggests a role for sex hormones [86], as seen in other ocular inflammatory conditions, such as dry eyes syndrome [87]. Estrogen and progesterone receptors have been reported to be overexpressed by eosinophils and other inflammatory cells in the conjunctiva of VC patients [88].

Differential diagnosis

The differential diagnosis for VC must include all causes of allergic conjunctivitis [89]. Although a classic case of VC may be easily recognized, milder cases may be less obvious. Further testing may be necessary to aid in the diagnosis.

VC and AKC may be difficult to distinguish. The onset of AKC is often in the late teen years and it may persist for many years. AKC is also a bilateral disease with seasonal variations, though an association with warmer climates is less pronounced than with VC [28]. Signs and symptoms are similar to those associated with VC, including itching, burning, tearing, mucous discharge, Horner's points, corneal vascularization and ulceration, keratoconus, and pseudogerontoxon [15]. Eyelids of individuals presenting with AKC often exhibit chronic blepharitis, eczema, and secondary skin infections. In contrast to VC, AKC tends to affect the inferior palpebral conjunctiva and cause smaller papillae. AKC can cause conjunctival scarring and cicatrization, with foreshortening of the lower fornix. Neovascularization of cornea in AKC tends to be deeper, and the corneal complications are potentially blinding. In general, AKC is a more serious disease.

Seasonal allergic conjunctivitis is the most common allergic conjunctivitis. Also known as hay fever conjunctivitis, it tends to present with bilateral itching, injection, and tearing. The better-known allergens that cause SAC are pollens from ragweed, grass and trees, animal dander, and house dust. These allergens dissolve in the tear film and traverse the conjunctival epithelium to contact IgE-primed mast cells, resulting in degranulation of mast cells and release of inflammatory mediators. Rapid onset of conjunctivitis and of an allergic rhinitis or sinusitis after exposure to the allergen is characteristic of SAC. Corneal changes are rare in SAC.

Giant papillary conjunctivitis (GPC) is believed to result from allergens on foreign bodies in direct contact with the conjunctiva. Though most widely associated with contact lenses, other irritants, such as exposed sutures and ocular prosthetics, may also cause GPC. Patients typically complain of itching, tearing, and foreign body sensation while contact lenses are worn. Giant papillae, similar to that seen in VC, can develop on the superior tarsal conjunctiva, and patients will describe a sense that the upper lid is catching the contact lens and displacing it upwards. The upper tarsal papillary response and mucus production can appear identical to VC; however, GPC will resolve with removal of the contact lens or the inciting agent.

Drug hypersensitivity can also produce a conjunctivitis that resembles VC. Common inciting agents include atropine, topical anesthetics, antibiotics, phenylephrine, glaucoma therapy, and various drug vehicles. The papillary conjunctival response tends to be less impressive and more commonly affects the inferior. Follicles tend to be more common in this condition.

Trachoma causes changes in the upper tarsal conjunctiva and superior corneoscleral limbus, which could initially appear similar to VC. In contrast to VC, however, trachoma is an infectious follicular conjunctivitis that can result in conjunctival scarring and visually significant corneal opacification. Conjunctival scraping will not contain eosinophils. VC and trachoma can present in the same patient, however, especially as these two conditions are prevalent in the same climates [90,91].

Laboratory evaluation

While the diagnosis of VC is largely clinical, laboratory testing can be helpful in differentiating VC from other forms of ocular allergy and in elucidating its various disease mechanisms [92].

Allergy testing

Allergy testing, such as skin-prick or RAST testing [36,48], have been used to identify specific triggers of VC, especially in patients with systemic allergy or atopy or in patients with a persistent disease course. However, the relatively low yield of such tests may limit their usefulness and hence they are not routinely recommended [3,13,28,30,31,89,93]. Interestingly, the tarsal form of the disease appears to be more frequently associated with allergic sensitization in both tests [3].

Conjunctival examination

Although rarely necessary, conjunctival scrapings and biopsy specimens can facilitate the diagnosis of an ocular allergic process. Because eosinophils and eosinophilic granules are not normally present in human conjunctiva, Giemsa-stained conjunctival scrapings can indicate the presence of an allergic process [48]. A conjunctival biopsy specimen can be examined by electron microscopy to identify and count mast cells, basophils, and eosinophils [48]. Light microscopy also can be used to visualize cellular infiltration, but may not be as accurate in identifying degranulated mast cells [37].

Tear evaluation

Cytologic examination of tear fluid is relatively quick and noninvasive. The presence of neutrophils, lymphocytes, and especially eosinophils in tear fluid suggests an allergic process. While no single inflammatory mediator can be considered specific for the diagnosis of VC [94], tear evaluations will continue to provide important clues into the pathogenesis of VC. In a study of tear IgA, low levels of total secretory IgA and high levels of house dust mite-specific secretory IgA were noted, suggesting local production and a possible link to a specific allergen in the pathogenesis of VC [95] that correlates to the Israeli study, which linked house dust mite allergen to increased VKC symptoms [96]. Proinflammatory cytokines, such as TNF-α, have been found to be significantly increased in tears of VC patients when compared with controls and severity of the disease [97].

Ocular challenge test

The conjunctiva can be challenged with dry allergens or solutions placed in the inferior conjunctival fornix, or with a contact lens saturated with the allergen applied to the cornea [98]. Then, the response can be clinically observed or the tears and conjunctival scrapings can be studied for released mediators or cellular response. This test is most often used experimentally to measure mediators such as histamine, tryptase, prostaglandins, or leukotrienes in the tear fluid at different time periods after a challenge with specific allergens. It is primarily used to evaluate the therapeutic efficacy of antiallergic agents, but can be used to assess responses to specific allergens in patients with VC [48].

Leonardi and colleagues [3] performed an ocular challenge test on 103 patients, who had previously undergone skin tests for the same allergens. Of the patients tested, 59% were positive for at least one allergen. Of the patients who were negative to skin or specific serum IgE tests, 42.4% were positive to ocular challenge.

Treatment

The treatment of VC is frequently challenging and may require a multidisciplinary approach. Despite the development of new medications, VC can still be debilitating for some patients. The currently available topical drugs are effective in treating acute phases of VC [99]. It is important to remember that for most patients, the disease is self-limited with good prognosis, and iatrogenic disease should be avoided. Steroids, which are very effective in controlling inflammation, can cause complications (cataract, glaucoma, secondary infection) and should be used sparingly.

Medical treatment options include mast cell stabilizers, immunosuppressives, corticosteroids, and antihistamines. In addition to medical therapy, the successful management of VC may also require general and sometimes surgical measures. It is also important to consider the possibility that other conditions, such as blepharitis and tear film insufficiency, may coexist with VC and that they should be treated accordingly. Education of young patients and their caregivers, regarding the prolonged and recurrent nature of the disease, is a critical step toward effective long-term management.

Avoidance of all known and potential allergens may be very beneficial to the patient and can be critical for long-term stability. In certain cases, an experienced allergist can use skin and serum RAST tests to identify specific inciting allergens and can provide the education and motivation necessary for a successful environmental control program. Sometimes these adjustments will include the removal of carpeting, installation of air-conditioning and air-filtering systems in the home heating system, as well as elimination of beloved pets. Nonspecific triggers, such as sun, wind, and salt water should also be avoided with the use of sunglasses, hats, and goggles [39]. The importance of these components of total care cannot be overemphasized. Less practical but potentially helpful is a move to cooler climates during the summer months [39].

Nonspecific and medical therapy

Cool compresses, ice packs, and chilled eye drops may provide some relief, perhaps from a vasoconstricting effect or some minor role in mast cell stabilization [100]. Artificial tears can dilute allergens and mediators in the tears and may also act as an eye wash [101]. Some patients experience relief when their eyes are closed, thus making occlusive therapies (patching, occlusive goggles, or a tarsorrhaphy) helpful in some situations [2], probably by minimizing contact with airborne allergens.

Eye rubbing should be strongly discouraged, as the mechanical trauma can cause release of mast cell mediators and worsen itching and inflammation [102,103]. Soft contact lenses may help protect the eye from the mechanical friction caused by the enlarged tarsal papillae. However, soft contact lens fitting can be difficult in these patients, and the increased susceptibility to infection in patients using topical corticosteroids may contraindicate their use [2].

Mast cell stabilizers

Mast cell stabilizers represent the mainstay of therapy for VC. These agents (cromolyn sodium, lodoxamide tromethamine, nedocromil sodium, and pemirolast potassium) are thought to limit the flux of calcium across the mast cell membrane, thus preventing degranulation and release of vasoactive substances. Mast cell stabilizer therapy, two to four times daily, should be initiated before seasonal occurrence and should continue throughout the affected season as first-line medical therapy.

Numerous studies have demonstrated the safety and effectiveness of cromolyn sodium, nedocromil, lodoxamide, and pemirolast in treating signs and symptoms of VC and SAC [36,104–110]. Additional studies suggest that mast cell stabilizers may act through other mechanisms. Cromolyn sodium reportedly inhibits the chemotaxis, activation, degranulation, and cytotoxicity of neutrophils, eosinophils, and monocytes [107,111]. Lodoxamide may exert antiallergic activity by reducing eosinophils in the conjunctiva [107]. Lodoxamide and cromolyn sodium may also have effects on Th2 cells, which have been implicated in the pathogenesis of VC [112].

A long-term comparison of nedocromil versus cromolyn sodium found that nedocromil 2% produced a more rapid and marked improvement in symptoms over cromolyn 2% and decreased the need for steroid rescue [113]. Lodoxamide 0.1% may have additional benefits over cromolyn sodium because of its anti-eosinophil action [114].

Antihistamines

Topical antihistamines, particularly those which block H1 receptors, can be useful as adjunctive therapy in mild to moderate cases of VC or in adult patients who have experienced significant improvement in symptomology since adolescence [39,86]. Topical antihistamines have been shown to reduce signs and symptoms of ocular allergy, in particular the severe itching that plagues many patients [115]. Newer agents, such as olopatadine, ketotifen, azelastine, and epinastine purportedly combine the effects of anti-H1 activity with mast-cell stabilization. However, these additional effects have not yet been validated clinically.

Systemic therapy with oral antihistamines (cetirizine, loratadine, ketotifen, oxatomide) may be beneficial given the chronicity of the disease and the potential for patients to become sensitized to preservatives in some commercial topical preparations. Patients with significant itching may benefit from hydroxyzine (25 mg–50 mg or more at bedtime), which may break the cycle of itching and scratching [2]. However, systemic antihistamines can cause or exacerbate tear film insufficiency, in which case patients should be aggressively treated with artificial tears.

Despite the symptomatic benefits experienced by select patients, both topical and systemic antihistamines often are ineffective in severe cases of VC.

Nonsteroidal anti-inflammatory drugs

Signs and symptoms of VC have been reported to improve with the addition of oral aspirin (1.5 g–4 g a day), although routine administration at these high doses could produce serious side effects, especially given that many VC patients are children [116,117].

Topical nonsteroidal anti-inflammatory drugs, such as ketorolac, diclofenac, and pronoprofen, have been shown to reduce itching, ICAM-1 expression, and tryptase levels in tears associate with ocular allergy [118–120]; however their use is now limited because of the availability of newer treatment options.

Corticosteroids

Moderate to severe cases of VC that are unresponsive to mast cell stabilizers and antihistamines may necessitate the short-term use of topical corticosteroids. Corneal involvement at any stage warrants the consideration of corticosteroid therapy.

Bonini and colleagues [13] reported that 85% of patients in their long-term cohort of 195 VC patients required steroids at some point during the course of the disease. Corticosteroids diminish the signs and symptoms of ocular allergy by stabilizing capillary permeability, decreasing the influx of inflammatory cells, and inhibiting the activation and degranulation of inflammatory cells [100]. They are particularly helpful in the treatment of VC and AKC but are seldom used for GPC or SAC.

Allansmith [121] found that "pulse" therapy with topical dexamethasone (1%) given every 2 hours, eight times daily and gradually tapered over days to weeks, to be effective for breakthrough attacks of VC inflammation.

In the absence of corneal involvement, low-absorption corticosteroids, such as fluorometholone, loteprednol, and rimexolone, should be tried first. Dose and frequency are determined based on the level of inflammation, with a gradual taper occurring over 2 weeks. Only after first-line therapy fails should more potent agents like prednisolone, dexamethasone, or betamethasone be considered [39]. Supratarsal injection of short- or intermediate-acting corticosteroids has also been reported to confer relief in severe VC [122].

Active corneal signs may necessitate the initial use of prednisolone. It is critical to recognize even the mildest forms of corneal disease, as delay in treatment could result in poor visual outcome. Although pathognomonic for VC, shield ulcers often begin as a mild, nonspecific subepithelial "haze."

Long-term maintenance, topical steroid therapy should be avoided given the potential complications, including glaucoma, formation of cataracts, and increased susceptibility to infections. Corticosteroid therapy has been associated with 2% to 7% of VC patients developing glaucoma and 14% developing cataracts [3,13,20].

Immunosuppressive agents

Cyclosporine, an immunosuppressive drug commonly used to prevent organ-graft rejection, has demonstrated efficacy in controlling ocular inflammation. Cyclosporine works primarily by blocking Th2 lymphocyte proliferation and IL-2 production [123]. It also inhibits histamine release from mast cells and basophils and reduces IL-5 production, which may limit the infiltration of eosinophils into the conjunctiva [20,124,125]. Leonardi and colleagues [126,127] suggest that cyclosporine shows particular effectiveness in VC by reducing conjunctival fibroblast proliferation and IL-1β production.

Cyclosporine 1% to 2% ophthalmic emulsions in olive or castor oil have been shown to be effective in the treatment of VC [128–134]. Leonardi and colleagues demonstrated that cyclosporine 2% used four times a day over 2 weeks significantly decreased signs and symptoms as well as tear levels of ECP in VC patients. Several groups have examined the effectiveness of cyclosporine at concentrations as low as 0.05%, but results at these levels have been equivocal. Spadavecchia and colleagues [135] suggest that 1% may be the lower bound for effective dosage as demonstrated in their cohort of school-age children. Leonardi and colleagues [57] found cyclosporine to have a significant steroid sparing effect, allowing VC to be controlled with mast cell stabilizers alone.

Unlike corticosteroids, cyclosporine has not been associated with lens changes or increases in intraocular pressure [133,136]. However, many patients complain of burning and irritation associated with current formulations. Other adverse events, such as bacterial or viral infections, are rare.

At present, topical cyclosporine is commercially available in the United States only as a 0.05% emulsion (Restasis). Higher concentrations must be formulated by hospital pharmacies. In Europe, phase III clinical trials have been completed for a new cyclosporine preparation, Vekacia, which is indicated for the treatment of VC. In May 2007, Vekacia also received "Orphan Drug" status by the United States Food and Drug Administration for the treatment of VC.

Other medical therapies

Lambiase and colleagues [79] have shown that montelukast, a sulfidopeptide receptor antagonist, when used for asthma treatment, also improves signs and symptoms of coexisting VC. Another immunosuppressive, Tacrolimus (FK-506), showed promise in treating VC in patients who had failed conventional therapy. However, controlled trials of this new ophthalmic application are yet to be completed [137]. Mitomycin-C has also been reported to confer benefit on VC patients [138]. Topical sirolimus has potential for topical potency, but has yet to be tested [139].

Surgical therapy

Conjunctival transposition or autografts have been performed with limited effect. Cryotherapy of the tarsal conjunctiva often provides temporary relief, possibly by decreasing the number of inflammatory cells and reducing the inflammatory mediators released; however, the papillae and symptoms usually return. Bonini and colleagues [13] have noted that cryogenic surgery performed to reduce papillary excrescences may result in a pemphigoid-like appearance throughout the conjunctiva. Belfair and colleagues [140] have recently described the use of CO_2 laser in removing giant papillae in refractory VC. However, the long-term effectiveness of this modality is unclear. In general, conjunctival surgery is rarely required and should be avoided.

Corneal shield ulcers may respond to bandage soft contact lenses, patching, and tarsorrhaphy, in addition to the medical therapy described. Cases that do not respond to conservative measures or exhibit inflammatory deposits in the ulcer base may require surgical intervention.

Surgical debridement and superficial keratectomy can aid in the re-epithelialization of the cornea [22,141]. Daily debridement of the ulcer may promote more rapid healing. One study demonstrated rapid re-epithelialization of three central corneal lesions from VC that were treated with excimer laser phototherapeutic keratectomy. This was performed after active inflammation was controlled and the inflammatory plaque overlying the shield ulcer was removed [142].

Cameron has proposed a classification system for shield ulcers based on their clinical characteristics, response to treatment, and complications. Grade 1 ulcers had a clear base, responded favorably to medical treatment, and re-epithelialized with minimal scarring. Grade 2 ulcers had visible inflammatory debris in the base, responded poorly to medical therapy alone, and demonstrated delayed re-epithelialization with complications, such as bacterial keratitis. Grade 2 patients showed dramatic response to scraping the base of the ulcer, with re-epithelialization occurring by 1 week. Grade 3 ulcers had elevated plaque formation and responded best to surgical therapy [22].

Solomon and colleagues [62] have also reported successful re-epithelialization of the cornea after surgical scraping of vernal plaques in patients who had been nonresponsive to maximal medical therapy. Sridhar and colleagues [143] demonstrated additional benefits in combining amniotic membrane grafting with surgical debridement in a small group of VC patients. Sangwan and colleagues [144] suggest that limbal stem cell transplantation may also have promise in severe cases of VC.

Phototherapeutic keratectomy also might be useful in removing superficial corneal scars. Penetrating keratoplasty might be necessary for deeper and visually compromising corneal scars. Restoring optical clarity of the cornea would be especially critical in a young child at risk for developing amblyopia. The chronic surrounding inflammation and the tendency toward trophic erosions can make corneal transplantation particularly challenging in this young population.

Treatment of secondary infections

Secondary infection of the trophic ulcers is always a risk, especially with steroid use. These require the standard scraping and culturing of the cornea in an attempt to isolate the organism and aggressive antimicrobial therapy. A lateral tarsorrhaphy may be helpful if re-epithelialization continues to be delayed after sterilization of the ulcer.

Hyposensitization and immunotherapy

Specific inciting allergens have been identified to correlate with VC, such as house dust mite that appears to be associated with increased VC symptoms [96], but systemic desensitization immunotherapy may be helpful in patients who are particularly sensitive to a limited number of allergens [145]. However, results are often disappointing. The effectiveness of immunotherapy for chronic ocular allergy differs from other forms of allergies, such as allergic rhinitis, asthma, and seasonal or perennial allergic conjunctivitis.

Prognosis

VC is most often a self-limiting disease, usually resolving within 2 to 10 years. Permanent conjunctival scarring is rare unless surgery was performed or unless the disease transforms into AKC. Although corneal changes, such as pannus, subepithelial scarring, astigmatism, keratoconus, and marginal corneal degeneration may be permanent, VC rarely results in diminished visual acuity that is not correctable by semirigid contact lenses or surgery. In their long-term follow-up of 195 VC patients, Bonini and colleagues [13] report that 6% of patients develop a visual impairment owing to corneal damage. Bonini and colleagues [13] also report that the size of the giant papillae is directly related to the probability of the persistence or worsening of symptoms, and that the bulbar forms of VC have a worse long-term prognosis than the tarsal forms.

References

[1] Buckley RJ. Vernal keratoconjunctivitis. Int Ophthalmol Clin 1988;28(4):303–8.
[2] Brody JM, Foster CS. Vernal conjunctivitis. In: Pepose JS, Holland GN, Wilhelmus KR, editors. Ocular infection and immunity. St. Louis (MO): Mosby-YearBook; 1996. p. 367–75.
[3] Leonardi A, Busca F, Motterle L, et al. Case series of 406 vernal keratoconjunctivitis patients: a demographic and epidemiological study. Acta Ophthalmol Scand 2006;84(3): 406–10.
[4] Bogacka E. [Epidemiology of allergic eye diseases]. Pol Merkur Lekarski 2003;14(84):714–5 [in Polish].
[5] Resnikoff S, Luzeau R, Filliard G, et al. Impression cytology with transfer in xerophthalmia and conjunctival diseases. Int Ophthalmol 1992;16(6):445–51.
[6] O'Shea JG. A survey of vernal keratoconjunctivitis and other eosinophil-mediated external eye diseases amongst Palestinians. Ophthalmic Epidemiol 2000;7(2):149–57.
[7] Ukponmwan CU. Vernal keratoconjunctivitis in Nigerians: 109 consecutive cases. Trop Doct 2003;33(4):242–5.

[8] Ajaiyeoba AI. Prevalence of atopic diseases in Nigerian children with vernal kerato-conjunctivitis. West Afr J Med 2003;22(1):15–7.

[9] Uchio E, Kimura R, Migita H, et al. Demographic aspects of allergic ocular diseases and evaluation of new criteria for clinical assessment of ocular allergy. Graefes Arch Clin Exp Ophthalmol 2007;246(2):291–6.

[10] Montan PG, Ekstrom K, Hedlin G, et al. Vernal keratoconjunctivitis in a Stockholm ophthalmic centre–epidemiological, functional, and immunologic investigations. Acta Ophthalmol Scand 1999;77(5):559–63.

[11] Bonini S, Bonini S, Lambiase A, et al. Vernal keratoconjunctivitis: a model of 5q cytokine gene cluster disease. Int Arch Allergy Immunol 1995;107(1–3):95–8.

[12] Smolin G, O'Connor CR. Atopic diseases affecting the eye. In: Smolin G, editor. Ocular immunology. Philadelphia: Lea and Febiger; 1981.

[13] Bonini S, Bonini S, Lambiase A, et al. Vernal keratoconjunctivitis revisited: a case series of 195 patients with long-term follow-up. Ophthalmology 2000;107(6):1157–63.

[14] Sacchetti M, Baiardini I, Lambiase A, et al. Development and testing of the quality of life in children with vernal keratoconjunctivitis questionnaire. Am J Ophthalmol 2007;144(4): 557–63.

[15] Trocme SD, Raizman MB, Bartley GB. Medical therapy for ocular allergy. Mayo Clin Proc 1992;67(6):557–65.

[16] Bonini S, Sacchetti M, Mantelli F, et al. Clinical grading of vernal keratoconjunctivitis. Curr Opin Allergy Clin Immunol 2007;7(5):436–41.

[17] Leonardi A, De Dominicis C, Motterle L. Immunopathogenesis of ocular allergy: a schematic approach to different clinical entities. Curr Opin Allergy Clin Immunol 2007;7(5):429–35.

[18] Foster CS. Immunologic disorders of the conjunctiva, cornea, and sclera. In: Albert DM, Jakobiec FA, editors. Principles and practice of ophthalmology. Philadelphia: W.B. Saunders; 1994. p. 190–217.

[19] Gedik S, Akova YA, Gur S. Secondary bacterial keratitis associated with shield ulcer caused by vernal conjunctivitis. Cornea 2006;25(8):974–6.

[20] Tabbara KF. Ocular complications of vernal keratoconjunctivitis. Can J Ophthalmol 1999; 34(2):88–92.

[21] Buckley RJ. Vernal keratopathy and its management. Trans Ophthalmol Soc U K 1981; 101(Pt 2):234–8.

[22] Cameron JA. Shield ulcers and plaques of the cornea in vernal keratoconjunctivitis. Ophthalmology 1995;102(6):985–93.

[23] Neumann E, Gutmann MJ, Blumenkranz N, et al. A review of four hundred cases of vernal conjunctivitis. Am J Ophthalmol 1959;47(2):166–72.

[24] Cameron JA, Mullaney PB. Amblyopia resulting from shield ulcers and plaques of the cornea in vernal keratoconjunctivitis. J Pediatr Ophthalmol Strabismus 1997;34(4):261–2.

[25] Jeng BH, Whitcher JP, Margolis TP. Pseudogerontoxon. Clin Experiment Ophthalmol 2004;32(4):433–4.

[26] Shuler JD, Levenson J, Mondino BJ. Inferior corneal ulcers associated with palpebral vernal conjunctivitis. Am J Ophthalmol 1988;106(1):106–7.

[27] Cameron JA, Al-Rajhi AA, Badr IA. Corneal ectasia in vernal keratoconjunctivitis. Ophthalmology 1989;96(11):1615–23.

[28] Bielory L. Allergic diseases of the eye. Med Clin North Am 2006;90(1):129–48.

[29] Bielory L, Goodman PE, Fisher EM. Allergic ocular disease. A review of pathophysiology and clinical presentations. Clin Rev Allergy Immunol 2001;20(2):183–200.

[30] Bielory L. Allergic and immunologic disorders of the eye. Part I: immunology of the eye. J Allergy Clin Immunol 2000;106(5):805–16.

[31] Bielory L. Allergic and immunologic disorders of the eye. Part II: ocular allergy. J Allergy Clin Immunol 2000;106(6):1019–32.

[32] Abelson MB, Baird RS, Allansmith MR. Tear histamine levels in vernal conjunctivitis and other ocular inflammations. Ophthalmology 1980;87(8):812–4.

[33] Bonini S, Bonini S, Schiavone M, et al. Conjunctival hyperresponsiveness to ocular histamine challenge in patients with vernal conjunctivitis. J Allergy Clin Immunol 1992; 89(1 Pt 1):103–7.

[34] Allansmith MR, Baird RS, Greiner JV. Vernal conjunctivitis and contact lens-associated giant papillary conjunctivitis compared and contrasted. Am J Ophthalmol 1979;87(4):544–55.

[35] Allansmith MR, Baird RS. Percentage of degranulated mast cells in vernal conjunctivitis and giant papillary conjunctivitis associated with contact-lens wear. Am J Ophthalmol 1981;91(1):71–5.

[36] Foster CS. Evaluation of topical cromolyn sodium in the treatment of vernal keratoconjunctivitis. Ophthalmology 1988;95(2):194–201.

[37] Henriquez AS, Kenyon KR, Allansmith MR. Mast cell ultrastructure. Comparison in contact lens-associated giant papillary conjunctivitis and vernal conjunctivitis. Arch Ophthalmol 1981;99(7):1266–72.

[38] Irani AM, Butrus SI, Tabbara KF, et al. Human conjunctival mast cells: distribution of MCT and MCTC in vernal conjunctivitis and giant papillary conjunctivitis. J Allergy Clin Immunol 1990;86(1):34–40.

[39] Leonardi A. Vernal keratoconjunctivitis: pathogenesis and treatment. Prog Retin Eye Res 2002;21(3):319–39.

[40] Bonini S, Bonini S, Bucci MG, et al. Allergen dose response and late symptoms in a human model of ocular allergy. J Allergy Clin Immunol 1990;86(6 Pt 1):869–76.

[41] Bonini S, Bonini S. IgE and non-IgE mechanisms in ocular allergy. Ann Allergy 1993;71(3): 296–9.

[42] Abelson MB, Soter NA, Simon MA, et al. Histamine in human tears. Am J Ophthalmol 1977;83(3):417–8.

[43] Butrus SI, Ochsner KI, Abelson MB, et al. The level of tryptase in human tears. An indicator of activation of conjunctival mast cells. Ophthalmology 1990;97(12):1678–83.

[44] Fukagawa K, Saito H, Azuma N, et al. Histamine and tryptase levels in allergic conjunctivitis and vernal keratoconjunctivitis. Cornea 1994;13(4):345–8.

[45] Abelson MB, Leonardi A, Smith L, et al. Histaminase activity in patients with vernal keratoconjunctivitis. Ophthalmology 1995;102(12):1958–63.

[46] Leonardi A, Radice M, Fregona IA, et al. Histamine effects on conjunctival fibroblasts from patients with vernal conjunctivitis. Exp Eye Res 1999;68(6):739–46.

[47] Leonardi A, DeFranchis G, De Paoli M, et al. Histamine-induced cytokine production and ICAM-1 expression in human conjunctival fibroblasts. Curr Eye Res 2002;25(3):189–96.

[48] Butrus SI, Abelson MB. Laboratory evaluation of ocular allergy. Int Ophthalmol Clin 1988;28(4):324–8.

[49] Tabbara KF. Tear tryptase in vernal keratoconjunctivitis. Arch Ophthalmol 2001;119(3): 338–42.

[50] Leonardi A, Brun P, Di Stefano A, et al. Matrix metalloproteases in vernal keratoconjunctivitis, nasal polyps and allergic asthma. Clin Exp Allergy 2007;37(6):872–9.

[51] Kumagai N, Fukuda K, Fujitsu Y, et al. Expression of functional ICAM-1 on cultured human keratocytes induced by tumor necrosis factor-alpha. Jpn J Ophthalmol 2003;47(2):134–41.

[52] Kumagai N, Fukuda K, Nishida T. Synergistic effect of TNF-alpha and IL-4 on the expression of thymus- and activation-regulated chemokine in human corneal fibroblasts. Biochem Biophys Res Commun 2000;279(1):1–5.

[53] Kumagai N, Fukuda K, Ishimura Y, et al. Synergistic induction of eotaxin expression in human keratocytes by TNF-alpha and IL-4 or IL-13. Invest Ophthalmol Vis Sci 2000; 41(6):1448–53.

[54] Kumagai N, Fukuda K, Fujitsu Y, et al. Synergistic effect of TNF-alpha and either IL-4 or IL-13 on VCAM-1 expression by cultured human corneal fibroblasts. Cornea 2003;22(6):557–61.

[55] Trocme SD, Kephart GM, Allansmith MR, et al. Conjunctival deposition of eosinophil granule major basic protein in vernal keratoconjunctivitis and contact lens-associated giant papillary conjunctivitis. Am J Ophthalmol 1989;108(1):57–63.

[56] Udell IJ, Gleich GJ, Allansmith MR, et al. Eosinophil granule major basic protein and Charcot-Leyden crystal protein in human tears. Am J Ophthalmol 1981;92(6):824–8.

[57] Leonardi A, Borghesan F, Faggian D, et al. Eosinophil cationic protein in tears of normal subjects and patients affected by vernal keratoconjunctivitis. Allergy 1995;50(7):610–3.

[58] Tomassini M, Magrini L, Bonini S, et al. Increased serum levels of eosinophil cationic protein and eosinophil-derived neurotoxin (protein X) in vernal keratoconjunctivitis. Ophthalmology 1994;101(11):1808–11.

[59] Trocme SD, Gleich GJ, Zieske JD. Eosinophil granule major basic protein inhibition of corneal epithelial wound healing. Invest Ophthalmol Vis Sci 1994;35(7):3051–6.

[60] Trocme SD, Kephart GM, Bourne WM, et al. Eosinophil granule major basic protein deposition in corneal ulcers associated with vernal keratoconjunctivitis. Am J Ophthalmol 1993;115(5):640–3.

[61] Trocme SD, Hallberg CK, Gill KS, et al. Effects of eosinophil granule proteins on human corneal epithelial cell viability and morphology. Invest Ophthalmol Vis Sci 1997;38(3): 593–9.

[62] Solomon A, Zamir E, Levartovsky S, et al. Surgical management of corneal plaques in vernal keratoconjunctivitis: a clinicopathologic study. Cornea 2004;23(6):608–12.

[63] Foster CS. The pathophysiology of ocular allergy: current thinking. Allergy 1995; 50(21 Suppl):6–9 [discussion: 34–8].

[64] Maggi E, Biswas P, Del Prete G, et al. Accumulation of Th-2-like helper T cells in the conjunctiva of patients with vernal conjunctivitis. J Immunol 1991;146(4):1169–74.

[65] Fujishima H, Takeuchi T, Shinozaki N, et al. Measurement of IL-4 in tears of patients with seasonal allergic conjunctivitis and vernal keratoconjunctivitis. Clin Exp Immunol 1995; 102(2):395–8.

[66] Leonardi A, DeFranchis G, Zancanaro F, et al. Identification of local Th2 and Th0 lymphocytes in vernal conjunctivitis by cytokine flow cytometry. Invest Ophthalmol Vis Sci 1999;40(12):3036–40.

[67] Nishimura A, Campbell-Meltzer R, Chute K, et al. Genetics of allergic disease: evidence for organ-specific susceptibility genes. Int Arch Allergy Immunol 2001;124(1–3):197–200.

[68] Ono SJ, Nakamura T, Miyazaki D, et al. Chemokines: roles in leukocyte development, trafficking, and effector function. J Allergy Clin Immunol 2003;111(6):1185–99 [quiz: 1200].

[69] Abu El-Asrar AM, Struyf S, Al-Kharashi SA, et al. Chemokines in the limbal form of vernal keratoconjunctivitis. Br J Ophthalmol 2000;84(12):1360–6.

[70] Ono SJ. Vernal keratoconjunctivitis: evidence for immunoglobulin E-dependent and immunoglobulin E-independent eosinophilia. Clin Exp Allergy 2003;33(3):279–81.

[71] Lambiase A, Normando EM, Vitiello L, et al. Natural killer cells in vernal keratoconjunctivitis. Mol Vis 2007;13:1562–7.

[72] Wardlaw AJ, Hay H, Cromwell O, et al. Leukotrienes, LTC4 and LTB4, in bronchoalveolar lavage in bronchial asthma and other respiratory diseases. J Allergy Clin Immunol 1989; 84(1):19–26.

[73] Drazen JM, Israel E, O'Byrne PM. Treatment of asthma with drugs modifying the leukotriene pathway. N Engl J Med 1999;340(3):197–206.

[74] Bisgaard H, Ford-Hutchinson AW, Charleson S, et al. Detection of leukotriene C4-liked immunoreactivity in tear fluid from subjects challenged with specific allergen. Prostaglandins 1984;27(3):369–74.

[75] Proud D, Sweet J, Stein P, et al. Inflammatory mediator release on conjunctival provocation of allergic subjects with allergen. J Allergy Clin Immunol 1990;85(5):896–905.

[76] Woodward DF, Ledgard SE. Effect of LTD4 on conjunctival vasopermeability and blood-aqueous barrier integrity. Invest Ophthalmol Vis Sci 1985;26(4):481–5.

[77] Bisgaard H, Ford-Hutchinson AW, Charleson S, et al. Production of leukotrienes in human skin and conjunctival mucosa after specific allergen challenge. Allergy 1985;40(6):417–23.

[78] Spada CS, Woodward DF, Hawley SB, et al. Leukotrienes cause eosinophil emigration into conjunctival tissue. Prostaglandins 1986;31(4):795–809.

[79] Lambiase A, Bonini S, Rasi G, et al. Montelukast, a leukotriene receptor antagonist, in vernal keratoconjunctivitis associated with asthma. Arch Ophthalmol 2003;121(5):615–20.

[80] Ono SJ, Abelson MB. Allergic conjunctivitis: update on pathophysiology and prospects for future treatment. J Allergy Clin Immunol 2005;115(1):118–22.

[81] Allam JP, Klein E, Bieber T, et al. Transforming growth factor-beta1 regulates the expression of the high-affinity receptor for IgE on CD34 stem cell-derived CD1a dendritic cells in vitro. J Invest Dermatol 2004;123(4):676–82.

[82] Hu Y, Matsumoto Y, Dogru M, et al. The differences of tear function and ocular surface findings in patients with atopic keratoconjunctivitis and vernal keratoconjunctivitis. Allergy 2007;62(8):917–25.

[83] Fujishima H, Takeyama M, Takeuchi T, et al. Elevated levels of substance P in tears of patients with allergic conjunctivitis and vernal keratoconjunctivitis. Clin Exp Allergy 1997;27(4):372–8.

[84] Lambiase A, Bonini S, Bonini S, et al. Increased plasma levels of nerve growth factor in vernal keratoconjunctivitis and relationship to conjunctival mast cells. Invest Ophthalmol Vis Sci 1995;36(10):2127–32.

[85] Lambiase A, Bonini S, Micera A, et al. Increased plasma levels of substance P in vernal keratoconjunctivitis. Invest Ophthalmol Vis Sci 1997;38(10):2161–4.

[86] Bonini S, Coassin M, Aronni S, et al. Vernal keratoconjunctivitis. Eye 2004;18(4):345–51.

[87] Kramer P, Lubkin V, Potter W, et al. Cyclic changes in conjunctival smears from menstruating females. Ophthalmology 1990;97(3):303–7.

[88] Bonini S, Lambiase A, Schiavone M, et al. Estrogen and progesterone receptors in vernal keratoconjunctivitis. Ophthalmology 1995;102(9):1374–9.

[89] Bielory L. Differential diagnoses of conjunctivitis for clinical allergist-immunologists. Ann Allergy Asthma Immunol 2007;98(2):105–14 [quiz: 114–7, 152].

[90] McMoli TE, Assonganyi T. Limbal vernal kerato-conjunctivitis in Yaounde, Cameroon. A clinico- immunology study. Rev Int Trach Pathol Ocul Trop Subtrop Sante Publique 1991;68:157–70 [in English, French].

[91] Dawson CR, Juster R, Marx R, et al. Limbal disease in trachoma and other ocular chlamydial infections: risk factors for corneal vascularisation. Eye 1989;3(Pt 2):204–9.

[92] Bielory L, Dinowitz M, Rescigno R. Ocular allergic diseases: differential diagnosis, examination techniques and testing. J Toxicol Cutaneous Ocul Toxicol 2002;21:329–51.

[93] Leonardi A, Battista MC, Gismondi M, et al. Antigen sensitivity evaluated by tear-specific and serum-specific IgE, skin tests, and conjunctival and nasal provocation tests in patients with ocular allergic disease. Eye 1993;7(Pt 3):461–4.

[94] Leonardi A, Borghesan F, Faggian D, et al. Tear and serum soluble leukocyte activation markers in conjunctival allergic diseases. Am J Ophthalmol 2000;129(2):151–8.

[95] Inada N, Shoji J, Hoshino M, et al. Evaluation of total and allergen-specific secretory IgA in tears of allergic conjunctival disease patients. Jpn J Ophthalmol 2007;51(5):338–42.

[96] Mumcuoglu YK, Zavaro A, Samra Z, et al. House dust mites and vernal keratoconjunctivitis. Ophthalmologica 1988;196(4):175–81.

[97] Leonardi A, Brun P, Tavolato M, et al. Tumor necrosis factor-alpha (TNF-alpha) in seasonal allergic conjunctivitis and vernal keratoconjunctivitis. Eur J Ophthalmol 2003;13(7):606–10.

[98] Spector SL, Perhach JL, Rohr AS, et al. Pharmacodynamic evaluation of azelastine in subjects with asthma. J Allergy Clin Immunol 1987;80(1):75–80.

[99] Mantelli F, Santos MS, Pettiti T, et al. Systematic review and meta-analysis of randomised clinical trials on topical treatments for vernal keratoconjunctivitis. Br J Ophthalmol 2007; 91(12):1656–61.

[100] Abelson MB, Schaefer K. Conjunctivitis of allergic origin: immunologic mechanisms and current approaches to therapy. Surv Ophthalmol 1993;38(Suppl):115–32.

[101] Hingorani M, Lightman S. Therapeutic options in ocular allergic disease. Drugs 1995;50(2): 208–21.

[102] Greiner JV, Peace DG, Baird RS, et al. Effects of eye rubbing on the conjunctiva as a model of ocular inflammation. Am J Ophthalmol 1985;100(1):45–50.

[103] Raizman MB, Rothman JS, Maroun F, et al. Effect of eye rubbing on signs and symptoms of allergic conjunctivitis in cat-sensitive individuals. Ophthalmology 2000;107(12):2158–61.

[104] Alexander M. Comparative therapeutic studies with Tilavist. Allergy 1995;50(21 Suppl): 23–9 [discussion: 34–8].

[105] Abelson MB, Berdy GJ, Mundorf T, et al. Pemirolast potassium 0.1% ophthalmic solution is an effective treatment for allergic conjunctivitis: a pooled analysis of two prospective, randomized, double-masked, placebo-controlled, phase III studies. J Ocul Pharmacol Ther 2002;18(5):475–88.

[106] Bonini S, Barney NP, Schiavone M, et al. Effectiveness of nedocromil sodium 2% eyedrops on clinical symptoms and tear fluid cytology of patients with vernal conjunctivitis. Eye 1992;6(Pt 6):648–52.

[107] Bonini S, Schiavone M, Bonini S, et al. Efficacy of lodoxamide eye drops on mast cells and eosinophils after allergen challenge in allergic conjunctivitis. Ophthalmology 1997;104(5): 849–53.

[108] Blumenthal M, Casale T, Dockhorn R, et al. Efficacy and safety of nedocromil sodium ophthalmic solution in the treatment of seasonal allergic conjunctivitis. Am J Ophthalmol 1992; 113(1):56–63.

[109] el Hennawi M. A double blind placebo controlled group comparative study of ophthalmic sodium cromoglycate and nedocromil sodium in the treatment of vernal keratoconjunctivitis. Br J Ophthalmol 1994;78(5):365–9.

[110] Kjellman NI, Stevens MT. Clinical experience with Tilavist: an overview of efficacy and safety. Allergy 1995;50(21 Suppl):14–22 [discussion: 34–8].

[111] Kay AB, Walsh GM, Moqbel R, et al. Disodium cromoglycate inhibits activation of human inflammatory cells in vitro. J Allergy Clin Immunol 1987;80(1):1–8.

[112] Avunduk AM, Avunduk MC, Kapicioglu Z, et al. Mechanisms and comparison of antiallergic efficacy of topical lodoxamide and cromolyn sodium treatment in vernal keratoconjunctivitis. Ophthalmology 2000;107(7):1333–7.

[113] Verin PH, Dicker ID, Mortemousque B. Nedocromil sodium eye drops are more effective than sodium cromoglycate eye drops for the long-term management of vernal keratoconjunctivitis. Clin Exp Allergy 1999;29(4):529–36.

[114] Caldwell DR, Verin P, Hartwich-Young R, et al. Efficacy and safety of lodoxamide 0.1% vs cromolyn sodium 4% in patients with vernal keratoconjunctivitis. Am J Ophthalmol 1992; 113(6):632–7.

[115] Azevedo M, Castel-Branco MG, Oliveira JF, et al. Double-blind comparison of levocabastine eye drops with sodium cromoglycate and placebo in the treatment of seasonal allergic conjunctivitis. Clin Exp Allergy 1991;21(6):689–94.

[116] Abelson MB, Butrus SI, Weston JH. Aspirin therapy in vernal conjunctivitis. Am J Ophthalmol 1983;95(4):502–5.

[117] Chaudhary KP. Evaluation of combined systemic aspirin and cromolyn sodium in intractable vernal catarrh. Ann Ophthalmol 1990;22(8):314–8.

[118] Tinkelman DG, Rupp G, Kaufman H, et al. Double-masked, paired-comparison clinical study of ketorolac tromethamine 0.5% ophthalmic solution compared with placebo eyedrops in the treatment of seasonal allergic conjunctivitis. Surv Ophthalmol 1993;38(Suppl):133–40.

[119] Ballas Z, Blumenthal M, Tinkelman DG, et al. Clinical evaluation of ketorolac tromethamine 0.5% ophthalmic solution for the treatment of seasonal allergic conjunctivitis. Surv Ophthalmol 1993;38(Suppl):141–8.

[120] Leonardi A, Busato F, Fregona IA, et al. Anti-inflammatory and antiallergic effects of ketorolac tromethamine in the conjunctival provocation model. Br J Ophthalmol 2000; 84(11):1228–32.

[121] Allansmith MR. Vernal conjunctivitis. In: Duane's clinical ophthalmology, volume 4. Philadelphia: JB Lippincott; 1992.

[122] Holsclaw DS, Whitcher JP, Wong IG, et al. Supratarsal injection of corticosteroid in the treatment of refractory vernal keratoconjunctivitis. Am J Ophthalmol 1996;121(3):243–9.

[123] Lightman S. Therapeutic considerations: symptoms, cells and mediators. Allergy 1995; 50(21 Suppl):10–3 [discussion: 34–8].

[124] Sperr WR, Agis H, Czerwenka K, et al. Effects of cyclosporin A and FK-506 on stem cell factor-induced histamine secretion and growth of human mast cells. J Allergy Clin Immunol 1996;98(2):389–99.

[125] Casolaro V, Spadaro G, Patella V, et al. In vivo characterization of the anti-inflammatory effect of cyclosporin A on human basophils. J Immunol 1993;151(10):5563–73.

[126] Leonardi A, Borghesan F, DePaoli M, et al. Procollagens and inflammatory cytokine concentrations in tarsal and limbal vernal keratoconjunctivitis. Exp Eye Res 1998;67(1): 105–12.

[127] Leonardi A, DeFranchis G, Fregona IA, et al. Effects of cyclosporin A on human conjunctival fibroblasts. Arch Ophthalmol 2001;119(10):1512–7.

[128] BenEzra D, Pe'er J, Brodsky M, et al. Cyclosporine eyedrops for the treatment of severe vernal keratoconjunctivitis. Am J Ophthalmol 1986;101(3):278–82.

[129] Bleik JH, Tabbara KF. Topical cyclosporine in vernal keratoconjunctivitis. Ophthalmology 1991;98(11):1679–84.

[130] Holland EJ, Olsen TW, Ketcham JM, et al. Topical cyclosporin A in the treatment of anterior segment inflammatory disease. Cornea 1993;12(5):413–9.

[131] Kaan G, Ozden O. Therapeutic use of topical cyclosporine. Ann Ophthalmol 1993;25(5): 182–6.

[132] Kilic A, Gurler B. Topical 2% cyclosporine A in preservative-free artificial tears for the treatment of vernal keratoconjunctivitis. Can J Ophthalmol 2006;41(6):693–8.

[133] Pucci N, Novembre E, Cianferoni A, et al. Efficacy and safety of cyclosporine eyedrops in vernal keratoconjunctivitis. Ann Allergy Asthma Immunol 2002;89(3):298–303.

[134] Secchi AG, Tognon MS, Leonardi A. Topical use of cyclosporine in the treatment of vernal keratoconjunctivitis. Am J Ophthalmol 1990;110(6):641–5.

[135] Spadavecchia L, Fanelli P, Tesse R, et al. Efficacy of 1.25% and 1% topical cyclosporine in the treatment of severe vernal keratoconjunctivitis in childhood. Pediatr Allergy Immunol 2006;17(7):527–32.

[136] Perry HD, Donnenfeld ED, Kanellopoulos AJ, et al. Topical cyclosporin A in the management of postkeratoplasty glaucoma. Cornea 1997;16(3):284–8.

[137] Vichyanond P, Tantimongkolsuk C, Dumrongkigchaiporn P, et al. Vernal keratoconjunctivitis: result of a novel therapy with 0.1% topical ophthalmic FK-506 ointment. J Allergy Clin Immunol 2004;113(2):355–8.

[138] Akpek EK, Hasiripi H, Christen WG, et al. A randomized trial of low-dose, topical mitomycin-C in the treatment of severe vernal keratoconjunctivitis. Ophthalmology 2000; 107(2):263–9.

[139] Buech G, Bertelmann E, Pleyer U, et al. Formulation of sirolimus eye drops and corneal permeation studies. J Ocul Pharmacol Ther 2007;23(3):292–303.

[140] Belfair N, Monos T, Levy J, et al. Removal of giant vernal papillae by CO_2 laser. Can J Ophthalmol 2005;40(4):472–6.

[141] Ozbek Z, Burakgazi AZ, Rapuano CJ. Rapid healing of vernal shield ulcer after surgical debridement: a case report. Cornea 2006;25(4):472–3.

[142] Cameron JA, Antonios SR, Badr IA. Excimer laser phototherapeutic keratectomy for shield ulcers and corneal plaques in vernal keratoconjunctivitis. J Refract Surg 1995; 11(1):31–5.

[143] Sridhar MS, Sangwan VS, Bansal AK, et al. Amniotic membrane transplantation in the management of shield ulcers of vernal keratoconjunctivitis. Ophthalmology 2001;108(7): 1218–22.

[144] Sangwan VS, Murthy SI, Vemuganti GK, et al. Cultivated corneal epithelial transplantation for severe ocular surface disease in vernal keratoconjunctivitis. Cornea 2005;24(4):426–30.

[145] Bousquet J, Michel FB. Advances in specific immunotherapy. Clin Exp Allergy 1992; 22(10):889–96.

ELSEVIER
SAUNDERS

Immunol Allergy Clin N Am
28 (2008) 83–103

IMMUNOLOGY
AND ALLERGY
CLINICS
OF NORTH AMERICA

Giant Papillary Conjunctivitis

Peter C. Donshik, MD[a],*, William H. Ehlers, MD[a], Mark Ballow, MD[b]

[a]University of Connecticut Health Center, 263 Farmington Avenue, Farmington,
CT 06030, USA
[b]Division of Allergy and Immunology, Department of Pediatrics, State University of
New York at Buffalo (SUNY Buffalo), Women and Children's Hospital of Buffalo,
219 Bryant Street, Buffalo, NY 14222, USA

Giant papillary conjunctivitis (GPC) was first noted by Spring [1] in 1974. He reported a papillary reaction, similar to that seen in allergic conditions, on the upper tarsal conjunctiva in soft contact lenses wearers. The condition has been described in detail by Allansmith and coworkers [2]. This syndrome, although predominantly associated with soft contact lens wear, has been reported in patients with rigid lenses, ocular prostheses, exposed sutures following ocular surgery, extruded scleral buckle, filtering blebs, band keratopathy, corneal foreign bodies, limbal dermoids, and cyanoacrylate tissue adhesives [2–13]. This condition is also known as "contact lens–induced papillary conjunctivitis."

Signs and symptoms

Contact lens wearers with GPC report a variety of symptoms, including decreased lens tolerance, increased lens awareness, excessive lens movement, increased mucus production associated with ocular irritation, redness, burning, and itching. These patients almost invariably have coated contact lenses, and they often report mucus accumulating in the inner canthus on awakening in the morning. On examination, the upper tarsal conjunctiva may show inflammation and papules, which are usually larger than 0.3 mm. It is important to note that in the very early stages of GPC, the

Portions of this article appeared in Donshik DC. Giant papillary conjunctivitis. Trans Am Ophthalmol Soc 1994;92:687–744; with permission; and Donshik PC, Ehlers WH. Giant papillary conjunctivitis. Immunology and Allergy Clinics 1997;17:53–73; with permission.

* Corresponding author. 47 Jolley Drive, Bloomfield, CT 06002.
 E-mail address: pdonshik@drdonshik.com (P.C. Donshik).

symptoms may precede the signs, with only tarsal injection being present. It is essential to question patients at each visit to elicit reports of symptoms consistent with GPC that they may consider to be normal contact lens discomfort.

Biomicroscopy of the normal tarsal conjunctiva reveals a moist, pink mucous membrane with a vascular arcade that appears as fine vessels radiating perpendicular to the tarsal margin. This appearance has been described as a satin appearance in which the surface is smooth and devoid of papillae. One may also see a fine, uniform papillary appearance with small papules (4–8 per milliliter) that are best detected after the instillation of fluorescein. In some normal individuals, the papules may not be uniform in size, but even the larger papules are less than 0.3 mm [2].

Allansmith and coworkers [2] quantified the distribution of normal findings and reported that in non–contact lens wearers 24% of subjects had a tarsal conjunctiva that could be classified as having a satin appearance, 69% had a uniform papillary appearance, and 7% had a nonuniform appearance. Papules greater than 1 mm were not present in normal non–contact lens wearers (Fig. 1). Korb and colleagues [14], however, reported that a small number (0.6%) of normal individuals who do not wear contact lenses did have a papillary reaction of 0.3 mm on the upper tarsal conjunctiva. On the basis of these findings, a papillary reaction greater than 0.3 mm

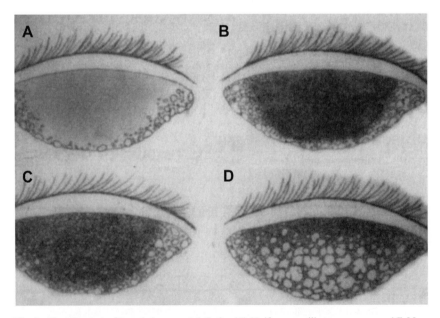

Fig. 1. Classification of tarsal changes. (*A*) Satin. (*B*) Uniform papillary appearance. (*C*) Non-uniform papillary appearance. (*D*) Giant papillary appearance. (*From* Allansmith MR, Korb DR, Greiner JV, et al. Giant papillary conjunctivitis in contact lens wearers. Am J Ophthalmol 1977;82:697–708; with permission.)

is generally considered abnormal and consistent with the diagnosis of GPC when accompanied by the appropriate symptoms.

In patients with GPC, the upper tarsal conjunctiva undergoes progressive changes that begin with nonspecific signs of inflammation and progress to the development of the characteristic papillary reaction that give this entity its name. For convenience of classification and treatment, this progression has been divided into stages, described later. The best method of examining a patient with suspected GPC is to have them remove their lenses and examine the conjunctiva and cornea under low and high power at the slit lamp biomicroscope. The presence of bulbar conjunctival injection, superior corneal pannus, or corneal opacities should be noted. The upper lid is then inverted for examination of the tarsal conjunctiva. The presence and location of hyperemia, abnormal tarsal vascular patterns, and papules should be recorded, along with any evidence of subconjunctival scarring. Fluorescein is then instilled into the cul-de-sac, and the patient is asked to blink several times to distribute the dye. The lid is again everted, and using the blue cobalt filter of the slit lamp, the tarsal conjunctiva is re-examined for the presence of a papillary reaction. The fluorescein-stained tear film outlines the presence of the papillary reaction, and the sterile 2% solution seems to give the best definition of the papules. One can then easily appreciate the pattern of the papillary reaction and estimate the size of the papules.

It is important to note the size of the papules and their location, and the presence of apical scarring or apical staining. This process is facilitated by dividing the redundant upper tarsal conjunctiva into three zones (Fig. 2). Zone 1 is the area along the tarsal border, zone 3 is the area along the lid margin, and zone 2 is the central area of the tarsal plate. The area

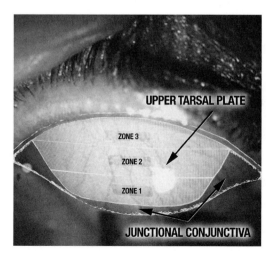

Fig. 2. Zones of the superior tarsal conjunctiva. (*From* Donshik PC, Elhers WG. Giant papillary conjunctivitis. Immunology and Allergy Clinics of North America 1997;17:53–73; with permission.)

along the medial and temporal aspects of the tarsal plate and the area along the superior border of the plate have been called transitional zones because one often sees a papillary reaction in normal individuals in these areas that can be quite large, and they are not considered pathologic and should be disregarded in assessing the condition of the upper tarsal plate.

Stages of giant papillary conjunctivitis

For purposes of classification and treatment, the signs and symptoms of GPC can be classified into four stages [2].

Stage 1: preclinical giant papillary conjunctivitis

In this early stage, the symptoms consist of minimal mucus discharge, usually noted on awakening, and occasional itching noted after lens removal. The lenses are often mildly coated. Examination of the upper tarsal conjunctiva may reveal a normal appearance, or there may be mild hyperemia, but a normal vascular pattern is usually visible (Fig. 3).

Stage 2: mild giant papillary conjunctivitis

This stage is characterized by increased mucus production with associated itching, increased lens awareness, and coating of the contact lenses. Occasionally, patients may note mild blurring of vision. Examination of the upper tarsal conjunctiva reveals mild to moderate injection and thickening of the conjunctiva with some loss of the normal vascular pattern. Although the superficial vessels are typically obscured, the deeper vessels are still visible. A papillary reaction is observed, and although there is variability in size, some of the papules measure 0.3 mm or more. At this stage some of the papules may begin to coalescence because several adjacent papules are

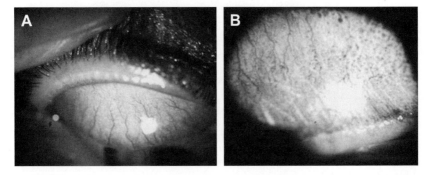

Fig. 3. Stage 1 giant papillary conjunctivitis. (*A*) Minimal hyperemia of the upper tarsal plate. (*B*) Papillary reaction in same patient (fluorescein instilled and photographed with cobalt filter).

elevated by thickening of the underlying tissue. These early changes may be difficult to detect with white light alone; however, the use of fluorescein dye and cobalt illumination greatly enhances the ability to detect these changes (Fig. 4).

Stage 3: moderate giant papillary conjunctivitis

As this condition progresses, itching and mucus formation have increased and lens coating is more prominent. Patients may find it difficult to keep their lenses clean and lens awareness is also increased, often resulting in a significant reduction in wearing time. There may be excessive lens movement with each blink that often results in fluctuating and blurred vision. At this stage, examination of the upper tarsal conjunctiva shows marked injection and thickening, and the normal vascular pattern is further obscured (Fig. 5). The papules on the tarsal conjunctiva have increased in size and number and are now becoming elevated. The apices of the papules may appear whitened from subconjunctival scarring and fibrosis and often exhibit staining with fluorescein dye.

Stage 4: severe giant papillary conjunctivitis

At this stage patients are usually completely unable to wear their lenses. Discomfort begins shortly after insertion of their lenses, which quickly become coated and cloudy. In addition to excessive lens movement, the lenses often fail to center properly. Mucus secretion is increased, sometimes so that the patients' eyelids can occasionally stick together in the morning. The thickening of the upper tarsal conjunctiva has progressed to the point where the normal vascular pattern is totally obscured (Fig. 6). Papules on

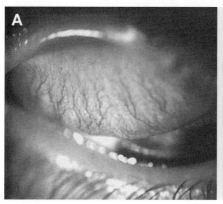
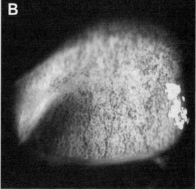

Fig. 4. Stage 2 giant papillary conjunctivitis. (*A*) Injection and thickening of the conjunctiva. (*B*) Enlargement and elevation of papillary reaction (fluorescein instilled and photographed with cobalt filter).

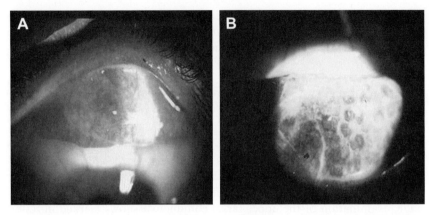

Fig. 5. Stage 3 giant papillary conjunctivitis. (*A*) Marked injection, thickening, and obscuration of the normal vascular pattern of the upper tarsal plate. (*B*) Papules are between 0.5 and 1 mm in size (fluorescein instilled and photographed with cobalt filter).

the upper tarsal conjunctiva are large (sometimes 1 mm or larger) and may have flattened apices. Fluorescein staining and subconjunctival scarring may also be present.

Although four stages have been described that illustrate the progression of both the signs and symptoms of GPC, individual variation is very common, and there may be a discrepancy between the severity of the signs and the symptoms. Some patients may have fairly severe symptoms with only early tarsal changes, whereas some asymptomatic patients or patients with minimal symptoms are found to have impressive inflammatory changes

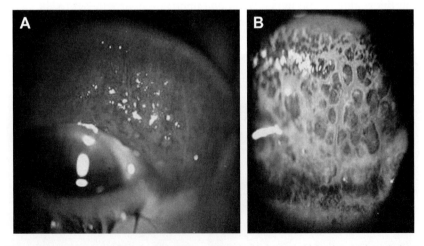

Fig. 6. Stage 4 giant papillary conjunctivitis. (*A*) Marked injection, thickening, and total obscuration of the normal vascular pattern. (*B*) Large papules with apical staining (fluorescein instilled and photographed with cobalt filter). (*From* Donshik PC, Ehlers WH. Giant papillary conjunctivitis. Immunology and Allergy Clinics of North America 1997;17:53–73; with permission.)

on examination of the tarsal conjunctiva. GPC is usually bilateral, but approximately 10% of patients have unilateral or markedly asymmetric signs and symptoms. In approximately 50% of the unilateral cases, an obvious reason for the asymmetry can be found, such as asymmetric coating of the lenses or a poor fit to explain the disparity between the manifestations of the disease in the two eyes; however, in the other half, no specific cause can be found [15].

The signs and symptoms of GPC can be present in both soft hydroxyethyl methacrylate (HEMA)–based hydrogels and rigid contact lens wearers; however, both the signs and symptoms occur sooner in patients wearing soft lenses than those wearing rigid lenses [2,16,17]. The tarsal conjunctival findings are usually similar in patients wearing soft or hard contact lenses. Korb and colleagues [18,19] have shown that in wearers of soft contact lenses the papules usually form first in the zones of the tarsal conjunctiva that are nearest the upper margin of the tarsal plate (zones 1 and 2) and then progress to all 3 zones. In rigid gas-permeable contact lens wearers, however, the papules usually form in the zones nearest the eyelid margin (zone 3 and then zone 2) and tend to remain more localized.

Silicone hydrogel contact lenses were introduced into the United States in 1999. Presently, there are six different silicone hydrogel contact lenses available in the United States. These contact lenses have high oxygen trans-missibility compared with conventional HEMA-based contact lenses, which is a benefit to the cornea. In addition to differences in their oxygen transmissibility, these lenses also vary in their modulus or stiffness, and their surface characteristics. GPC has been associated with use of these lenses, especially the first-generation silicone hydrogel contact lenses. In addition to the typical generalized pattern seen in HEMA-based contact lenses, a localized GPC presentation has been reported with silicone hydrogel lenses, and occurs more frequently than the generalized form [20]. The localized presentation involves the presence of papillae in one or two areas of the tarsal conjunctiva (Fig. 7), whereas in the generalized condition, the papillae

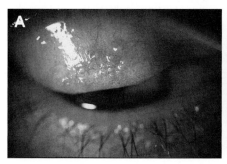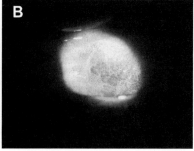

Fig. 7. Localized giant papillary conjunctivitis in a patient wearing silicone hydrogel contact lenses. (A) White light showing the localized papillary reaction. (B) Localized reaction with fluorescein and cobalt filter.

occurred in all three zones. The papules in the localized GPC associated with silicone hydrogels usually occur in zones 2 and 3 (but can also be seen in zone 1), which is similar to the pattern seen with rigid contact lens wearers [21].

Epidemiology

Although GPC can occur with any type of contact lens, it is most often associated with wearing soft lenses. In a study of 221 patients, 85% were wearing soft contact lenses, whereas 15% were wearing rigid lenses [22]. The onset of GPC seems to occur sooner with soft lenses than rigid lenses. Allansmith and colleagues [2] reported an average interval of 10 months for the development of GPC in soft lens wearers, compared with an average of 8.5 years for wearers of rigid lenses. In a study of 221 patients with GPC, however, those wearing soft daily wear contact lenses had been wearing the same brand of lenses for an average of 19.9 months, whereas the patients wearing rigid gas-permeable lenses averaged 21.6 months before developing GPC, and patients wearing polymethyl methacrylate lenses wore them for longer than 90 months [22]. If one considers the total time that patients had been wearing lenses, soft daily wear contact lens patients wore their soft lenses (a variety of brands) an average of 87.4 months before being diagnosed with GPC, patients wearing rigid gas-permeable lenses had worn their lenses an average of 129.8 months, and polymethyl methacrylate wearers averaged 205.5 months of lens wear. This study confirmed the impression that the development of GPC does occur sooner in wearers of soft lenses than in those with rigid lenses (silicone hydrogels were not involved in this study). The study also reported that the signs and symptoms associated with GPC seemed to be more severe in soft lens wearers than in rigid gas-permeable lens wearers [22].

Because GPC is believed to have an immunologic basis, researchers have studied the occurrence of other atopic conditions in patients with GPC. The estimated frequency of hay fever and allergic rhinitis in the general population is considered to be 15% to 20%; reported studies have varied on the incidence of allergies in patients with GPC. Friedlaender [5] reported an incidence of 12%, whereas Donshik [22] reported an incidence of over 26%. In addition, patients with allergies seem to have more severe signs and symptoms of GPC than patients who do not have allergies [22]. The presence or absence of other allergic conditions does not seem to have any effect, however, on the ultimate management of patients with GPC or their ability to continue to contact lens wear [22].

The US Food and Drug Administration has divided soft contact lenses into four groups based on water content and ionic properties of the lens material. There is some debate as to whether silicone hydrogel lenses should have a separate classification, but as of this writing they are currently sorted into several of the existing groups. All types and brands of soft lenses have been associated with the occurrence of GPC. When a large study compared the various lens groups to determine the relationship between lens group and the development of GPC, the contact lenses in Food and Drug Administration group 1 (low water content, nonionic lenses) and group 4 (high water content, ionic lenses) seem to be similar in the severity of the signs and symptoms, and the length of time to onset of GPC. When group 1 contact lenses were compared with group 3 (low water content, ionic lenses), however, patients wearing group 3 contact lenses were found to have more severe signs and symptoms and a shorter time to onset of GPC [22]. The relatively small number of patients in group 2 lenses in this study prevented meaningful comparison with the other groups.

The incidence of GPC among silicone hydrogel contact lens wearers is probably equal to or less than with HEMA-based contact lenses. Silicone hydrogel contact lens wearers, however, are more likely to develop localized GPC than generalized GPC. Contact lens wearers who develop localized GPC seem to have milder symptoms than those associated with generalized GPC. Lens discomfort, blurred vision, secretions, itching, lens awareness, and the need to clean lenses were reported less often in patients with localized GPC compared with patients with generalized GPC. In addition, the incidence of unilateral GPC was greater in localized GPC patients, whereas bilateral GPC was greater in patents that developed generalized GPC. In a study of 124 patients who developed GPC while wearing silicone hydrogels contact lenses, the mean time in lenses before developing GPC was similar for the localized and generalized forms of GPC; and somewhat less than the time reported for HEMA-based hydrogels [21].

Histopathology

When the histopathology of GPC patients is studied, it must be remembered that even asymptomatic lens wearers can have histologic and morphologic changes of the upper tarsal conjunctiva [23,24]. In patients with GPC, however, the changes in the tarsal conjunctiva are more severe [25].

Although studies have found the concentration of inflammatory cells in the conjunctival epithelium of patients with GPC ($44,000/mm^3$) is similar to that found in normal individuals ($55,000/mm^3$) [26], there is a definite difference in the distribution of the various types of inflammatory cells. In normal conjunctival tissue, neutrophils and lymphocytes are present only in the epithelium and the substantia propria, whereas mast cells and plasma cells are present in the substantia propria but not in the epithelium. Basophils and eosinophils are not normally found in either the epithelium or the substantia propria. Conjunctival biopsies from patients with GPC, however, found mast cells in the epithelium, and eosinophils were found in the epithelium and substantia propria. Basophils were also found in the epithelium and substantia propria.

It must also be remembered that although the inflammatory cell density is similar in normal conjunctiva and conjunctiva from GPC patients, the total conjunctival mass for GPC patients is twice that found in normal individuals. This increase in tissue mass is seen clinically as the thickening of the conjunctiva and the formation of papules. Individuals with GPC also have double the total number of inflammatory cells compared with individuals without GPC [23].

The histologic appearance of conjunctiva from patients with GPC is very similar to that seen in vernal conjunctivitis, lending support for an immunologic basis for GPC [27,28]. Differences have been found, however, in inflammatory markers in the tears. Tear histamine levels in patients with vernal conjunctivitis are markedly elevated, averaging four times higher than those associated with GPC [29]. Histamine is released predominantly from the mast cells, which are slightly more numerous in vernal conjunctivitis than in GPC, although the difference is not statistically significant [27]. Studies have also found that the percentage of degranulated mast cells is similar in the epithelium and stroma in patients with vernal conjunctivitis and GPC [26,30]. It is possible that the measured differences in histamine levels in GPC and vernal conjunctivitis are related to a difference in either the presence of histaminase or in the mechanism that controls histamine release. Two types of mast cells with different neutroprotease composition, MCt and MCtc, have been reported [31–34]. The MCt cells contain tryptase, but not chymase, and their granules are characterized by discrete scrolls. This is the predominant mast cell in the alveoli of the lung and the small intestines, and they seem to be dependent on the presence of functional T lymphocytes. The MCtc mast cells contain both tryptase and chymase and are not dependent on T lymphocytes for normal growth. MCtc cells are the predominant type in the skin and small intestinal submucosa, and their granules are characterized by grading and lattice substructures.

The normal conjunctival epithelium is devoid of mast cells, whereas the substantia propria contains an average of $11,054/mm^3$. The predominant mast cell in normal conjunctival tissue is the MCtc cells (mast cells containing tryptase and chymase) [35]. In patients with allergic conjunctivitis, and in asymptomatic wearers of soft contact lenses, mast cells are found in the substantia propria but not in the epithelium. Patients with vernal conjunctivitis and GPC have mast cells present in both the epithelium and substantia propria, but in patients with vernal conjunctivitis, MCt mast cells are present in the substantia propria and they are not found in patients with GPC or allergic conjunctivitis. This contrast may help explain the clinical difference between these two conditions.

Elevated levels of other inflammatory markers are found in the tears of patients with GPC. Tear immunoglobulins, specifically IgE, IgG, and in the more severe cases IgM, have been found in the tears of patients with active GPC [17]. These tear immunoglobulins are locally produced by the external eye and are not elevated in an asymptomatic contact lens wearer. The levels seen in GPC patients are related to the severity of symptoms, and after contact lens wear has been discontinued and the inflammation resolves, the tear immunoglobulins levels in patients with GPC return to normal levels within 1 to 2 weeks, despite the persistence of the tarsal papillary reaction [17]. Levels of complement factors, including C3, Factor B, and C3 anaphylatoxin, are also elevated in tears of GPC patient [36]. Decay-accelerating factor, a complement regulatory protein that inhibits C3 amplification convertase, is decreased in patients with GPC and may be responsible for enhancing complement activation [37]. Tear lactoferrin levels are increased in GPC patients, whereas tear lysozyme levels seem to remain normal [38,39]. The elevated levels of tear immunoglobulins and inflammatory mediators, which are also found in vernal conjunctivitis, further support an immunologic cause of GPC.

Eotaxin, a chemokine that attracts eosinophils, is elevated in patients with contact lens–induced GPC. The levels are correlated with the severity of the papillary reaction. Because eosinophils are important cells in allergic reactions, their presence in GPC is additional evidence of an immunologic cause of GPC, and may play a role in papillary formation [40]. It is interesting to note, however, that eotaxin levels were not found to be elevated in chronic GPC secondary to ocular prosthesis [41].

Neutrophilic chemotactic factor (NCF) has been detected in the tears of GPC patients at 15 times the level found in the tears of normal individuals. Asymptomatic contact lens wearers also have elevated levels of NCF, but the levels are only three times higher than normal levels [42]. NCF is released from injured conjunctival tissue, and the factor released is not related to interleukin-1, complement compound C5a, or leukotriene B4 [43]. When injected into normal tarsal conjunctiva of rabbits, NCF can create tarsal injection and a papillary reaction that is similar to that seen in GPC (Fig. 8). Histologic analysis of the conjunctiva from these rabbits

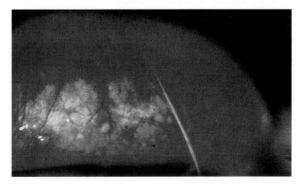

Fig. 8. Upper tarsal conjunctiva of rabbit after injection of neutrophilic chemotactic factor. A papillary reaction can be observed.

shows infiltration of neutrophils, eosinophils, and plasma cells. The specific source of this factor has not yet been determined.

Leukotriene C4 has also been reported to be elevated in the tears of patients with GPC. This mediator's actions on ocular tissues may be in part responsible for conjunctival injection and edema, increased mucoid secretions, and the papillary reaction that occurs in GPC [44].

The elevated levels of tear immunoglobulins, inflammatory mediators, and chemotactic factors (also found in vernal conjunctivitis) provide further evidence of an immunologic basis of GPC.

Coated contact lenses

Contact lenses rapidly develop a complex coating of various substances after insertion onto the eye. Within 30 minutes after lens insertion, 50% of the contact lens is coated, and by 8 hours, approximately 90% of the surface of the lens is coated [45,46]. Even with the best of cleaning regimens, using surfactants and enzymatic treatment, only 75% of the coating is removed. New coating material is constantly built on the surface of the contact lens [47]. Coated contact lenses are a constant feature of GPC, and as the syndrome progresses, lens coating increases. Patients find it increasingly difficult to keep their lenses clean [48]. Lenses with higher water content tend to accumulate more coating than lenses with lower water content [49–51]. Glyceryl methylmethacrylate contact lenses have been shown to accumulate less calcium deposits than HEMA contact lenses, and it is believed that these lenses may tend to coat less than HEMA lenses [52]. Silicone hydrogel contact lenses deposit less lysozyme and total protein than HEMA-based hydrogels but are more prone to lipid deposition [53,54]. Studies have shown that the nature of the deposits on lenses of patients with GPC and asymptomatic individuals are similar [55–60]. Although coating does not necessarily lead to the occurrence of GPC, patients with GPC accumulate more coating on their contact lenses than do patients who do not have GPC [48,61].

There are no morphologic or biochemical findings that can differentiate the coating on the contact lenses of patients who have GPC from that on the lenses of those who do not have GPC [48]. When coated contact lenses from GPC patients are placed on the eyes of rhesus monkeys, however, the monkeys develop injection, thickening, and a papillary reaction on the upper tarsal conjunctiva, which resembles that seen in GPC (Fig. 9) [62]. In addition, elevated levels of IgE and IgG have been found in the tears of these monkeys who were wearing the coated contact lenses. A biopsy of the tarsal plate shows a cellular infiltrate consisting of eosinophils and plasma cells, which are similar to the infiltrates observed in biopsies from patients with GPC [62]. Contact lenses worn by patients who did not have GPC and new unworn contact lenses did not elicit the inflammatory, histologic, or immunologic changes when placed on the eyes of monkeys. It is

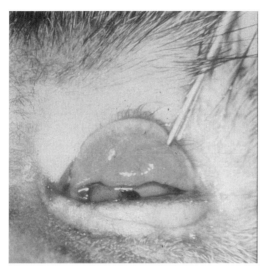

Fig. 9. Upper tarsal conjunctiva of rhesus monkey after being fitted with contact lens from a patient with giant papillary conjunctivitis. Note the marked tarsal injection, thickening, and papillary reaction.

believed this animal model shows the development of GPC secondary to coated contact lenses, and strongly suggests that an antigen does exist on the coated contact lens that can simulate the inflammatory reaction seen clinically as GPC.

Pathophysiology

Although the cause of GPC is unknown, many factors seem to influence its development. The morphologic and histologic similarities between GPC and vernal conjunctivitis have led many investigators to believe that these conditions share a common pathophysiology [27]. Whether GPC is a purely immunologic disease or whether mechanical trauma or irritation are contributing factors is a matter of ongoing debate. The authors' hypothesis of the pathophysiology of contact lens–associated GPC is as follows. Contact lenses become coated and this coating serves as an antigen stimulus. This stimulation causes the production of tear immunoglobulins, IgE, IgG, and in severe cases IgM. The complement system is also activated by the formation of C3 anaphylatoxin. C3 anaphylatoxin, in addition to IgE and some classes of IgG, can interact with mast cells and basophils, resulting in the release of vasoactive amines. The coated contact lens also cause conjunctival trauma, which results in the release of NCF and other inflammatory mediators, which attract eosinophils, mast cells, and basophils, and lymphocytes and plasma cells to the conjunctiva. These cells interact with IgG, IgE, and C3a, resulting in the release of additional inflammatory mediators including vasoactive amines, which are responsible for initiating the complex of symptoms. The increased proteins in the tear film result in further coating on the contact lenses, perpetuating the cycle of events. Lactoferrin, a potent inhibitor of C3a, has been found to be decreased in the tears of patients with GPC; this results in an increased formation of C3a, also found to be elevated in the tears of patients with GPC. This cascade of events is shown graphically in Fig. 10. In addition, tear film clearance is delayed, and this delay in tear clearance can prolong the presence of inflammatory mediators and may aggravate the coating of the contact lens [63].

It is possible that in localized GPC secondary to silicone hydrogels, the stiffer modulus of the contact lens itself, the edge design, or the fitting characteristics of these lenses may induce trauma to the conjunctiva, resulting in the release of NCF, which in itself may be important in the development of the clinical picture seen in the localized form of GPC. The generalized form is associated with a reaction to the coated contact lens similar to that occuring with HEMA-based contact lenses.

Treatment

On the basis of the authors' hypothesis, a rational approach to the treatment of GPC can be undertaken. Therapy can either be directed at decreasing the coating on the contact lens, which decreases the antigen load and trauma to the conjunctival surface, or it can involve modulation

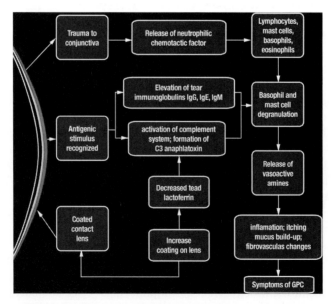

Fig. 10. Flow chart outlining pathophysiology of giant papillary conjunctivitis. (*From* Donshik PC. Giant papillary conjunctivitis. Trans Am Ophthalmol Soc 1994;92:687–744; with permission.)

of the immune reaction. The modalities that are available to decrease the coating of contact lenses are improved cleaning, decreased wearing time, or a change in the contact lens material or design [64–71]. Methods that are available to modulate the immune response are the use of topical corticosteroids, topical nonsteroidal anti-inflammatory agents, and mast cell stabilizers.

In a study of 221 patients with GPC [22], the authors found that if contact lens wear was not discontinued, but the cleaning regimen was changed, only 50% were able to continue wearing their contact lenses. If the patients decreased their wearing time, only 20% were able to continue wearing their lenses, and if they just replaced their contact lenses, 78% of patients could continue wearing their lenses. If patients discontinued wearing their contact lenses for 3 to 4 weeks and then were refitted with a new contact lens, however, 94% were able to continue wearing their lenses. If one looked at the different types of lenses used in refitting patients after a period of discontinuing contact lens wear, refitting the patients with the same type of lens only resulted in a success rate of 68%. Refitting to a rigid gas-permeable lens resulted in a success rate of 82%, and changing to a glyceryl methylmethacrylate resulted in an 81% success rate; however, using a frequent replacement or disposable lens resulted in a 91% success rate. It seems that the most successful lens modality to refit patients with GPC is the use of a frequent replacement or a disposable contact lens worn on a daily wear basis.

Studies reported in the literature on modulating the immune response have consisted mainly of the use of mast cell stabilizers [72–74]. Kruger and colleagues [75] reported that 14 (70%) of 20 patients with moderate to severe GPC who had a return of symptoms after changing their contact lens (patients first treated with a combination of improved lens care and refitting with a contact lens of a different design or polymer) were able to continue wearing their contact lenses when treated with topical cromolyn sodium. There have also been reports of nonsteroidal anti-inflammatory agents being effective in the management of GPC [76]. The use of topical steroids has not been widely advocated because the potential complications of glaucoma and cataracts outweigh the potential benefits of keeping individuals in contact lenses. Loteprednol etabonate (a soft steroid) has been reported to be beneficial in treating the signs and symptoms of GPC over a 4-week period; however, the long-term beneficial effects of this drug have not been investigated [77,78]. On the basis of these studies, the following regimen for the management of GPC is suggested.

Treatment for stage 1: preclinical giant papillary conjunctivitis

Patients who have minimal lens changes with minimal or no symptoms can often be managed by decreasing the replacement interval of their contact lenses. If the patient wears conventional hydrogel contact lenses they should be replaced at least twice a year. Another alternative is to use frequent replacement or disposable lenses, with replacement intervals of 2 weeks to 3 months. In addition to daily lens cleaning and disinfection, preferably with hydrogen peroxide and unpreserved saline solution, enzymatic cleaning once or twice a week should be used if lenses are replaced at intervals greater than 2 weeks. Because they are at higher risk, these patients should be followed two to three times a year and instructed to consult their physician at the initiation of any of the symptoms associated with GPC.

Treatment for stage 2: mild giant papillary conjunctivitis

Patients with early lens changes and mild symptoms are best managed by the use of frequent replacement daily wear lenses with a replacement cycle of 2 to 4 weeks. For patients wearing soft HEMA lenses, another alternative is to change to a lens of a non-HEMA material. The use of an enzymatic cleaner once or twice a week is then required, and these lenses can be replaced every 4 to 6 months. These patients are at high risk and should be followed four times a year.

Treatment for stage 3: moderate giant papillary conjunctivitis

Patients with moderate signs and symptoms should stop wearing their contact lenses for approximately 4 weeks. At that time, patients should be re-evaluated to ascertain that there is no evidence of keratitis and to ensure that the apical staining of the tarsal papules has resolved. In the authors' experience, these patients do well with frequent replacement or disposable contact lenses worn on a daily wear basis and replaced every 1 to 2 weeks. These lenses require daily cleaning and disinfection, preferably with hydrogen peroxide and unpreserved saline. Newly introduced daily disposable contact lenses should be effective in the management of patients in stage 3. Another option is to refit these patients with rigid gas-permeable lenses. They should be followed at 3-month intervals.

Treatment for stage 4: severe giant papillary conjunctivitis

Patients with severe GPC require discontinuation of their contact lenses for a minimum of 4 weeks. During this time, the inflammatory reaction should resolve; however, if apical staining of the papules was noted at the time of diagnosis, the tarsal plate must be re-examined to ensure that staining has resolved. The cornea also has to be free of punctate staining noted with fluorescein instillation. The papillary reaction of the tarsal plate will probably be unchanged. Injection and inflammation of the tarsal conjunctiva often diminishes, but may not totally be eliminated during this time. In the authors' experience, these patients are best managed by fitting them with frequent replacement or disposable contact lenses worn on a daily wear basis and replaced at 1-week intervals; however, it may be necessary for the patient to change their lenses after 2 or 3 days. These contact lenses require the daily use of a cleaner and disinfection with hydrogen peroxide and unpreserved saline solution. The recently introduced daily disposable lenses are very effective in managing patients in stage 4. As in stage 3, another option is to refit these patients with rigid gas-permeable lenses. These patients, as in stage 3, need to be followed frequently while they wear their new lenses.

Although frequent-replacement contact lenses seem to offer a treatment option, the frequency of replacement is important. In a study of patients wearing frequent-replacement daily wear contact lenses who replaced their contact lenses between 1 day and 12 weeks, the incidence of GPC in those patients replacing their contact lenses 4 weeks or longer was 36%, whereas patients who replaced their contact lenses less than 4 weeks had an incidence of 4.5%. GPC was not reported in any patient who wore a daily disposable contact lens. In patients who are at high risk of developing GPC, replacing contact lenses at intervals of 1 day to 2 weeks seems to offer the best strategy in keeping these patients in contact lenses [79].

The treatment of GPC in patients wearing silicone hydrogel contact lenses is still evolving. If patients are wearing their lenses overnight, they should be switched to a daily wear schedule, the type or brand of silicone hydrogel should be changed, and they should be instructed to replace their lenses more frequently. If they still have signs and symptoms related to GPC, then they should be refitted to a non–silicone hydrogel that is replaced daily or at 1 to 2 weeks. If the signs and symptoms of GPC recur after being managed with the previously mentioned recommendations, the use of topical mast cell stabilizers four times a day or combination mast cell stabilizer-antihistamines twice daily can be considered. If this is to be effective, the eye has to be free of inflammation (ie, the contact lenses have to be discontinued for 3–4 weeks) and the previous contact lenses have to be replaced with new and clean contact lenses.

Summary

If GPC is under control, patients are able to maintain a wearing schedule that is satisfactory to their lifestyle without the recurrence of the symptoms associated with this syndrome. The upper tarsal inflammation in the form of injection usually resolves; however, the papules either remain unchanged or over time may slowly decrease in diameter and height. In some patients, however, the tarsal conjunctiva remains thickened, with a significant papillary reaction but without inflammation, for years after the onset of GPC; yet, they are still be able comfortably to wear their contact lenses. Patients have to be instructed at the first onset of excessive mucus, coating of the contact lens, or increased contact lens awareness to contact their ophthalmologist. With proper lens care, frequent lens replacement, and continued follow-up care, over 90% of patients with GPC can continue in contact lenses.

References

[1] Spring TF. Reaction to hydrophilic lenses. Med J Aust 1974;1(12):449–50.
[2] Allansmith MR, Korb DR, Greiner JV, et al. Giant papillary conjunctivitis in contact lens wearers. Am J Ophthalmol 1977;83(5):697–708.
[3] Carlson AN, Wilhelmus KR. Giant papillary conjunctivitis associated with cyanoacrylate glue. Am J Ophthalmol 1987;104(4):437–8.
[4] Douglas JP, Lowder CY, Lazorik R, et al. Giant papillary conjunctivitis associated with rigid gas permeable contact lenses. CLAO J 1988;14(3):143–7.
[5] Friedlaender MH. Some unusual nonallergic causes of giant papillary conjunctivitis. Trans Am Ophthalmol Soc 1990;88:343–9 [discussion: 349–51].
[6] Greiner JV. Papillary conjunctivitis induced by an epithelialized corneal foreign body. Ophthalmologica 1988;196(2):82–6.
[7] Heidemann DG, Dunn SP, Siegal MJ. Unusual causes of giant papillary conjunctivitis. Cornea 1993;12(1):78–80.
[8] Jolson AS, Jolson SC. Suture barb giant papillary conjunctivitis. Ophthalmic Surg 1984; 15(2):139–40.
[9] Nirankari VS, Karesh JW, Richards RD. Complications of exposed monofilament sutures. Am J Ophthalmol 1983;95(4):515–9.
[10] Robin JB, Regis-Pacheco LF, May WN, et al. Giant papillary conjunctivitis associated with an extruded scleral buckle: case report. Arch Ophthalmol 1987;105(5):619.
[11] Skrypuch OW, Willis NR. Giant papillary conjunctivitis from an exposed Prolene suture. Can J Ophthalmol 1986;21(5):189–92.
[12] Srinivasan BD, et al. Giant papillary conjunctivitis with ocular prostheses. Arch Ophthalmol 1979;97(5):892–5.
[13] Sugar A, Meyer RF. Giant papillary conjunctivitis after keratoplasty. Am J Ophthalmol 1981;91(2):239–42.
[14] Korb DR, Allansmith MR, Greiner JV, et al. Prevalence of conjunctival changes in wearers of hard contact lenses. Am J Ophthalmol 1980;90(3):336–41.
[15] Palmisano PC, Ehlers WH, Donshik PC. Causative factors in unilateral giant papillary conjunctivitis. CLAO J 1993;19(2):103–7.
[16] Allansmith MR. Pathology and treatment of giant papillary conjunctivitis. I. The U.S. perspective. Clin Ther 1987;9(5):443–50.
[17] Donshik PC, Ballow M. Tear immunoglobulins in giant papillary conjunctivitis induced by contact lenses. Am J Ophthalmol 1983;96(4):460–6.
[18] Korb DR, Allansmith RM, Greiner JV, et al. Biomicroscopy of papillae associated with hard contact lens wearing. Ophthalmology 1981;88(11):1132–6.
[19] Korb DR, Allansmith MR, Greiner JV, et al. Biomicroscopy of papillae associated with wearing of soft contact lenses. Br J Ophthalmol 1983;67(11):733–6.
[20] Skotnitsky C, Sankaridurg PR, Sweeney DF, et al. General and local contact lens induced papillary conjunctivitis (CLPC). Clin Exp Optom 2002;85(3):193–7.
[21] Skotnitsky CC, Naduvilath TH, Sweeney DF, et al. Two presentations of contact lens-induced papillary conjunctivitis (CLPC) in hydrogel lens wear: local and general. Optom Vis Sci 2006;83(1):27–36.
[22] Donshik PC. Giant papillary conjunctivitis. Trans Am Ophthalmol Soc 1994;92:687–744.
[23] Greiner JV, Covington HI, Allansmith MR. Surface morphology of the human upper tarsal conjunctiva. Am J Ophthalmol 1977;83(6):892–905.
[24] Greiner JV, Covington HJ, Korb DR, et al. Conjunctiva in asymptomatic contact lens wearers. Am J Ophthalmol 1978;86(3):403–13.

[25] Greiner JV, Covington HI, Allansmith MR. Surface morphology of giant papillary conjunctivitis in contact lens wearers. Am J Ophthalmol 1978;85(2):242–52.

[26] Allansmith MR, Korb DR, Greiner JV. Giant papillary conjunctivitis induced by hard or soft contact lens wear: quantitative histology. Ophthalmology 1978;85(8):766–78.

[27] Allansmith MR, Baird RS, Greiner JV. Vernal conjunctivitis and contact lens-associated giant papillary conjunctivitis compared and contrasted. Am J Ophthalmol 1979;87(4): 544–55.

[28] Collin HB, Allansmith MR. Basophils in vernal conjunctivitis in humans: an electron microscopic study. Invest Ophthalmol Vis Sci 1977;16(9):858–64.

[29] Abelson MB, Soter NA, Simpon M, et al. Histamine in human tears. Am J Ophthalmol 1977; 83(3):417–8.

[30] Allansmith MR, Baird RS. Percentage of degranulated mast cells in vernal conjunctivitis and giant papillary conjunctivitis associated with contact-lens wear. Am J Ophthalmol 1981; 91(1):71–5.

[31] Craig SS, Schechter NM, Schwartz LB. Ultrastructural analysis of human T and TC mast cells identified by immunoelectron microscopy. Lab Invest 1988;58(6):682–91.

[32] Schwartz LB, Irani AA, Roller K, et al. Quantitation of histamine, tryptase, and chymase in dispersed human T and TC mast cells. J Immunol 1987;138(8):2611–5.

[33] Irani AM, Craig SS, Del Belois G, et al. Deficiency of the tryptase-positive, chymase-negative mast cell type in gastrointestinal mucosa of patients with defective T lymphocyte function. J Immunol 1987;138(12):4381–6.

[34] Irani AA, Schechter NM, Craig SS, et al. Two types of human mast cells that have distinct neutral protease compositions. Proc Natl Acad Sci U S A 1986;83(12):4464–8.

[35] Irani AM, Burtus I, Tabbar KF, et al. Human conjunctival mast cells: distribution of MCT and MCTC in vernal conjunctivitis and giant papillary conjunctivitis. J Allergy Clin Immunol 1990;86(1):34–40.

[36] Ballow M, Donshik PC, Mendelson L. Complement proteins and C3 anaphylatoxin in the tears of patients with conjunctivitis. J Allergy Clin Immunol 1985;76(3):473–6.

[37] Szczotka LB, Cocuzzi E, Medof ME. Decay-accelerating factor in tears of contact lens wearers and patients with contact lens-associated complications. Optom Vis Sci 2000; 77(11):586–91.

[38] Ballow M, Donshik PC, Rapacz P, et al. Tear lactoferrin levels in patients with external inflammatory ocular disease. Invest Ophthalmol Vis Sci 1987;28(3):543–5.

[39] Rapacz P, Tedesco J, Donshik PC, et al. Tear lysozyme and lactoferrin levels in giant papillary conjunctivitis and vernal conjunctivitis. CLAO J 1988;14(4):207–9.

[40] Moschos MM, Eperon S, Guex-Crosier Y. Increased eotaxin in tears of patients wearing contact lenses. Cornea 2004;23(8):771–5.

[41] Sarac O, Erdener I, Irkec M, et al. Tear eotaxin levels in giant papillary conjunctivitis associated with ocular prosthesis. Ocul Immunol Inflamm 2003;11(3):223–30.

[42] Elgebaly SA, Donshik PC, Rahhal F, et al. Neutrophil chemotactic factors in the tears of giant papillary conjunctivitis patients. Invest Ophthalmol Vis Sci 1991;32(1):208–13.

[43] Ehlers WH, Fishman JB, Donshik BC, et al. Neutrophil chemotactic factors derived from conjunctival epithelial cells: preliminary biochemical characterization. CLAO J 1991; 17(1):65–8.

[44] Irkec MT, Orhan M, Erdener U. Role of tear inflammatory mediators in contact lens-associated giant papillary conjunctivitis in soft contact lens wearers. Ocul Immunol Inflamm 1999;7(1):35–8.

[45] Fowler SA, Allansmith MR. Evolution of soft contact lens coatings. Arch Ophthalmol 1980; 98(1):95–9.

[46] Fowler SA, Allansmith MR. The surface of the continuously worn contact lens. Arch Ophthalmol 1980;98(7):1233–6.

[47] Fowler SA, Allansmith MR. The effect of cleaning soft contact lenses: a scanning electron microscopic study. Arch Ophthalmol 1981;99(8):1382–6.

[48] Fowler SA, Greiner JV, Allansmith MR. Soft contact lenses from patients with giant papillary conjunctivitis. Am J Ophthalmol 1979;88(6):1056–61.

[49] Fowler SA, Korb DR, Allansmith MR. Deposits on soft contact lenses of various water contents. CLAO J 1985;11(2):124–7.

[50] Hosaka S, et al. Analysis of deposits on high water content contact lenses. J Biomed Mater Res 1983;17(2):261–74.

[51] Hind HW, Szekely IJ. Wetting and hydration of contact lenses. Contacto. The Contact Lens J 1959;3:65–8.

[52] Levy B. Calcium deposits on glyceryl methyl methacrylate and hydroxyethyl methacrylate contact lenses. Am J Optom Physiol Opt 1984;61(9):605–7.

[53] Jones L, et al. Lysozyme and lipid deposition on silicone hydrogel contact lens materials. Eye Contact Lens 2003;29(1 Suppl):S75–9 [discussion: S83–4; S192–4].

[54] Santos L, et al. The influence of surface treatment on hydrophobicity, protein adsorption and microbial colonisation of silicone hydrogel contact lenses. Cont Lens Anterior Eye 2007;30(3):183–8.

[55] Gudmundsson OG, et al. Identification of proteins in contact lens surface deposits by immunofluorescence microscopy. Arch Ophthalmol 1985;103(2):196–7.

[56] Barr JT, et al. Protein and elemental analysis of contact lenses of patients with superior limbic keratoconjunctivitis or giant papillary conjunctivitis. Optom Vis Sci 1989;66(3): 133–40.

[57] Caroline PJ, et al. Microscopic and elemental analysis of deposits on extended wear soft contact lenses. CLAO J 1985;11(4):311–6.

[58] Lowther GE, Hilbert JA. Deposits on hydrophilic lenses: differential appearance and clinical causes. Am J Optom Physiol Opt 1975;52(10):687–92.

[59] Hovding G, Seland JH. Deposits on hydrophilic bandage lenses: a scanning electronmicroscopic and x-ray microanalytic study. Acta Ophthalmol (Copenh) 1984;62(6):849–58.

[60] Matas BR, Spencer WH, Hayes TL. Scanning electron microscopy of hydrophilic contact lenses. Arch Ophthalmol 1972;88(3):287–95.

[61] Conrads H. [Scanning electron microscope investigations on soft contact lenses (author's transl)]. Klin Monatsbl Augenheilkd 1975;167(6):846–55 [in German].

[62] Ballow M, et al. Immune responses in monkeys to lenses from patients with contact lens induced giant papillary conjunctivitis. CLAO J 1989;15(1):64–70.

[63] Chang SW, Chang CJ. Delayed tear clearance in contact lens associated papillary conjunctivitis. Curr Eye Res 2001;22(4):253–7.

[64] Bucci FA Jr, et al. Comparison of the clinical performance of the Acuvue disposable contact lens and CSI lens in patients with giant papillary conjunctivitis. Am J Ophthalmol 1993; 115(4):454–9.

[65] Donshik PC, et al. Treatment of contact lens-induced giant papillary conjunctivitis. CLAO J 1984;10(4):346–50.

[66] Farkas P, Kassalow TW, Farkas B. Clinical management and control of giant papillary conjunctivitis secondary to contact lens wear. J Am Optom Assoc 1986;57(3):197–200.

[67] Mackie IA, Wright P. Giant papillary conjunctivitis (secondary vernal) in association with contact lens wear. Trans Ophthalmol Soc U K 1978;98(1):3–9.

[68] Molinari JF. The clinical management of giant papillary conjunctivitis. Am J Optom Physiol Opt 1981;58(10):886–91.

[69] Cho MH, Norden LC, Chang FW. Disposable extended wear soft contact lenses for the treatment of giant papillary conjunctivitis. South J Optom 1988;41:9–12.

[70] Molinari JF. Giant papillary conjunctivitis: a review of management and a retrospective clinical study. Clin Eye Vis Care 1991;3:1–5.

[71] Strulowitz L, Brudno J. The management and treatment of giant papillary conjunctivitis with disposables. Contact Lens Spectrum 1989;9:45–6.

[72] Lustine T, Bouchard CS, Cavanagh HD. Continued contact lens wear in patients with giant papillary conjunctivitis. CLAO J 1991;17(2):104–7.

[73] Meisler DM, et al. Cromolyn treatment of giant papillary conjunctivitis. Arch Ophthalmol 1982;100(10):1608–10.

[74] Molinari JF. Giant papillary conjunctivitis management in hydrogel contact lens wearers. Trans Br Contact Lens Assoc 1982;5:94–9.

[75] Kruger CJ, Ehlers WH, Donshik PC, et al. Treatment of giant papillary conjunctivitis with cromolyn sodium. CLAO J 1992;18(1):46–8.

[76] Wood TS, Stewart RH, Bowman RW, et al. Suprofen treatment of contact lens-associated giant papillary conjunctivitis. Ophthalmology 1988;95(6):822–6.

[77] Bartlett JD, Howes JF, Ghormley NR, et al. Safety and efficacy of loteprednol etabonate for treatment of papillae in contact lens-associated giant papillary conjunctivitis. Curr Eye Res 1993;12(4):313–21.

[78] Asbell P, Howes J. A double-masked, placebo-controlled evaluation of the efficacy and safety of loteprednol etabonate in the treatment of giant papillary conjunctivitis. CLAO J 1997;23(1):31–6.

[79] Porazinski AD, Donshik PC. Giant papillary conjunctivitis in frequent replacement contact lens wearers: a retrospective study. CLAO J 1999;25(3):142–7.

ELSEVIER
SAUNDERS

Immunol Allergy Clin N Am
28 (2008) 105–117

IMMUNOLOGY
AND ALLERGY
CLINICS
OF NORTH AMERICA

Contact Lenses and Associated Anterior Segment Disorders: Dry Eye Disease, Blepharitis, and Allergy

Michael A. Lemp, MD[a,b,]*, Leonard Bielory, MD[c]

[a]*Georgetown University School of Medicine, 3900 Reservoir Road NW,
Washington, DC 20007, USA*
[b]*George Washington University School of Medicine, 2150 Penn Avenue NW,
Washington, DC 20005, USA*
[c]*UMDNJ-New Jersey Medical School, 90 Bergen Street, DOC Suite 4700,
Newark, NJ 07103, USA*

The tear film is a dynamic structure consisting of three major components (lipid, aqueous, and mucin), which overlies the cornea and conjunctiva and is bounded by the lid margins. It is essential to maintain the cornea and conjunctiva in a normal state; it provides moisture, lubrication, and oxygen necessary for corneal and conjunctival epithelial respiration and forms a smooth surface interfacing with air to provide a clear image of incoming light to subserve vision. In addition, it serves as a pathway for movement of cytokines and other proteins secreted by the lacrimal glands, which act on the surface epithelium to direct and regulate normal cell proliferation, differentiation, maturation, and exfoliation to maintain the homeostatic state of the ocular surface and to facilitate cellular response to injury [1].

The ocular surface cells, lacrimal glands, and eyelids form a tightly regulated functional unit linked by a neural pathway from the sensory fibers of the ophthalmic division of the fifth cranial nerve, which innervate the ocular surface epithelium [2]. From these nerves afferent impulses run to the central nervous system from which efferent fibers course to the cornea, conjunctiva, lacrimal glands, meibomian glands of the eyelids, and the orbicularis muscle of the eyelids. Efferent nerve signals regulate lacrimal gland secretion of water, electrolytes, and over 300 immunologically active proteins. Many of these small molecular weight proteins are cytokines, which act on receptors on surface cells regulating cellular functions. In addition, efferent neural fibers also innervate the meibomian glands of the eyelid and the goblet cells

* Corresponding author. 4000 Cathedral Avenue NW, 828 B, Washington, DC 20016.
  E-mail address: malemp@lempdc.com (M.A. Lemp).

of the conjunctival. The presence of an intact neural pathway that mediates these functions is essential for the maintenance of a normal ocular surface.

The structure of tears is thought to be that of a two- or three-layered film consisting of an inner transmembrane mucin layer (MUC1 and MUC4) derived from the epithelial cells similar to the mucin in the bronchial linings. Overlying this is a thicker aqueous layer, the product of the lacrimal glands and possible transconjunctival fluid transport. Within this layer is a gradient of highly hydrated loose mucin (MUC5-AC), which forms a "blanket" protecting the ocular surface and stabilizing the tear film. Other mucin-soluble and gel-forming mucins include MUC7 and MUC16, whose function may be related to surface morphology [3]. The outermost covering of tears is a thin lipid layer, the product of the meibomian glands of the eyelid. This functions to limit evaporative loss of tears [4]. The interaction of these components contributes to the meta-stability of the tear film between blinks.

In the recent report of the International Dry Eye Workshop a new definition and classification system was issued [5–10].

Dry eye is a multifactorial disease of the tears and ocular surface that results in symptoms of discomfort, visual disturbance, and tear film instability with potential damage to the ocular surface. It is accompanied by increased osmolarity of the tear film and inflammation of the ocular surface.

Two major etiopathogenic types of dry eye disease (DED) are recognized: an aqueous-deficient type in which there is a deficiency of the secretion of the lacrimal glands, and an evaporative type in which the meibomian glands of the

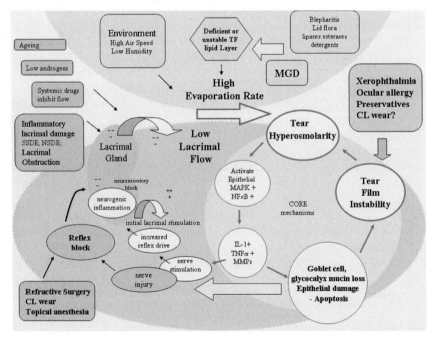

eyelid are dysfunctional resulting in a quantitative and qualitative change in secretion of the evaporation-sparing lipids of the tear film. In practice, about two thirds of patients present with both forms of the disease. There are a number of risk factors associated with the development of DED: age; female gender; a decrease in bioavailable androgen; systemic autoimmune disease, such as Sjögren's syndrome; collagen vascular disease, such as rheumatoid arthritis, lupus, and scleroderma; environmental stress including dry and windy climatic conditions; sustained video display terminal use; long air travel; neurologic sensory loss in the ocular surface; and decreased blinking.

Regardless of the initiating factor or group of factors, the final common expression of disease is breakdown in the homeostatic mechanisms operative at the tear-ocular surface interface resulting in instability of the tear film, an increase in the osmolarity of the tear film with damage to the ocular surface, and sensory and visual disturbances (Fig. 1).

Fig. 1. Mechanisms of dry eye [10]. The core mechanisms of dry eye are driven by tear hyperosmolarity and tear film instability. The cycle of events is shown on the right of the figure. Tear hyperosmolarity causes damage to the surface epithelium by activating a cascade of inflammatory events at the ocular surface and a release of inflammatory mediators into the tears. Epithelial damage involves cell death by apoptosis, a loss of goblet cells, and disturbance of mucin expression leading to tear film instability. This instability exacerbates ocular surface hyperosmolarity and completes the vicious circle. Tear film instability can be initiated without the prior occurrence of tear hyperosmolarity, by several etiologies including xerophthalmia, ocular allergy, topical preservative use, and contact lens wear. The epithelial injury caused by dry eye stimulates corneal nerve endings, leading to symptoms of discomfort; increased blinking; and, potentially, compensatory reflex lacrimal tear secretion. Loss of normal mucins at the ocular surface contributes to symptoms by increasing frictional resistance between the lids and globe. During this period, the high reflex input has been suggested as the basis of a neurogenic inflammation within the gland. The major causes of tear hyperosmolarity are reduced aqueous tear flow, resulting from lacrimal failure, or increased evaporation from the tear film. This is indicated by the arrow at the top-center of the figure. Increased evaporative loss is favored by environmental conditions of low humidity and high air flow and may be caused clinically, in particular, by meibomian gland dysfunction (MGD), which leads to an unstable tear film lipid layer. The quality of lid oil is modified by the action of esterases and lipases released by normal lid commensals, whose numbers are increased in blepharitis. Reduced aqueous tear flow is caused by impaired delivery of lacrimal fluid into the conjunctival sac. It is unclear whether this is a feature of normal ageing, but it may be induced by certain systemic drugs, such as antihistamines and antimuscarinic agents. The most common cause is inflammatory lacrimal damage, which is seen in autoimmune disorders, such as Sjögren's syndrome and in non-Sjögren dry eye (NSDE). Inflammation causes both tissue destruction and a potentially reversible neurosecretory block. A receptor block may also be caused by circulating antibodies to the M3 receptor. Inflammation is favored by low tissue androgen levels. Also, tear delivery may be obstructed by cicatricial conjunctival scarring or reduced by a loss of sensory reflex drive to the lacrimal gland from the ocular surface. Eventually, the chronic surface damage of dry eye leads to a fall in corneal sensitivity and a reduction of reflex tear secretion. Various etiologies may cause dry eye acting at least in part by the mechanism of reflex secretory block, including refractive surgery (LASIK dry eye); contact lens wear; and the chronic abuse of topical anesthetics. Individual etiologies often cause dry eye by several interacting mechanisms. Further details may be found in the text. CL, contact lens; IL, interleukin; MMP, matrix metalloproteases; SSDE, Sjogren syndrome dry eye; TF, tear film; TNF, tumor necrosis factor.

More severe forms of dry eye are associated with a systemic autoimmune disease (eg, Sjögren's syndrome, in which there is heavy lymphocytic cell infiltration with severe inflammation of the lacrimal glands, ocular surface, and associated structures, such as the meibomian glands of the eyelids). In the most severe cases vision-threatening complications, such as scleritis, corneal ulcers, and secondary bacterial infection, can occur. There is recent evidence that even in milder forms of aqueous tear deficiency, there is subclinical inflammation suggesting a commonality of disease processes [1].

Evaporative tear deficiency is most commonly associated with dysfunction of the meibomian glands of the eyelid. The term "blepharitis" is applied to various inflammatory conditions of the eyelids, some of which are infectious (eg, chalazia) and some noninfectious (eg, atopic blepharitis). The pathogenesis of a discrete category of blepharitis, meibomian gland dysfunction (posterior blepharitis, meibomitis), remains poorly explained. Meibomian gland dysfunction is, however, an extremely common condition; its prevalence increases with advancing age and is associated with the presence of androgen insufficiency and aqueous tear deficiency [11].

DED is widely prevalent. In its severe form, as keratoconjunctivitis sicca, it is part of a more systemic autoimmune process, Sjögren's syndrome, which is estimated to involve 4 million people in the United States. Epidemiologic studies have reported a DED prevalence of 13% to 15% in people 65 and older [12–14]. Recent studies estimate that over 9 million persons in the United States are afflicted with moderate to severe DED [15]. Based on these data and clinical studies, DED can be estimated to involve 40 to 60 million Americans. It is more common in women and involves large numbers of people from the third decade of life onward. This includes the prime age groups for contact lens wear.

Contact lenses represent a foreign body placed in the preocular tear film environment. Contact lenses have a number of effects on the ocular surface and the tear film. The effects of contact lenses on the cornea include hypoxia, a slight elevation in corneal temperature, microtrauma to the cornea, a reduction in corneal metabolic rate, a decrease in the mitotic rate of the epithelium, increased epithelial fragility, compromised junctional integrity, and an increase in lactate [16]. Despite these changes patients with a normal ocular surface accommodate to the presence of a contact lens with remarkable success.

In addition, contact lenses have been shown to have a number of effects on the tear film. Contact lenses disrupt the tear film by thinning and breakup of the film, increasing evaporative tear loss probably by a disruptive effect on the tear lipid layer [17,18]. Soft contact lenses have been shown to allow evaporation of fluid from corneal tissue, actually drawing fluid out of the cornea [19]. It is thought that only about 10% of the normal volume of tears is necessary to maintain the ocular surface. In a patient with an adequate volume of tears and normal meibomian gland secretion, the presence of a contact lens represents a tolerable stress on the tear film. In the absence of these normal adaptive reservoirs, a contact lens can induce a clinically apparent dry eye state. The condition contact lens–induced dry eye is estimated to occur in 20% to 30% of soft contact lens wearers, and in over 80% of rigid contact lens wearers [20]. Both rigid and soft lenses create a thinned tear film at the lens edge; this is reported to affect adversely mucin spreading and lipid layer reformation. Moreover, the tear film overlying the lens is thinner than a normal tear film leading to more rapid breakup of the prelens tear film. The presence of a contact lens, rigid or soft, represents a stress to the tear film that in a predisposed patient can lead to contact lens–induced dry eye [21].

Recognizing marginal dry eye disease

Because patients who have pre-existing abnormalities of the tear film and ocular surface are at greater risk for contact lens failure, such as discomfort leading to discontinuance of contact lens wear and the development of contact lens–induced dry eye, it is important to screen candidates for contact lens wear before fitting. Screening tests generally identify subjects with abnormalities. Screening tests for dry eye syndrome can include the following, but they have been noted to have limited predictive values.

Dry eye questionnaires
Tear film breakup time
Schirmer test (and similar tests)
Ocular surface staining
Lid margin examination
Tear clearance test
Ocular Protection Index

Although tear osmolarity has been considered the gold standard for the diagnosis of dry eye, the lack of a readily available instrument for measuring this property of tears in a reproducible manner has left clinicians with a number of clinical tests that, taken together, can usually diagnose moderate to severe dry eye conditions. The diagnosis of early or mild dry eye can be more difficult because symptoms usually precede signs and more subtle measures are necessary. In this regard, the use of patient questionnaires has assumed importance in identifying dry eye subjects. These include an assessment of subjective complaints (eg, dryness, grittiness, sandiness, itching, burning, photophobia, and other complaints). In addition, frequency and intensity of symptoms, effect of environmental conditions, limitation of activities because of ocular symptoms, frequency of medications, symptoms of dry mouth, and other questions are included. Frequently used subjective instruments include the McMonnies Dry Eye Questionaire, the Ocular Surface Disease Index, the Dry Eye Questionnaire, and the NEI-VFQ. Although these have been criticized because of a lack of correlation with clinical signs of dry eye, they have power to identify early to moderate dry eye patients who lack many signs of more advanced cases. The use of one of these patient-administered questionnaires by practitioners can be a very useful tool in recognizing patients who are at higher risk for developing contact lens intolerance. The Dry Eye Workshop report recognizes the potential role of tear osmolarity as a diagnostic tool of choice in DED and recent reports of a new tear collecting system and technology for measuring tear osmolarity on nanoliter samples of tears opens the way to a new clinically relevant method of diagnosing DED, which may change the diagnostic and disease management paradigm [8].

Tear film breakup time (BUT) is a global test for tear film instability [8]. In this test a small amount of 1% sodium fluorescein is instilled in the conjunctival cul-de-sac, and the patient is instructed to blink for 30 seconds and then to stare ahead without blinking. While the examiner is scanning the corneal surface with the broad beam and cobalt blue filter of the slit lamp, the appearance of the first randomly distributed dry spot is noted (usually with a stop watch or in a more sophisticated setting with a video camera with on-screen timer). BUT is usually measured three times in a row and averaged. In normal subjects the BUT is usually in excess of 10 seconds. Using the more sophisticated video recording technology, referent values of 7 seconds have been reported [22]. The test is exquisitely sensitive to the testing methods, such as the amount of fluorescein instilled, width of the interpalpebral fissure, intensity of the light source, and the patient's ability to cooperate and not blink prematurely. With practice, however, standard conditions of measurement can be achieved with reasonably reproducible results. To determine accurately a normal range of BUT under one's testing conditions, perform the test on a series of normal subjects. This test is a useful screening test.

The Schirmer test is the most widely used test to measure aqueous tear production because of its ease of performance, cost, and availability. It has been criticized for lack of reproducibility and discrimination in identifying dry eye. A commercial filter paper strip with a notch is bent and inserted over the lower lid margin at the junction of the middle and outer third of the lid. The patient is instructed to close the eye (both eyes are measured at once); the strip is removed at 5 minutes and the length of wetting of the strip from the notch is measured. Values less than 5 mm of wetting are considered suggestive of aqueous tear deficiency (ATD). This test can be performed after instillation of a topical anesthetic (which abolishes sensory input from the conjunctiva and cornea but not the lids and lashes). Most practitioners, however, consider a Schirmer test performed without anesthetic to be more predictive. The degree of stimulation with insertion of the strips and ambient test conditions can lead to variation in results but serially consistent values below 5 mm of wetting at 5 minutes are highly suggestive of ATD. A variant of this test is the phenol red thread test that uses a thread impregnated with phenol red (which undergoes a color change on contact with tears). Insertion of the thread is thought to cause less reflex tearing. Either of these tests should be part of a contact lens screening evaluation. One should also realize that ocular allergy does not preclude the concomitant development of tear film abnormalities because many patients have intrinsic defects noted in metalloproteinases or because of use of oral antihistamines with their antimuscarinic binding [23].

Ocular surface staining is a commonly used test to measure damage to the ocular surface that is a hallmark of dry eye. There are three stains in use: (1) sodium fluorescein (1%); (2) rose Bengal (1%); and (3) lissamine green B. Fluorescein stains breaks in the corneal epithelium and is best seen using the cobalt blue filter. Rose Bengal stains epithelial cells that are unprotected by an intact mucin layer. Lissamine green B is thought to have staining patterns similar to rose Bengal but causes less irritation and takes slightly longer to become apparent, about 2 to 3 minutes after instillation. Rose Bengal and lissamine green B are more easily visualized on the conjunctival surface with a scleral background [24]. Although the presence of staining is an important sign of dry eye, it is a relatively late sign.

Examination of the lid margins is an important part of an evaluation for dry eye. As noted earlier, evaporative tear deficiency resulting from meibomian gland dysfunction is an extremely common condition and recognition can be subtle. Suggestive signs include increased vascularity of the lid margin and pouting or closure of the meibomian gland openings. Some of these changes are seen with aging and are not pathognomonic. Expression of meibom from the glands is a more reliable sign. With the fingernail pressed onto the lid about 1 mm from the glands openings, it is possible to express lipid from several glands above the fingernail. Normal secretion is clear; in meibomian gland dysfunction the secretion becomes cloudy or coagulated, like toothpaste. This alteration in lipid secretion is characteristic of meibomian gland dysfunction that causes excessive evaporative tear loss.

A newer measure of aqueous tear production is fluorescein tear clearance. In this test 5 μL of 1% fluorescein is instilled in the conjunctival sac. One-minute Schirmer tests are performed at 10-minute intervals. Persistent fluorescein staining of the strips indicates delayed tear turnover and, by inference, decreased aqueous tear production.

The Ocular Protection Index is a new concept based on measuring the BUT and the interblink interval (IBI) [25]. It is based on the idea that an early sign of dry eye is the breakup of the tear film before initiation of the next blink, exposing the ocular surface to drying. By measuring the IBI and BUT a ratio or index (BUT/IBI) can be created; this Ocular Protection Index is equal to or greater than 1 in normals and below 1 in dry eye patients. Although this concept is still new, it provides an easily performed test that should yield valuable information to identify dry eye patients.

Evaluation of the lids looking for abnormalities of lid structure, closure, and blink rate is essential in identifying poor candidates for contact lens wear. The tests listed are by no means exhaustive but rather provide a short list of practical measurements to identify potential contact lens problem patients.

Contact lens wear in patients with dry eye

It is possible for patients with mild to moderate dry eye successfully to wear contact lenses. To improve the chances for success it is necessary to modify the normal fitting and care process. In this regard supplementation of normal tears (and replacement of evaporative tear loss) is accomplished by the use of tear substitutes. Most artificial tear products in multiuse bottles contain preservatives to prevent contamination by microbes. These preservatives can be toxic to the ocular surface; their use in conjunction with soft contact lenses is not recommended. Preservative-free artificial tear can be used safely with soft and rigid lenses. In addition, the newer "transiently preserved" preparations are also compatible with contact lenses.

Although all contact lenses cause increased evaporative tear loss, certain types of soft lenses are thought to demonstrate less of a desiccating effect in patients with dry eye. It is recommended to fit patients with a hydrogel lens from Group I of the United States Food and Drug Administration lens categories. These lenses have less than 50% water content and are nonionic. This guideline is based on reports that higher water content lenses dehydrate more than lower water content ones.

A study investigated the use of using a hydrogel lens (Proclear) composed of omafilacon A combined with a synthetic analogue of the naturally occurring phospholipid, phosphatidylcholine. The resultant surface resembles that of the cell membrane of mammalian cells and is thought to be biomimetic. Initial studies reported that these lenses were resistant to dehydration and deposit formation [21]. A subsequent clinical trial demonstrated that the use of these lenses in patients with mild to moderate dry eyes resulted in a decrease in ocular staining, and an increase in comfort and wearing time [26]. Similar results have been reported with hioxofilocon contact lenses [27].

The silicone hydrogel lenses with low water content and high oxygen transmissibility are expected to show less dehydration than hydrogel lenses. One clinical study, however, did not demonstrate any difference in comfort and dryness between silicone hydrogel lenses and hydrogel lenses [28].

With careful management and patient compliance it is possible to achieve clinical success for contact lens wear in a motivated patient with dry eye. In patients with moderate to severe dry eye, those patients with Schirmer tests of 2 mm or less, more than mild ocular staining, or signs of clinically apparent surface inflammation, contact lens wear is contraindicated. The risk for serious, sight-threatening problems, such as infection, is too high. Contact lens–induced changes in tear flow, evaporative tear loss, the development of lens deposits that predispose to bacterial attachment, and the loss of antimicrobial ocular defense mechanisms in dry eye render the patient at risk for infection. The presence of a chronic infectious condition, such as blepharitis, is a contraindication to lens wear. Contact lens wear is contraindicated in all patients with Sjögren's syndrome (with the exception of special situations in which therapeutic contact lenses are used).

The use of therapeutic contact lenses in dry eye

Although the previous discussion has focused on identification of patients at risk for contact lens–induced dry eye and its attendant dangers, contact lenses have been used in patients with dry eye in certain clinical situations. Scleral lenses have been used for over 50 years to manage severely dry eyes. They reduce the frictional forces of the upper lid on the cornea and can act as a reservoir for instilled fluid. With the advent of newer materials with greater oxygen transmissibility, there has been renewed interest in both rigid scleral lenses and semiscleral soft lenses. The use of rigid scleral lenses is generally confined to severely desiccated eyes not amenable to other forms of therapy.

Hydrogel bandage lenses can be very useful in the management of a number of recalcitrant ocular surface disease states associated with dry eye. Because they provide a moist covering to the cornea and serve as an interface between the upper lid protecting the cornea from the frictional forces of the upper lid, they have found a place in the management of (1) filamentary keratitis; (2) mucin-deficient states, such as ocular pemphigoid, erythema multiforme, and chemical burns; (3) exposure keratitis; and (4) persistent epithelial defects [29]. Caution is urged, however, in their use. A small amount of lid movement is necessary to ensure that the lens does not become stuck to the surface. In addition, supplementation of tears is essential to maintain the moisture to facilitate healing. The use of prophylactic anti-infective medications is controversial because long-term use may encourage the emergence of resistant organisms. Because bandage lenses are frequently in place for extended periods and ocular surface defense mechanisms are compromised in dry eye, the presence of a contact lens (even a high D/k, highly oxygen-permeable) represents an increased risk for infection. The presence of chronic blepharitis (untreated) is a contraindication. Close monitoring of the patient after insertion and careful counseling to be alert for early signs of infection are essential to minimize the risks inherent in this form of therapy. Bandage lenses used with care represent an important adjunct in the management of difficult ocular surface disease problems.

Contact lenses of contemporary design and composition can be used in patients with mild to moderate dry eye with careful attention to identification of patients at higher risk for developing problems and appropriate modification of tear supplementation and wearing schedule. In certain difficult ocular surface disease states the use of contact lenses can be an important tool in successfully treating these conditions, but careful monitoring and patient counseling is essential to minimize the risk for infection.

The use of contact lenses in a patient with ocular allergy

Up to 40% of the population suffers from allergic rhinitis and 80% to 90% of these patients also have some form of ocular allergy [30]. It is common for patients with ocular allergy to present for contact lens evaluation to correct ametropia. In addition, in certain conditions associated with allergy (eg, keratoconus and vernal conjunctivitis), contact lenses form an important therapeutic modality. It is important to recognize that certain features of ocular allergy alter the ocular response to contact lenses and care must be exercised to avoid complications. Ocular allergy can take different forms, including nonspecific allergic conjunctivitis, seasonal and perennial conjunctivitis, atopic conjunctivitis, vernal conjunctivitis, drug-induced allergic conjunctivitis, and contact lens–associated giant papillary conjunctivitis. This last condition develops in some contact lens wearers and an allergic response has been implicated in its pathogenesis.

Contact lenses and allergic reactions

In patients with various forms of allergic rhinoconjunctivitis, contact lenses play a dual role in instigating a progressive ocular condition, such as giant papillary conjunctivitis, or can be used in a treatment paradigm. The contact lens can act as a barrier or as an antigen depot, extending their exposure to the ocular surface. It is important to realize that the contact lens materials are in themselves inert plastics not capable of eliciting and allergic response. It has been demonstrated, however, that contact lenses are, within minutes of insertion, coated with a biofilm consisting of proteins and possibly lipid components [31]. This biofilm is an important adaptive phenomenon promoting comfort. The biofilm acts as a base for subsequent deposit formation consisting of denatured proteins, mucins, calcium, and lipids. A lens coated attracts bacteria that can contribute to increased surface inflammation. Antigens can bind directly to the coated surface.

Managing contact lens wear in the patient with ocular allergy

There are three key elements in successful contact lens wear in the presence of ocular allergy. First, in patients with seasonal allergies, avoid lens wear during these times of allergic response. As earlier studies of soft contact lenses tolerance in atopic versus nonatopic during the course of a year have shown, 58% of atopics had experienced symptoms compared with 33% of nonatopics ($P = .034$). Detection of eosinophils and neutrophils in the conjunctival scrapings at the first examination seemed to predict poor contact lens tolerance. History of an atopic condition increased fivefold the risk of experiencing various external eye symptoms during the prolonged use of contact lenses [32]. Similarly, in another study investigating whether underlying rhinoconjunctivitis contributed to contact lens intolerance, 76% of those with allergy exhibited intolerance compared with 60% of those with no allergy. Furthermore, the frequency of seasonal exacerbation of eye symptoms when using contact lenses was significantly higher in subjects with allergy compared with those without allergy (spring, 49% versus 19%, $P < .0001$; summer, 35% versus 20%, $P < .001$; fall, 27% versus 12%, $P < .0001$). The chronic use of continuous-wear contact lenses in patients with allergic rhino-conjunctivitis seems to contribute to contact lenses intolerance [33]. Interestingly, comfort noted between the newer soft silicone and increased gas permeability reflected a higher satisfaction of comfort (56%) than rigid gas permeable lens (14%), whereas 63% of nonatopic and only 47% of atopic subjects described their lenses as very comfortable to wear [34].

Second, make sure that patients use a regular effective lens cleaning regimen. The use of enzymatic cleansers to remove deposits and limit further deposit formation is important in reducing allergy-enhancing events. An alternative strategy is the use of daily disposable lenses to achieve the same result. In a study evaluating the impact of daily disposable lenses versus patient's standard chronic wear lenses, 67% reported that the 1-day disposable lenses provided improved comfort compared with the lenses they wore before the study, compared with 18% agreeing that the new pair of habitual lenses provided improved comfort, suggesting that the use of 1-day disposable lenses may be an effective strategy for managing allergy-suffering contact lens wearers [35]. Certain lens materials have fewer tendencies to accumulate deposits, although the evidence for this is less than convincing. Because avoidance of significant lens deposits is a critical feature, the use of extended-wear lenses is contraindicated.

Third, the use of topical antiallergic medications while lenses are in place is not recommended. Although it is possible to use these agents after lens removal but if the condition is symptomatic enough to require pharmacologic treatment, a better course is to discontinue lens wear until the allergic condition is under control with topical agents. There are ongoing clinical investigations comparing two allergy drops for enhancing comfort and performance of contact lens wear (epinastine and olopatadine) (http://clinicaltrials.gov/show/NCT00489398, accessed October 21, 2007). In addition, there are actual studies to evaluate the efficacy and safety of an antiallergy drug, antihistamine, and mast stabilizing agent (ketotifen) with a contact lens compared with placebo in preventing ocular itching associated with allergic conjunctivitis. The primary outcome is ocular itching; conjunctival, ciliary, and episcleral redness; chemosis and mucus discharge; tearing; and lid swelling (http://clinicaltrials.gov/show/NCT00445874, accessed September 26, 2007). It is important to note that the use of topical vasoconstrictors has been associated with hypoxia of the ocular surface epithelium.

Summary of contact lens use in patient with ocular allergy

Contact lenses should be used with caution in patients with ocular allergy. In patients with seasonal allergy, avoid contact lens use during seasonal flare-ups. Patients with allergy need to have clean lenses with minimal deposit buildup; to this end, patients should use daily wear lenses with rigid disinfecting and cleaning techniques. Alternatively, they should use daily disposable lenses [36]. When such individuals wear contact lenses, a special set of circumstances arises that increases the risk of ocular infection. The risk is greatest if the lenses are soft and provide for little tear exchange beneath their surface. Under such circumstances, limited tear flow allows for a greater buildup of lens deposits and metabolic wastes, while permitting increased tear evaporation from the lens surface [37–39].

Avoid the use of topical antiallergy agents while lenses are in place, in particular vasoconstrictor agents, until studies demonstrate that concomitant use with specific agents is not deleterious. Extended-wear contact lenses are contraindicated in patients with ocular allergy. In general, the use of contact lenses is contraindicated in patients with vernal conjunctivitis.

With careful attention to recognizing the patient with ocular allergy, regular monitoring, and patient compliance to lens care, successful contact lens wear can be achieved in most patients with ocular allergy [36].

References

[1] Holly FJ, Lemp MA. Tear physiology and dry eye. Surv Ophthalmol 1977;22:69–87.
[2] Stern ME, Beuerman RW, Fox RI, et al. The pathology of dry eye: the interaction between the ocular surface and lacrimal glands. Cornea 1998;17(6):584–9.
[3] Gipson IK, Hori Y, Argueso P. Character of ocular surface mucins and their alteration in dry eye disease. Ocul Surf 2004;2(2):131–48.
[4] Bron AJ, Tiffany JM. The contribution of meibomian gland dysfunction to dry eye. Ocul Surf 2004;2(2):149–64.
[5] Research in dry eye: report of the Research Subcommittee of the International Dry Eye WorkShop (2007). Ocul Surf 2007;5(2):179–93.
[6] Management and therapy of dry eye disease: report of the Management and Therapy Subcommittee of the International Dry Eye WorkShop (2007). Ocul Surf 2007;5(2):163–78.
[7] Design and conduct of clinical trials: report of the Clinical Trials Subcommittee of the International Dry Eye WorkShop (2007). Ocul Surf 2007;5(2):153–62.
[8] Methodologies to diagnose and monitor dry eye disease: report of the Diagnostic Methodology Subcommittee of the International Dry Eye WorkShop (2007). Ocul Surf 2007;5(2):108–52.
[9] The epidemiology of dry eye disease: report of the Epidemiology Subcommittee of the International Dry Eye WorkShop (2007). Ocul Surf 2007;5(2):93–107.
[10] The definition and classification of dry eye disease: report of the Definition and Classification Subcommittee of the International Dry Eye WorkShop (2007). Ocul Surf 2007;5(2):75–92.
[11] Sullivan DA, Sullivan BD, Ullman MD, et al. Androgen influence on the meibomian gland. Invest Ophthalmol Vis Sci 2004;41:3732–42.
[12] Jacobsson LT, Axell TE, Hansen, et al. Dry eyes or mouth: an epidemiological study in Swedish adults, with special reference to primary Sjögren's syndrome. J Autoimmun 1989;2(4):521–7.
[13] Schein OD, Munoz B, Tielsch JM, et al. Prevalence of dry eye among the elderly. Am J Ophthalmol 1997;124(6):723–8.
[14] Schein OD, Munoz B, Tielsch JM. Estimating the prevalence of dry eye among elderly Americans: SEE Project. Invest Ophthalmol Vis Sci 1996;37:S636.
[15] Hamano H, Kaufman HE. The physiology of the cornea and contact lens applications. New York: Churchill Livingstone; 1987.
[16] Hamano H. The change of precorneal tear film by the application of contact lenses. Contact Intraocul Lens Med J 1981;7(3):205–9.
[17] Holden BA, Sweeney DF, Seger RG. Epithelial erosions caused by thin high water content lenses. Clin Exp Optom 1986;69:103–7.

[18] Guillon JP. Tear film structure on contact lenses. In: Holly FJ, editor. The preocular tear film in health, disease, and contact lens wear. Lubbock (TX): Dry Eye Institute; 1986. p. 914–39.
[19] Solomon J. Causes and treatments of peripheral corneal desiccation. Contact Lens Forum 1986;11(6):30–6.
[20] Tomlinson A. Tear film changes with contact lens wear. In: Tomlinson A, editor. Complications of contact lens wear. St. Louis (MO): Mosby; 1992. p. 157–94.
[21] Hall B, Jones S, Young G, et al. The on-eye dehydration of Proclear compatibles lenses. CLAO J 1999;25(4):233–7.
[22] Abelson MB, Ousler GW, Nally L. Alternative reference values for tear film break up time in normal and dry eye populations. Adv Exp Med Biol 2002;506(Pt B):1121–5.
[23] Bielory L. Ocular allergy and dry eye syndrome. Curr Opin Allergy Clin Immunol 2004;4(5): 421–4.
[24] Nichols KK, Mitchell GL, Zadnik K. The repeatability of clinical measurements of dry eye. Cornea 2004;23(3):272–85.
[25] Ousler GW, Emory TB, Welch D, et al. Factors that influence the Inter-Blink Interval (IBI) as measured by the Ocular Protection Index (OPI). Invest Ophthalmol Vis Sci 2002;43(12): 56.
[26] Lemp MA, Caffery B, Lebow K, et al. Omafilcon A (Proclear) soft contact lenses in a dry eye population. CLAO J 1999;25(1):40–7.
[27] Riley C, Chalmers RL, Pence N. The impact of lens choice in the relief of contact lens related symptoms and ocular surface findings. Cont Lens Anterior Eye 2005;28(1):13–9.
[28] Fonn D, Dumbleton K. Dryness and discomfort with silicone hydrogel contact lenses. Eye Contact Lens 2003;29(Suppl 1):S101–4 [discussion: S115–8, S192–4].
[29] Lemp MA. Contact lenses and the dry-eye patient. Int Ophthalmol Clin 1986;26(1):63–71.
[30] Skoner DP. Allergic rhinitis: definition, epidemiology, pathophysiology, detection, and diagnosis. J Allergy Clin Immunol 2001;108(Suppl 1):S2–8.
[31] Fowler SA, Allansmith MR. Evolution of soft contact lens coatings. Arch Ophthalmol 1980; 98:95–9.
[32] Kari O, Haahtela T. Is atopy a risk factor for the use of contact lenses? Allergy 1992; 47(4 Pt 1):295–8.
[33] Kumar P, Elston R, Black D, et al. Allergic rhinoconjunctivitis and contact lens intolerance. CLAO J 1991;17(1):31–4.
[34] Kari O, Teir H, Huuskonen R, et al. Tolerance to different kinds of contact lenses in young atopic and non-atopic wearers. CLAO J 2001;27(3):151–4.
[35] Hayes VY, Schnider CM, Veys J. An evaluation of 1-day disposable contact lens wear in a population of allergy sufferers. Cont Lens Anterior Eye 2003;26(2):85–93.
[36] Lemp MA. Contact lenses and associated anterior segment disorders: dry eye, blepharitis, and allergy. Ophthalmol Clin North Am 2003;16(3):463–9.
[37] Lemp MA. Is the dry eye contact lens wearer at risk? Yes. Cornea 1990;9(Suppl 1):S48–50 [discussion: S54].
[38] Stapleton F, Stretton S, Papas E, et al. Silicone hydrogel contact lenses and the ocular surface. Ocul Surf 2006;4(1):24–43.
[39] Porazinski AD, Donshik PC. Giant papillary conjunctivitis in frequent replacement contact lens wearers: a retrospective study. CLAO J 1999;25(3):142–7.

ELSEVIER
SAUNDERS

Immunol Allergy Clin N Am
28 (2008) 119–136

IMMUNOLOGY
AND ALLERGY
CLINICS
OF NORTH AMERICA

Ocular Manifestations of Blistering Diseases

Samih Elchahal, MD[a], Eric R. Kavosh, MD[b],
David S. Chu, MD[a],*

[a]Institute of Ophthalmology and Visual Science, UMDNJ–New Jersey Medical School,
Doctors Office Center, 90 Bergen Street, Suite 1600, Newark, NJ 07103, USA
[b]Department of Medicine, UMDNJ–New Jersey Medical School, University Hospital,
150 Bergen Street, UH-1248, Newark, NJ 07103, USA

Autoimmune blistering diseases with ocular-surface manifestations belong to a group of systemic entities characterized by autoantibodies against the epithelial basement membrane zone (BMZ) of conjunctiva. The specific tissue components targeted by these autoantibodies and the characteristic patterns of mucocutaneous involvement differentiate these diseases. The autoimmune activity in mucous membrane pemphigoid (MMP), linear immunoglobulin A disease (LAD), and epidermolysis bullosa acquisita (EBA) occurs at a subepithelial location, whereas ocular pemphigus vulgaris (OPV) exhibits intraepithelial activity.

Mucous membrane pemphigoid

Clinical features

MMP is an idiopathic systemic disorder that manifests on the eyes primarily through scarring of the conjunctiva in a progressive, chronic nature. This condition, characterized by antibody tissue–specific antigen-mediated (type-2 hypersensitivity) reaction, is rare, with estimates in the ophthalmic population ranging from 1 in 8000 to 1 in 46,000 [1,2]. Typical presentation involves a patient in the fifth or sixth decade of life who has bilateral ocular and mucocutaneous lesions, although the disease can present at other times.

* Corresponding author.
  E-mail address: chuda@umdnj.edu (D.S. Chu).

No racial or geographic predispositions have been found; however, women are estimated as being 1.5 to 5 times more frequently affected than men [3]. Several human leukocyte antigens (HLAs) including HLA-DR2, HLA-DR4, and HLA-DQw7 (DQB1*0301) have been associated with creating increased susceptibility to the disease [4–6].

The diagnosis of MMP should be considered in patients who present with blistering, erosive, scarring conjunctivitis, with or without other associated mucocutaneous involvement. Although these lesions may be found on initial examination, the disease typically presents insidiously, with nonspecific complaints of bilateral red eyes, itching, burning, foreign-body sensation, or tearing—all of which are common symptoms and findings of chronic conjunctivitis. The disease is usually bilateral; however, asymmetrical presentation is not uncommon. Slit-lamp examination may reveal papillary conjunctivitis associated with diffuse conjunctival hyperemia, followed by formation of subconjunctival bullae, which may rupture, leading to ulceration and pseudomembrane formation [1,2]. Fibrosis and retraction of subepithelial tissue leads to fornix foreshortening and flattening of the plica semilunaris (medial fold of redundant conjunctival that allows for unrestricted eye movement) and caruncle. Patients who have advanced disease exhibit symblepharon (conjunctival adhesions) formation—a sign typically seen inferiorly first—or ankyloblepharon (lid adhesions) involving the lateral canthi [7]. Entropion (eyelid inversion), lagophthalmos (incomplete eyelid closure), and lash metaplasia including distichiasis (eyelash growth arising from meibomian glands) and trichiasis (misdirected eyelash growth, usually toward the globe) may follow (Figs. 1 and 2) [1]. Patients commonly complain of dry eye symptoms, the etiology of which involves all three components of the tear film (mucin, aqueous, and lipid) because scarring destroys conjunctival goblet cells and obstructs lacrimal gland ductules and meibomian gland orifices. Eyelid involvement thus contributes to tear film dysfunction to create the keratopathy observed in MMP. In addition,

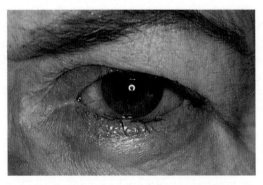

Fig. 1. A 70-year-old white woman who has MMP exhibits madarosis, entropion, and ocular surface inflammation.

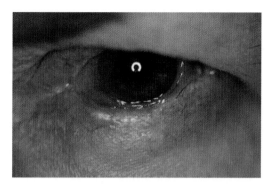

Fig. 2. One-year later, the patient in Fig. 1 exhibits active disease with progression of ocular surface disease.

depletion of limbal stem cells (perilimbal basal epithelial cells that replete the corneal epithelial cell layers through continuous proliferation) plays a recognized role in the development of vision-threatening keratopathy, presenting initially as small epithelial defects and ultimately as large corneal ulcerations with resultant total corneal surface keratinization and vascularization [8,9]. If bilateral, the associated corneal opacification may lead to blindness.

The differential diagnosis of MMP includes other autoimmune bullous diseases, including LAD, EBA, and OPV, chronic atopic keratoconjunctivitis, rosacea, scleroderma, paraneoplastic pemphigus, and scarring secondary to ocular trauma or irradiation. It is important that the clinician also consider drug-induced MMP, which occurs as a side effect of certain topically administered medications including several antiglaucoma medications such as pilocarpine hydrochloride, timolol maleate (Timoptic), epinephrine, echothiophate iodide, and medication preservatives such as benzalkonium chloride [10–12]. Drug-induced MMP can present similarly but has several differentiating characteristics including the lack of cutaneous lesions in the topical drug-induced form, and disease that does not progress after the causal medication has been discontinued [13].

Diagnostic studies

Histologic examination of the conjunctiva in MMP shows epithelial metaplasia as conjunctival squamous keratinization, parakeratosis, and scarcity of goblet cells. Subepithelial blister formation is constituted by a mixed dermal infiltrate of neutrophils, monocytes, macrophages, lymphocytes, and eosinophils [14,15]. Acute disease exacerbation is marked by neutrophilic and eosinophilic stromal infiltration, excessive mucous presence in the inferior fornix, and increased fibroblast and mast cell activity and proliferation [16,17]. Disruption of the BMZ includes redundancy and variation of basal laminar thickness, increased desmosome concentration, and disorganized collagen fibrils. The ensuing cicatrization yields an end result of conjunctival fibrosis [16,17].

Diagnosis of an autoimmune bullous disease is confirmed through immunofluorescent and immunoperoxidase laboratory techniques on conjunctival tissue biopsy samples. Perilesional skin biopsies are also diagnostically helpful because direct immunofluorescence testing exhibits characteristic linear immunoglobulin and complement (C3) deposition along conjunctival, buccal, or cutaneous tissue basement membranes in most cases [18–20]. A higher frequency of association is found in mucosal lesions compared with cutaneous lesions and with the immunoglobulin (Ig)G class of immunoglobulins over IgA and IgM, although sole IgA presence has also been documented [21,22]. Purely ocular MMP exhibits immune deposition in the upper lamina lucida, whereas mucocutaneous involvement is characterized by deposition in the lower lamina lucida and lamina densa [23–26]. Circulating autoantibodies used in indirect immunoelectron microscopy demonstrate regularly clustered lower lamina lucida and lamina densa immunostaining [27]. In addition, the sensitivity of detecting immune deposits increases from between 50% and 52% with immunofluorescence alone to 83% when labeled immunoperoxidase is used [21]. Various autoantibody targets have been described, including the beta 4 integrin subunit and laminin-5, suggesting that the clinical diagnosis of MMP encompasses various pathophysiologic disease entities [28–32]. Support for the antigenic role played by the beta 4 integrin subunit as a feature of MMP has been shown, with demonstrated presence of autoantibodies whose circulating levels may correspond to clinical disease improvement with intravenous immunoglobulin (IVIG) treatment [33,34].

Disease course and treatment

The course of MMP is variable among patients. Some experience limited disease and mild ocular scarring that remits following treatment, others follow an intermittent course, and approximately one third of patients experience chronic, progressive disease with only partial response to treatment, necessitating lifelong follow-up [35–37]. A multimodal approach to treatment is preferred to optimize patient response and minimize permanent disease sequelae.

Topical corticosteroids such as triamcinolone acetonide, fluocinonide, or clobetasol propionate may be used for limited acute and early-stage cases that present with ocular or oral lesions, although topical treatment alone is not adequately effective in stopping MMP progression [38]. Posterior lid margin conjunctival keratinization may respond to topical retinoid treatment [32]. When progressive conjunctival cicatrization is present, subconjunctival mitomycin C or steroid injection may be efficacious as a temporizing measure to slow disease progression [39].

In most cases, systemic treatment is required for acute exacerbations and chronic disease. In mild or moderate cases of MMP, first-line systemic treatment involves long-term use of immunoregulatory chemotherapy such as dapsone, unless the patient has a history of glucose-6-phosphate dehydrogenase deficiency or drug intolerance [35,36]. In contraindicated cases or in those who do not have adequate response to dapsone, cytotoxic agents such as mycophenolate mofetil (Cellcept), sulfasalazine, methotrexate, or azathioprine (Imuran) are used for suppression of conjunctival inflammatory activity and prevention of progressive cicatrization [35,36,40–43]. Persistent inflammation should prompt transition to treatment with cyclophosphamide (Cytoxan) [35,36]. In severe or extensive cases, cyclophosphamide treatment may be used along with a rapid systemic prednisone taper [35,36]. Monotherapy with systemic steroids should be avoided because they are not as effective as other immunosuppressive therapies and are associated with significant systemic toxicity when used at required doses [35,36]. In addition, disease relapse with tapering of steroid treatment supports their use as adjunct rather than sole treatment agents in patients refractory to immunosuppressive drug therapy. Immunosuppressive treatment should be continued for at least 1 year beyond the resolution of the episode of active inflammation, and patients should be routinely monitored for known side effects while on systemic immunosuppressive medications [35,36]. Additional immunosuppressive agents with exhibited efficacy include infliximab, daclizumab, and rituxamab [44,45]. Although IVIG therapy can be used in refractory cases or treatment-intolerant patients, it is also playing an increasing role as a primary systemic treatment of MMP. Increasing evidence shows that IVIG therapy can result in a decrease in circulating autoantibody against B4 through the treatment course [37,44–50]. IVIG is usually administered in dosages of approximately 2 to 3 g/kg per cycle, with each cycle lasting 3 to 5 consecutive days each month. Clinical improvement and disease remission has been shown to continue with increased time between cycles and a gradual tapering of IVIG [33]. On average, patients who had successful halting of disease progression had received an average of 32 cycles over 35 months [51]. The efficacy of IVIG at halting disease progression in patients unresponsive to traditional immunosuppressive treatments and its ability to avoid the limiting side effects of other agents have encouraged its use as a primary treatment for refractory disease.

To minimize disease reactivation or progression, surgical techniques should be preempted by medical control of inflammation and supplanted with perioperative systemic corticosteroids in patients because reconstructive surgery will be successful only with proper control of disease activity [1,52]. Nonpharmacologic options include therapeutic interventions to protect and maintain the ocular surface and address any eyelid or conjunctival cicatrization present [1,2,52,53]. In cases of advanced corneal keratinization or ulceration, one may perform amniotic membrane grafting, penetrating keratoplasty (PKP), or limbal stem cell transplantation (LSCT) to restore ocular surface integrity and to regain useful vision to a functionally blind eye, although surrounding host tissue disease can limit long-term success of these techniques [54,55]. As limbal stem cell deficiency is thought to be present in blistering diseases, LSCT is playing an increasing role in treatment as techniques are advanced [8,9,54–59]. When LSCT and PKP are unsuccessful, keratoprostheses offer another option for rehabilitation of vision [1,2,50,52–59].

Linear immunoglobulin A disease

Clinical features

LAD patients commonly complain of ocular symptoms including eye pain, dry eyes, foreign-body sensation, burning, or ocular discharge. Even in the absence of ocular complaints, slit-lamp examination may reveal fine conjunctival scarring, subconjunctival fibrosis, and subsequent inner canthal architecture loss, inferior forniceal foreshortening, trichiasis, entropion, and symblepharon formation with secondary corneal opacification. The ocular changes may be clinically indistinguishable from those of MMP. Because ocular involvement is common (~50% of LAD patients) and may be asymptomatic, all LAD patients should undergo ophthalmologic examination [60].

LAD is a rare disease characterized by circulating autoimmune antibodies to the epithelial BMZ, with the prevalence estimated to be 0.6 cases per 100,000 adults in Utah [61]. Internationally, estimates include incidences of 1 case per 250,000 individuals per year in southern England, and 0.13 cases per 250,000 individuals in France [62]. Association with HLA-B8 has been noted, and LAD patients present in a bimodal age distribution, with pediatric disease presenting at a mean age of 3.3 to 4.5 years and adult cases at a mean age of 52 years [63–66]. Male and female patients are equally affected and typically present with a lengthened prodrome of a pruritus or cutaneous burning sensation before emergence of lesions classically characterized as annular tense bullae, resembling a "string of pearls" or "cluster of jewels" surrounding a patch of erythematous skin [61]. Lesions typically involve the perioral region, perineum, and extremities. In addition, mucous membrane involvement is seen in adults, with oral, genital, and conjunctival lesions that can result in scarring. These lesions may appear gradually or, in drug-associated cases, more acutely [61,63,64].

Associations between LAD and various suspected etiologies include drug-induced (most commonly vancomycin hydrochloride) cases, which are more common in adults due to treatment with multiple medical therapies for comorbid conditions [67–69]. Other suspected drugs associated with one or several cases of LAD include captopril, amiodarone, and phenytoin [70–73]. Thus, the clinician should examine the presenting patient's medication regimen for possible iatrogenic causes. Other associations have been considered, including preceding illness, malignancy, and coexistence with other autoimmune disorders [61,64,69].

Diagnostic studies

Histopathologic examination of cutaneous blisters in LAD reveals characteristic findings including neutrophil alignment along the BMZ and subepidermal cleavage with inflammatory cells in the upper dermis. In some cases, neutrophilic microabscesses may form within the papillary ridges. Mature lesions reveal subepidermal blistering with a predominantly neutrophilic infiltrate, although eosinophils and monocytes may be present. In patients who have atypical presentations, additional testing including bacterial culture and Gram stain of blister fluid to rule out bullous impetigo and Tzanck smear to rule out herpesvirus infection may be diagnostically informative [60,61,64,66].

As in MMP, biopsy and immunofluorescent study are the predominant modalities used to confirm the diagnosis of LAD. Direct immunofluorescent assay of involved and spared areas of skin shows corresponding linear IgA (and less frequently IgG or IgM) and complement C3 deposition along the basement membrane [60,74]. Similar deposition is observed with analysis of conjunctival and oral mucosa in affected patients [60,74]. Addition of indirect immunofluorescence or direct immunoelectron microscopy techniques increases sensitivity, with the former identifying circulating anti-BMZ autoantibodies in approximately one half of LAD patients [60,74]. Circulating autoantibody titers are characteristically higher in children than in adults but are generally a low-frequency finding in both age groups. The use of immunoperoxidase in indirect and direct immunoelectron microscopy localizes immunoglobulin deposition to the lamina lucida and to the target antigen LAD-1, secreted by keratinocytes as a component of the anchoring filament [60,66,74]. Immunoblotting and immunoelectron microscopy studies show reactivity between LAD sera and several different antigenic targets [75,76]. Prediction of a particular patient's disease course or clinical response to treatment should take this intradisease variability into account because patients are less treatment responsive in cases in which type VII collagen is the molecular target antigen [64]. Because these diseases may present with indistinguishable clinical pictures, this would explain the variation in the clinical picture and therapeutic responses seen with LAD [75,76].

Disease course and treatment

LAD typically follows an exacerbating and remitting disease course, with the possibility of progression to blindness. Overall, remission occurs in 64% of children, usually within 2 years from symptomatic onset [61,66]. Adult patients experience less frequent (48%) remission and a more prolonged disease course lasting an average of 5 to 6 years [61–66]. Drug-induced cases typically resolve quickly with identification and withdrawal of the offending agent [67–73]. Although ocular and oral lesions may leave persistent scarring as in the case with MMP, cutaneous lesions usually heal without scarring. Involvement of the other gastrointestinal and genitourinary mucous membranes may coexist [60].

Localized treatment addresses the mucosal and cutaneous lesions, although bullae do not usually require specific care beyond hygienic dressings, with topical antibacterial agents such as mupirocin used for infected lesions. The use of dapsone or sulfapyridine is successful in most cases, and noticeable response to treatment may be seen within several days [61–64,77]. Treated disease lasting longer than a few weeks may benefit from adjunct therapy including prednisone, dicloxacillin, sulfamethoxypyridazine, and colchicine [77,78]. As in MMP, treatment of refractory cases with IVIG has shown efficacy [79–81]. Treatment of drug-induced LAD should begin with removal of the presumed causative agent. In cases of LAD induced by vancomycin, new lesions stop forming within approximately 2 weeks of cessation [67,68,82]. In persistent cases of drug-induced LAD, a short oral steroid course may be beneficial [60,61].

Epidermolysis bullosa acquisita

Clinical features

EBA is an autoimmune blistering disease of the skin and mucous membranes that is mediated by IgG autoantibodies against type VII collagen [83]. A small subset of EBA, however, is known to be due to IgA rather than to IgG [84]. Type VII collagen is a major component of the anchoring fibrils in the lamina densa of the epithelial basement membrane. There are three different phenotypes of this disease: mechanobullous, inflammatory, and cicatricial pemphigoid. The disease is rare, with an estimated annual incidence of 0.25 per 1 million in Western Europe [85]. The male-to-female ratio is 1:1.4, and it has been noted that patients of Korean descent have a higher predilection for EBA [86]. HLA-DR2 depicts hyperimmunity that is seen in EBA and in bullous forms of pemphigoid, pointing to an autoimmune etiology for these entities. Immunogenetic studies on EBA reveal that most black patients from the southeastern part of the United States have an association with HLA-DR2. Subsequent studies on a larger population of white patients failed to reveal any statistically significant HLA allele associations with EBA [87].

EBA typically presents in the third to fifth decade, with patients exhibiting various aspects of chronic conjunctivitis, symblepharon formation, keratitis, subepithelial corneal vesiculation, perforation, and possibly opacification. EBA presents with scarring blisters and milia at sites of trauma, such as elbows, knees, and buttocks and the dorsa of the hands and feet. The scarring nature of EBA can lead to nail destruction and hair loss [85,88]. EBA is most commonly non- or mildly inflammatory, manifested as tense vesicles and bullae. The blisters may be hemorrhagic and rupture easily, with subsequent erosion [89]. Other subsets of patients may also have mucosal involvement that can mimic MMP or can present with inflammatory blisters that mimic bullous pemphigoid. The blisters of patients who have the classic mechanobullous noninflammatory EBA resemble those in adult or child dystrophic epidermolysis bullosa because both disease processes involve type VII collagen [90]. These lesions can also mimic bullous lupus erythematosus and porphyria cutanea tarda in the elderly, whereas the inflammatory form of EBA can resemble bullous pemphigoid because these blisters are tense and widespread [91].

Despite frequent mucous membrane involvement in EBA, this is usually limited to oral mucosa, and is then termed the cicatricial pemphigoid form of EBA [89]. EBA can also involve the nasal, pharyngeal, ocular, and esophageal mucosa or, in children, the oral mucosa, genitals, and ocular mucosa, causing symblepharon formation. In very severe cases (most notably cases mediated by IgA), total blindness has been reported [92,93].

Diagnostic studies

Various tests are used to diagnose EBA, including direct and indirect immunofluorescence, fluorescent overlay antigen mapping, immunoelectron microscopy, Western immunoblotting, and enzyme-linked immunosorbent assay (ELISA) [94]. Laboratory tests including urine porphyrin levels and antinuclear antibody are used to exclude porphyria cutanea tarda and to search for evidence of bullous systemic lupus erythematosus, which is also characterized by antibodies directed against type VII collagen. To diagnose EBA, histopathology from the edge of a new blister, direct immunofluorescence on normal-appearing perilesional skin, and indirect immunofluorescence with the patient's serum on salt-split normal human skin substrate should be obtained [79]. The histopathology of EBA shows subepidermal blisters, with the epidermis remaining intact. In addition, there is a dermal infiltrate composed of monocytes and neutrophils, which is minimal in the classic form of EBA and more abundant in the inflammatory form [92]. Direct immunofluorescence reveals the immune-mediated disease process, with a thick band of IgG and, to a lesser extent, C3 deposited linearly at the BMZ [91]. Other immunoreactants such as IgM or IgA may also be seen. Indirect immunofluorescence demonstrates the presence of IgG antibodies directed toward type VII collagen and is used to differentiate EBA from bullous pemphigoid [95]. The IgG autoantibodies in patients who have bullous pemphigoid bind to the epidermal roof of salt-split skin, whereas the dermal floor pattern of indirect immunofluorescence on salt-split skin substrate is also found in sera of patients who have bullous systemic lupus erythematosus and antiepiligrin cicatricial pemphigoid [94]. In immunoblotting, circulating autoantibodies bind a dermal protein of 290 kDa identified as type VII collagen, whereas detection of anti-type VII collagen antibodies by ELISA uses fusion proteins corresponding to different portions of the noncollagenous domain of type VII collagen [96].

Although the precise role of autoantibodies against type VII collagen is unknown, it has been hypothesized that they disrupt the assembly of type VII collagen into anchoring fibrils and interfere with their interactions with other extracellular matrix molecules [97]. Lesional skin histology initially reveals edema within the papilla in addition to edema and vacuolar alteration along the dermal-epidermal junction. A subepidermal blister forms as the disease progresses. Neutrophilic inflammation along with eosinophils and monocytes within the dermis can be seen histologically, revealing little inflammatory infiltrate, unlike bullous pemphigoid [98]. The infiltrate can be found perivascularly, around follicles, and in the interstitium and can lead to fibrosis in older lesions. Autoantibodies to type VII collagen have also been found to activate complement in both in vivo and in vitro studies. The complement components C3, C5b, and the membrane attack complex have been found in patients who have EBA. Passive transfer of IgG into mice from a patient who had EBA was shown to induce dermal edema and a granulocytic infiltrate in the superficial dermis, with immune deposits at the BMZ localized by direct immunofluorescence and by direct immunoelectron microscopy to anchoring fibrils; however, no clinical disease was observed [99].

Disease course and treatment

EBA has a protracted course and is usually resistant to treatment. EBA persists for several years in most patients, and the likelihood of remission is unpredictable. The primary therapeutic choices include immunosuppressive or anti-inflammatory agents. Systemic immunosuppressive drugs including prednisone, azathioprine, cyclophosphamide, methotrexate, and cyclosporine are used in various dosages. A group of anti-inflammatory drugs including dapsone, sulfapyridine, and colchicine appear to be effective and may decrease inflammation because of their antineutrophil effect [100,101]. Children who have EBA respond better with dapsone and prednisone, whereas patients who have bullous systemic lupus erythematosus usually respond rapidly and completely to dapsone [102]. Photochemotherapy was reported to be effective in one study but resulted in only partial improvement in two of three patients in another study [103]. IVIG has also recently been reported to be effective as a sole therapeutic agent and when used in combination with other immunomodulatory agents such as rituxamab [93,97]. The basis for treatment with rituximab is to deplete pre-, immature, and mature B lymphocytes; cases of dramatically improved symptoms within a few weeks and a decrease in steroid requirements have been noted [97]. Of note, the patients who respond best to rituximab are those who have pemphigoid-type EBA [79].

Ocular pemphigus vulgaris

Clinical features

OPV is an autoimmune blistering disease localized to the skin and mucous membranes. The hallmark of the disease is acantholysis, and patients present with flaccid blisters on an erythematous base as opposed to the bulging, tense blisters seen in bullous pemphigoid [104]. The blisters may present with Nikolsky's sign (describing the separation of the epithelium with tangential pressure on the skin surface), which offers a moderately sensitive but highly specific tool for the diagnosis of pemphigus [105,106]. The skin lesions can be found on the trunk, groin, axilla, scalp, face, and other pressure points. Oral and mucosal lesions are seen in 80% to 90% of cases and may be the initial presentation, although the disease can present with an early urticarial, nonblistering phase. Affected mucosal surfaces include the conjunctiva, esophagus, vulva, cervix, anus, and larynx [104,106]. Ocular involvement in pemphigus vulgaris is rare, is limited to the conjunctiva and eyelids, and does not typically progress to scarring. Lid margin erosions can appear in lower and upper lids, and lid margin erosions in the medial aspect of the lower eyelid may be pathognomonic of OPV [107]. OPV does not appear to affect visual acuity, and patients have a full recovery without sequelae [108]. Even more uncommonly, eyes are affected by pemphigus erythematosus, a pemphigus variant characterized by erythematous and crusted lesions in seborrheic areas of the head and trunk. This difference is due to differential expression of the OPV and pemphigus erythematosus autoantigens desmoglein 3 and 1, respectively, throughout squamous epithelia, leading to a distinct antibody profile against targeted tissues [109].

Diagnostic studies

Perilesional biopsy demonstrating IgG deposits in the intracellular space with direct and indirect immunofluorescence confirms the diagnosis of OPV [106]. The pemphigus antigens include the desmosomal cadherins desmoglein 1 and 3 and the epithelial acetylcholine receptors alpha 9 and pemphaxin [110,111]. Direct immunofluorescence demonstrates in vivo intercellular deposits of antibodies, primarily IgG, on the surface of keratinocytes in and around lesions throughout the epidermis, with IgG1 and IgG4 as the most common subclasses [112]. Other immunoreactants such as complement C3 and IgM can be deposited less frequently than IgG [113]. This pattern of intracellular deposition throughout the dermis is not specific for OPV and may be seen in pemphigus vegetans, pemphigus foliaceus, and pemphigus erythematosus. Indirect immunofluorescence demonstrates the presence of circulating IgG autoantibodies that bind to the epidermis in 80% to 90% of patients who have OPV and that correlate with disease course [110]. Laboratory use of ELISA to reveal desmoglein 1 and 3 antibodies provides objective, quantitative, and reproducible data that allow differentiation of OPV from pemphigus foliaceus. Due to these diagnostic advantages, ELISA is likely to become a routine technique in diagnostic laboratories [114].

Histopathology demonstrates an intradermal blister, with changes consisting of intercellular edema with loss of intercellular attachments in the basal layer. The blisters are formed from suprabasal epidermal cells that subsequently separate from the basal cells that remain attached to the basement membrane [115]. Tumor necrosis factor alpha (TNF-α) and inter-leukin (IL)-6 are increased in serum and in blister fluid in patients who have OPV [110]. Along with IL-6 and IL-1, TNF-α is an important proinflamma-tory cytokine that mediates the blistering processes of pemphigus by activat-ing innate and acquired immune responses.

New developments in OPV reveal that IgG autoantibodies cause desmo-glein 3 dissociation from catenin, leading to abnormal cytoplasmic distribu-tion of g-catenin. G- and b-catenin play roles in the pathogenesis of OPV through genetic modification, which is thought to induce transcription of selected target genes [114].

Disease course and treatment

Systemic corticosteroid therapy is still the mainstay of treatment for OPV; however, various adverse effects limit its use, and steroid-sparing agents such as azathioprine, cyclophosphamide, cyclosporine, mycopheno-late, and dapsone are often used to avoid these adverse effects. Glucocorti-coids and immunosuppressive agents can induce remission in most pemphigus patients; however, the associated mortality remains at 5% to 15% as a result of side effects [116–118]. Rituximab has been shown to in-duce a prolonged clinical remission after a single course of four treatments in patients who have OPV in addition to pemphigus foliaceus. The response to rituximab suggests that it may be a valuable therapeutic option for refrac-tory OPV and warrants further studies to evaluate the risk-to-benefit ratio in patients who have OPV and are refractory to standard immunosuppressive therapy [110]. Etanercept has also proved to be efficacious in OPV and al-lows for easy tapering and discontinuation of treatment with prednisolone and azathioprine [109]. In patients who do not respond to conventional im-munosuppressants, IVIG appears to be an effective treatment alternative, even as monotherapy [107]. Its early use is of significant benefit in patients who may experience life-threatening complications from immunosuppres-sion. Blisters can heal approximately 3 weeks after the onset of therapy, although cases OPV may require skin grafting and cosmetic correction after immunosuppression has been optimized [113].

Summary

Addressing the ocular manifestations of autoimmune blistering diseases including MMP, EBA, LAD, and OPV frequently requires collaborative efforts among the dermatologist, the ophthalmologist, the immunologist, and other specialists. Although there is significant clinical overlap in muco-cutaneous involvement and underlying pathophysiology among this group of diseases, certain features aid in differentiating them: (1) primarily mucous membrane involvement, with scarring in MMP and without scarring in LAD; and (2) tense cutaneous blisters in areas of trauma in EBA versus flaccid blisters and acantholysis in OPV. Further, the commonalities in clinical presentation strongly emphasize the importance of tissue biopsy for diagnostic confirmation. To guide appropriate therapy, biopsy should preferably be performed early in the disease course after a treatment-resistant chronic conjunctivitis has been identified . Treatment with monoclonal antibodies such as infliximab, daclizumab, and rituxamab and treatment with IVIG play an increasing role in these diseases, with early initiation providing cessation of disease progression. Future directions in the diagnosis and treatment of these blistering diseases include further characterization of the target antigens initiating the autoimmune process and the development and commercialization of additional ELISAs and other tests. A focus on early initiation of existing immunoregulatory agents and the development of new agents bear the most promise for avoiding the morbidities of these chronic diseases.

References

[1] Nguyen QD, Foster CS. Cicatricial pemphigoid: diagnosis and treatment. Int Ophthalmol Clin 1996;36(1):41–60.

[2] Foster CS, Neumann R, Tauber J. Long-term results of systemic chemotherapy for ocular cicatricial pemphigoid. Doc Ophthalmol 1992;82(3):223–9.

[3] Casiglia J, Woo SB, Ahmed AR. Oral involvement in autoimmune blistering diseases. Clin Dermatol 2001;19(6):737–41.

[4] Ahmed AR, Foster S, Zaltas M, et al. Association of DQw7 (DQB1*0301) with ocular cicatricial pemphigoid. Proc Natl Acad Sci U S A 1991;88:11579–82.

[5] Bhol K, Udell I, Haider N, et al. Ocular cicatricial pemphigoid: a case report of monozygotic twins discordant for the disease. Arch Ophthalmol 1995;113:202–7.

[6] Chan LS, Wang T, Wang XS, et al. High frequency of HLA-DQB1*0301 allele in patients with pure ocular cicatricial pemphigoid. Dermatology 1994;189:99–101.

[7] Mutasim DF, Pelc NJ, Anhalt GJ. Cicatricial pemphigoid. Dermatol Clin 1993;11:499–510.

[8] Schwab IR. Cultured corneal epithelia for ocular surface disease. Trans Am Ophthalmol Soc 1999;97:891–986.

[9] Liesegang TJ. Conjunctival changes associated with glaucoma therapy: implications for the external disease consultant and the treatment of glaucoma. Cornea 1998;17(6):574–83.

[10] Butt Z, Kaufman D, McNab A, et al. Drug-induced ocular cicatricial pemphigoid: a series of clinico-pathological reports. Eye 1998;12(2):285–90.

[11] Fiore PM, Jacobs IH, Goldberg DB. Drug-induced pemphigoid: a spectrum of diseases. Arch Ophthalmol 1987;105(12):1660–3.

[12] Bhol KC, Dans MJ, Simmons RK, et al. The autoantibodies to alpha 6 beta 4 integrin of patients affected by ocular cicatricial pemphigoid recognize predominantly epitopes within the large cytoplasmic domain of human beta 4. J Immunol 2000;165(5):2824–9.

[13] Bernauer W, Broadway DC, Wright P. Chronic progressive conjunctival cicatrisation. Eye 1993;7:371–8.

[14] Sacks EH, Jakobiec FA, Wieczorek R, et al. Immunophenotypic analysis of the inflammatory infiltrate in ocular cicatricial pemphigoid: further evidence for a T cell-mediated disease. Ophthalmology 1989;96:236–43.

[15] Schaller J, Heiligenhaus A, Engelbrecht S, et al. Detection of eosinophil cationic protein in active ocular cicatricial pemphigoid. Abstracts for the 25th Annual Meeting of the European Society for Dermatological Research. J Invest Dermatol 1995;105:445–520.

[16] Hoang-Xuan T, Foster CS, Raizman MB, et al. Mast cells in conjunctiva affected by cicatricial pemphigoid. Ophthalmology 1989;96:1110–4.

[17] Bernauer W, Wright P, Dart JK, et al. The conjunctiva in acute and chronic mucous membrane pemphigoid: an immunohistochemical analysis. Ophthalmology 1993;100: 339–46.

[18] Kelly S, Wojnarowska F. The use of chemically split tissue in the detection of circulating anti-basement membrane zone antibodies in bullous pemphigoid and cicatricial pemphigoid. Br J Dermatol 1988;118:31–40.

[19] Leonard JN, Hobday CM, Haffenden GP, et al. Immunofluorescent studies in ocular cicatricial pemphigoid. Br J Dermatol 1988;118:209–17.

[20] Setterfield J, Bhogal B, Morgan P, et al. Clinical and immunopathological correlation in cicatricial pemphigoid: a study of 36 cases. British Society for Investigative Dermatology Annual Meeting, Oxford, April 6–7, 1995. British Journal of Dermatology 1995;132(4): 631–60.

[21] Power WJ, Neves RA, Rodriguez A, et al. Increasing the diagnostic yield of conjunctival biopsy in patients with suspected ocular cicatricial pemphigoid. Ophthalmology 1995; 102:1158–63.

[22] Sarret Y, Hall R, Cobo LM, et al. Salt-split human skin substrate for the immunofluorescent screening of serum from patients with cicatricial pemphigoid and a new method of immunoprecipitation with IgA antibodies. J Am Acad Dermatol 1991;24: 952–8.

[23] Bernard P, Prost C, Lecerf V, et al. Studies of cicatricial pemphigoid autoantibodies using direct immunoelectron microscopy and immunoblot analysis. J Invest Dermatol 1990;94:630–5.

[24] Fine JD, Neises GR, Katz SI. Immunofluorescence and immunoelectron microscopic studies in cicatricial pemphigoid. J Invest Dermatol 1984;82:39–45.

[25] Nieboer C, Boorsma DM, Woederman MJ. Immunoelectron microscopic findings in cicatricial pemphigoid: their significance in relation to epidermolysis bullosa acquisita. Br J Dermatol 1982;106:419–22.

[26] Prost C, Robin H, Caux F, et al. Direct immunoelectron microscopy on the conjunctiva in ocular cicatricial pemphigoid versus subepidermal autoimmune bullous dermatoses with ocular involvement: report of 10 cases. Abstracts for the 1996 Annual Meeting Society for Investigative Dermatology. J Invest Dermatol 1996;106:805–950.

[27] Bedane C, Prost C, Bernard P, et al. Cicatricial pemphigoid antigen differs from bullous pemphigoid antigen by its exclusive extracellular localization: a study by indirect immunoelectron microscopy. J Invest Dermatol 1991;97:3–9.

[28] Domloge-Hultsch N, Anhalt G, Gammon WR, et al. Antiepiligrin cicatricial pemphigoid: a subepithelial bullous disorder. Arch Dermatol 1994;130:1521–9.

[29] Domlodge-Hultsch N, Gammon W, Briggaman R, et al. Epiligrin, the major human keratinocyte integrin ligand, is a target in both an acquired autoimmune and an inherited subepidermal blistering skin disease. J Clin Invest 1992;90:1628–33.

[30] Hashimoto T, Murakami H, Senboshi Y, et al. Antiepiligrin cicatricial pemphigoid: the first case report from Japan. J Am Acad Dermatol 1996;34:940–2.

[31] Chan RY, Bhol K, Tesavibul N, et al. The role of antibody to human beta 4 integrin in conjunctival basement membrane separation: possible in vitro model for ocular cicatricial pemphigoid. Invest Ophthalmol Vis Sci 1999;40(10):2283–90.

[32] Herbort CP, Zografos L, Zwingli M, et al. Topical retinoic acid in dysplastic and metaplastic keratinization of corneoconjunctival epithelium. Graefes Arch Clin Exp Ophthalmol 1988;226(1):22–6.

[33] Letko E, Bhol K, Foster SC, et al. Influence of intravenous immunoglobulin therapy on serum levels of anti-beta 4 antibodies in ocular cicatricial pemphigoid. A correlation with disease activity. A preliminary study. Curr Eye Res 2000;21(2):646–54.

[34] Leverkus M, Hirako Y, Pas H, et al. Cicatricial pemphigoid with circulating autoantibodies to beta 4 integrin, bullous pemphigoid 180, and bullous pemphigoid 230. Br J Dermatol 2001;145:998–1004.

[35] Foster CS, Wilson LA, Ekins MB. Immunosuppressive therapy for progressive ocular cicatricial pemphigoid. Ophthalmology 1982;89(4):340–53.

[36] Foster CS, Ahmed AR. Intravenous immunoglobulin therapy for ocular cicatricial pemphigoid: a preliminary study. Ophthalmology 1999;106(11):2136–43.

[37] Heiligenhaus A, Shore JW, Rubin PA, et al. Long-term results of mucous membrane grafting in ocular cicatricial pemphigoid. Implications for patient selection and surgical considerations. Ophthalmology 1993;100(9):1283–8.

[38] Silverman S Jr, Gorsky M, Lozada-Nur F, et al. Oral mucous membrane pemphigoid: a study of sixty-five patients. Oral Surg Oral Med Oral Pathol Oral Radiol Endod 1986; 61:233–7.

[39] Celis Sanchez J, Lopez Ferrando N, Garcia Largacha M, et al. Subconjunctival mitomycin C for the treatment of ocular cicatricial pemphigoid. Arch Soc Esp Oftalmol 2002;77(9): 501–6.

[40] Fern AL, Jay JL, Young H, et al. Dapsone therapy for the acute inflammatory phase of ocular pemphigoid. Br J Ophthalmol 1992;76:332–5.

[41] Thorne JE, Jabs DA, Qazi FA, et al. Mycophenolate mofetil therapy for inflammatory eye disease. Ophthalmology 2005;112(8):1472–7.

[42] Marzano AV, Dassoni F, Caputo R. Treatment of refractory blistering autoimmune diseases with mycophenolic acid. J Dermatolog Treat 2006;17(6):370–6.

[43] Megahed M, Schmiedeberg S, Becker J, et al. Treatment of cicatricial pemphigoid with mycophenolate mofetil as a steroid-sparing agent. J Am Acad Dermatol 2001;45(2):256–9.

[44] Heffernan MP, Bentley DD. Successful treatment of mucous membrane pemphigoid with infliximab. Arch Dermatol 2006;142(10):1268–70.

[45] Papaliodis GN, Chu D, Foster CS. Treatment of ocular inflammatory disorders with daclizumab. Ophthalmology 2003;110(4):786–9.

[46] Rogers RS 3rd, Seehafer JR, Perry HO. Treatment of cicatricial (benign mucous membrane) pemphigoid with dapsone. J Am Acad Dermatol 1982;6:215–23.

[47] Schmidt E, Seitz CS, Benoit S, et al. Rituximab in autoimmune bullous diseases: mixed responses and adverse effects. Br J Dermatol 2007;156(2):352–6.

[48] Ahmed AR, Spigelman Z, Cavacini LA, et al. Treatment of pemphigus vulgaris with rituximab and intravenous immune globulin. N Engl J Med 2006;355(17):1772–9.

[49] Gurcan HM, Ahmed AR. Frequency of adverse events associated with intravenous immunoglobulin therapy in patients with pemphigus or pemphigoid. Ann Pharmacother 2007; 41(10):1604–10.

[50] Ahmed AR. Use of intravenous immunoglobulin therapy in autoimmune blistering diseases. Int Immunopharmacol 2006;6(4):557–78.

[51] Sami N, Letko E, Androudi S, et al. Intravenous immunoglobulin therapy in patients with ocular-cicatricial pemphigoid: a long-term follow-up. Ophthalmology 2004;111(7):1380–2.

[52] Schwab IR, Reyes M, Isseroff RR. Successful transplantation of bioengineered tissue replacements in patients with ocular surface disease. Cornea 2000;19(4):421–6.

[53] Neumann R, Tauber J, Foster CS. Remission and recurrence after withdrawal of therapy for ocular cicatricial pemphigoid. Ophthalmology 1991;98(6):858–62.

[54] Tsubota K, Satake Y, Ohyama M, et al. Surgical reconstruction of the ocular surface in advanced ocular cicatricial pemphigoid and Stevens-Johnson syndrome. Am J Ophthalmol 1996;122(1):38–52.

[55] Samson CM, Nduaguba C, Baltatzis S, et al. Limbal stem cell transplantation in chronic inflammatory eye disease. Ophthalmology 2002;109(5):862–8.

[56] Koizumi N, Inatomi T, Suzuki T, et al. Cultivated corneal epithelial stem cell transplantation in ocular surface disorders. Ophthalmology 2001;108(9):1569–74.

[57] Daya SM, Ilari FA. Living related conjunctival limbal allograft for the treatment of stem cell deficiency. Ophthalmology 2001;108(1):126–33.

[58] Tsai RJ, Li LM, Chen JK. Reconstruction of damaged corneas by transplantation of autologous limbal epithelial cells. N Engl J Med 2000;343(2):86–93.

[59] Tsubota K, Satake Y, Kaido M, et al. Treatment of severe ocular-surface disorders with corneal epithelial stem-cell transplantation. N Engl J Med 1999;340(22):1697–703.

[60] Aultbrinker EA, Starr MB, Donnenfeld ED. Linear IgA disease. The ocular manifestations. Ophthalmology 1988;95(3):340–3.

[61] Chorzelski TP, Jablonska S, Maciejowska E. Linear IgA bullous dermatosis of adults. Clin Dermatol 1991;9(3):383–92.

[62] Bernard P, Vaillant L, Labeille B, et al. Incidence and distribution of subepidermal autoimmune bullous skin diseases in three French regions. Bullous Diseases French Study Group. Arch Dermatol 1995;131(1):48–52.

[63] Collier PM, Wojnarowska F, Welsh K, et al. Adult linear IgA disease and chronic bullous disease of childhood: the association with human lymphocyte antigens Cw7, B8, DR3 and tumour necrosis factor influences disease expression. Br J Dermatol 1999;141(5):867–75.

[64] Wojnarowska F, Allen J, Collier P. Linear IgA disease: a heterogeneous disease. Dermatology 1994;189(Suppl 1):52–6.

[65] Jablonska S, Chorzelski TP, Rosinska D, et al. Linear IgA bullous dermatosis of childhood (chronic bullous dermatosis of childhood). Clin Dermatol 1991;9(3):393–401.

[66] Wojnarowska F, Marsden RA, Bhogal B, et al. Chronic bullous disease of childhood, childhood cicatricial pemphigoid, and linear IgA disease of adults. A comparative study demonstrating clinical and immunopathologic overlap. J Am Acad Dermatol 1988;19(5 Pt 1): 792–805.

[67] Klein PA, Callen JP. Drug-induced linear IgA bullous dermatosis after vancomycin discontinuance in a patient with renal insufficiency. J Am Acad Dermatol 2000;42 (2 Pt 2):316–23.

[68] Nousari HC, Kimyai-Asadi A, Caeiro JP, et al. Clinical, demographic, and immunohistologic features of vancomycin-induced linear IgA bullous disease of the skin. Report of 2 cases and review of the literature. Medicine (Baltimore) 1999;78(1):1–8.

[69] Onodera H, Mihm MC Jr, Yoshida A, et al. Drug-induced linear IgA bullous dermatosis. J Dermatol 2005;32(9):759–64.

[70] Friedman IS, Rudikoff D, Phelps RG, et al. Captopril-triggered linear IgA bullous dermatosis. Int J Dermatol 1998;37(8):608–12.

[71] Kuechle MK, Stegemeir E, Maynard B, et al. Drug-induced linear IgA bullous dermatosis: report of six cases and review of the literature. J Am Acad Dermatol 1994;30(2 Pt 1):187–92.

[72] Primka EJ 3rd, Liranzo MO, Bergfeld WF, et al. Amiodarone-induced linear IgA disease. J Am Acad Dermatol 1995;33(2 Pt 1):320–1.

[73] Acostamadiedo JM, Perniciaro C, Rogers RS 3rd. Phenytoin-induced linear IgA bullous disease. J Am Acad Dermatol 1998;38(2 Pt 2):352–6.

[74] Kelly SE, Frith PA, Millard PR, et al. A clinicopathological study of mucosal involvement in linear IgA disease. Br J Dermatol 1988;119:161–70.

[75] Darling TN, Cardenas AA, Beard JS, et al. A child with antibodies targeting both linear IgA bullous dermatosis and bullous pemphigoid antigens. Arch Dermatol 1995;131:1438–42.

[76] Zone JJ, Pazderka Smith E, Powell D, et al. Antigenic specificity of antibodies from patients with linear basement membrane deposition of IgA. Dermatology 1994; 189(Suppl 1):64–6.

[77] Pulimood S, Ajithkumar K, Jacob M, et al. Linear IgA bullous dermatosis of childhood: treatment with dapsone and cotrimoxazole. Clin Exp Dermatol 1997;22:90–1.

[78] Ang P, Tay YK. Treatment of linear IgA bullous dermatosis of childhood with colchicine. Pediatr Dermatol 1999;16(1):50–2.

[79] Segura S, Iranzo P, Martinez-de Pablo I, et al. High-dose intravenous immunoglobulins for the treatment of autoimmune mucocutaneous blistering diseases: evaluation of its use in 19 cases. J Am Acad Dermatol 2007;56(6):960–7.

[80] Letko E, Bhol K, Foster CS, et al. Linear IgA bullous disease limited to the eye: a diagnostic dilemma: response to intravenous immunoglobulin therapy. Ophthalmology 2000;107(8):1524–8.

[81] Kroiss MM, Vogt T, Landthaler M, et al. High-dose intravenous immune globulin is also effective in linear IgA disease. Br J Dermatol 2000;142(3):582.

[82] Caux FA, Giudice GJ, Diaz LA, et al. Autoimmune subepithelial blistering diseases with ocular involvement. Immunology and Allergy Clinics of North America 1997;17:139–59.

[83] Schattenkirchner S, Eming S, Hunzelmann N, et al. Treatment of epidermolysis bullosa acquisita with mycophenolate mofetil and autologous keratinocyte grafting. Br J Dermatol 1999;141(5):932–3.

[84] Vassileva S. Bullous systemic lupus erythematosus. Clin Dermatol 2004;22(2):129–38.

[85] Hughes AP, Callen JP. Epidermolysis bullosa acquisita responsive to dapsone therapy. J Cutan Med Surg 2001;5(5):397–9.

[86] Mihai S, Chiriac MT, Takahashi K, et al. The alternative pathway of complement activation is critical for blister induction in experimental epidermolysis bullosa acquisita. J Immunol 2007;178(10):6514–21.

[87] Liu Y, Shimizu H, Hashimoto T. Immunofluorescence studies using skin sections of recessive dystrophic epidermolysis bullosa patients indicated that the antigen of anti-p200 pemphigoid is not a fragment of type VII collagen. J Dermatol Sci 2003;32(2):125–9.

[88] Cox NH, Bearn MA, Herold J, et al. Blindness due to the IgA variant of epidermolysis bullosa acquisita, and treatment with osteo-odonto-keratoprosthesis. Br J Dermatol 2007;156(4):775–7.

[89] Yancey KB. The pathophysiology of autoimmune blistering diseases. J Clin Invest 2005;115(4):825–8.

[90] Chen M, Doostan A, Bandyopadhyay P, et al. The cartilage matrix protein subdomain of type VII collagen is pathogenic for epidermolysis bullosa acquisita. Am J Pathol 2007;170(6):2009–18.

[91] Trigo-Guzman FX, Conti A, Aoki V, et al. Epidermolysis bullosa acquisita in childhood. J Dermatol 2003;30(3):226–9.

[92] Kasperkiewicz M, Zillikens D. Rituximab (anti-CD20) for the treatment of autoimmune bullous diseases. Hautarzt 2007;58(2):115–6, 118–21.

[93] Letko E, Bhol K, Anzaar F, et al. Chronic cicatrizing conjunctivitis in a patient with epidermolysis bullosa acquisita. Arch Ophthalmol 2006;124:1615–8.

[94] Sadler E, Schafleitner B, Lanschuetzer C, et al. Treatment-resistant classical epidermolysis bullosa acquisita responding to rituximab. Br J Dermatol 2007;157(2):417–9.

[95] Sitaru C. Experimental models of epidermolysis bullosa acquisita. Exp Dermatol 2007;16(6):520–31.

[96] Ishii N, Yoshida M, Hisamatsu Y, et al. Epidermolysis bullosa acquisita sera react with distinct epitopes on the NC1 and NC2 domains of type VII collagen: study using immunoblotting of domain-specific recombinant proteins and postembedding immunoelectron microscopy. Br J Dermatol 2004;150(5):843–51.

[97] McCuin JB, Hanlon T, Mutasim DF. Autoimmune bullous diseases: diagnosis and management. Dermatol Nurs 2006;18(1):20–5.

[98] Hakki SS, Celenligil-Nazliel H, Karaduman A, et al. Epidermolysis bullosa acquisita: clinical manifestations, microscopic findings, and surgical periodontal therapy. A case report. J Periodontol 2001;72(4):550–8.

[99] Das JK, Sengupta S, Gangopadhyay AK. Epidermolysis bullosa acquisita. Indian J Dermatol Venereol Leprol 2006;72(1):86.

[100] Haufs MG, Haneke E. Epidermolysis bullosa acquisita treated with basiliximab, an interleukin-2 receptor antibody. Acta Derm Venereol 2001;81(1):72.

[101] Hallel-Halevy D, Nadelman C, Chen M, et al. Epidermolysis bullosa acquisita: update and review. Clin Dermatol 2001;19(6):712–8.
[102] Stein JA, Mikkilineni R. Epidermolysis bullosa acquisita. Dermatol Online J 2007;13(1):15.
[103] Suchniak JM, Diaz LA, Lin MS, et al. IgM-mediated epidermolysis bullosa acquisita. Arch Dermatol 2002;138(10):1385–6.
[104] Smith RJ, Manche EE, Mondino BJ. Ocular cicatricial pemphigoid and ocular manifestations of pemphigus vulgaris. Int Ophthalmol Clin 1997;37(2):63–75.
[105] Challacombe SJ, Setterfield J, Shirlaw P, et al. Immunodiagnosis of pemphigus and mucous membrane pemphigoid. Acta Odontol Scand 2001;59(4):226–34.
[106] Bhol KC, Rojas AI, Khan IU, et al. Presence of interleukin 10 in the serum and blister fluid of patients with pemphigus vulgaris and pemphigoid. Cytokine 2000;12(7):1076–83.
[107] Laforest C, Huilgol SC, Casson R, et al. Autoimmune bullous diseases: ocular manifestations and management. Drugs 2005;65(13):1767–79.
[108] Daoud YJ, Cervantes R, Foster CS, et al. Ocular pemphigus. J Am Acad Dermatol 2005;53(4):585–90.
[109] Tenner E. Ocular involvement in pemphigus vulgaris. J Am Acad Dermatol 2006;55(4):725; author reply 725–6.
[110] Michailidou EZ, Belazi MA, Markopoulos AK, et al. Epidemiologic survey of pemphigus vulgaris with oral manifestations in northern Greece: retrospective study of 129 patients. Int J Dermatol 2007;46(4):356–61.
[111] Bianciotto C, Herreras Cantalapiedra JM, Alvarez MA, et al. Conjunctival blistering associated with pemphigus vulgaris: report of a case. Arch Soc Esp Oftalmol 2005;80(6):365–8.
[112] Hall VC, Liesegang TJ, Kostick DA, et al. Ocular mucous membrane pemphigoid and ocular pemphigus vulgaris treated topically with tacrolimus ointment. Arch Dermatol 2003;139(8):1083–4.
[113] Merchant S, Weinstein M. Pemphigus vulgaris: the eyes have it. Pediatrics 2003;112(1 Pt 1):183–5.
[114] Palleschi GM, Giomi B, Fabbri P. Ocular involvement in pemphigus. Am J Ophthalmol 2007;144(1):149–52.
[115] Vaillant L. Bullous autoimmune diseases of the oral mucosa. Rev Stomatol Chir Maxillofac 1999;100(5):230–9.
[116] Bhol K, Tyagi S, Natarajan K, et al. Use of recombinant pemphigus vulgaris antigen in development of ELISA and IB assays to detect pemphigus vulgaris autoantibodies. J Eur Acad Dermatol Venereol 1998;10(1):28–35.
[117] Kavosh ER, Bielory L. Allergic disease of the eye. In: Mahmoudi M, editor. Allergy and asthma: practical diagnosis and management. 1st edition. New York: McGraw Hill; 2007. p. 21–31.
[118] Kavosh E, Bielory L. Letters to the editor. Allergy Asthma Proc 2007;28(5):606–7.

ELSEVIER
SAUNDERS

Immunol Allergy Clin N Am
28 (2008) 137–168

IMMUNOLOGY
AND ALLERGY
CLINICS
OF NORTH AMERICA

Dermatologic and Allergic Conditions of the Eyelid

Belle Peralejo, MD[a], Vincent Beltrani, MD[a,b,*],
Leonard Bielory, MD[c]

[a]*Department of Medicine, Division of Allergy, Immunology, and Rheumatology,
UMDNJ–New Jersey Medical School, 90 Bergen Street, Newark, NJ 07103, USA*
[b]*Department of Dermatology, Columbia University, HIP 12, New York, NY 10032, USA*
[c]*Department of Medicine, Pediatrics, Ophthalmology, and Visual Sciences,
UMDNJ–New Jersey Medical School, 90 Bergen Street, DOC Suite 4700,
Newark, NJ 07103, USA*

The skin, the largest organ of the body [1], is composed of three layers: the epidermis, dermis, and subcutaneous. The outermost layer (the epidermis) is composed of keratinocytes (squamous cells), melanocytes (pigment cells), and the immunologically active dendritic cells (antigen-presenting cells). The thickness of the epidermis varies, with increased thickness in areas exposed to friction, such as the palms and soles, and a thin epidermal layer, such as that found in the eyelids [2], to allow for easier movement and flexibility. The second layer of the skin (the dermis) is composed of blood vessels, nerves, glands (eccrine and sebaceous), and other accessory structures such as hair follicles of the eyelashes and eyelids. In addition, the dermis of the eyelid is rich in arteriovenous anastomoses. The innermost layer is the subcutaneous layer. The eyelid contains loose areolar tissue and little subcutaneous fat, important characteristics that allow easy mobility of the first two layers over the underlying muscle. The loose tissue, however, has great potential for accumulation of fluid, leading to periorbital edema.

Clinical diagnosis of lesions on the skin is primarily based on proper description of the lesions and their categorization according to appearance and evolution. Primary lesions are caused by the disease stimulus, whereas secondary lesions are later changes that occur due to evolution of the primary lesions [3]. Primary lesions include macules, papules, vesicles, bullae, pustules, wheals, plaques, and nodules. Secondary lesions consist of

---

* Corresponding author.
E-mail address: dermguys@hvc.rr.com (V. Beltrani).

scales, erosions, excoriations, ulcers, and lichenification. Primary and secondary lesions can occur together, in various combinations, and with evolving patterns that assist in the diagnosis of the disorder. Disease may be categorized according to the presenting primary lesions, but one should remember that diseases have "lives" and may evolve from one primary lesion to another and become associated with a variety of secondary lesions.

Seborrheic dermatitis

Seborrheic dermatitis (SD) is a common macular condition of skin that is commonly chronic and recurrent and characterized by symmetric erythematous inflammation with scaling that is often greasy and sometimes with crusting. When SD involves periocular tissue (the eyebrows and eyelids), it is known as seborrheic blepharitis. Other areas of predilection include the scalp, ears, sides of the nose, chest, axilla, and inguinal area. *Malassezia* (previously *Pityrosporum*) yeasts have been associated with the development of SD [4–6] through an altered immune response or as the result of hyperproliferation [4,5].

SD is common in the newborn (cradle cap) due to activation of sebaceous glands by maternal androgen stimulation. Endogenous androgens induce seborrhea in adolescence. Ocular complications of chronic seborrhea of the eyelids include hordeola (styes) and inflammation of the meibomian glands (meibomianitis) with secondary conjunctivitis (blepharoconjunctivitis). Uncontrolled severe SD has observed in HIV patients and may be the initial presentation prompting workup for HIV infection [7].

Treatment

SD is easily controlled with steroid creams, but this treatment does not cure the dermatitis, which recurs. On the eyelids, which are very thin, a mild steroid may be used sparingly, but due to the possibility of side effects from steroids, only short courses or steroid-sparing remedies have been used for safety. Calcineurin inhibitors (eg, Elidel, Protopic) are effective, but their safety in children younger than 2 years is controversial [8]. Saline compresses and baby shampoo wiped gently on the affected areas are safe and mild remedies used to help alleviate the scaling and crusting of blepharitis. Topical antifungal creams, shampoos, and lotions containing selenium sulfide and zinc pyrithione have been used, with some improvement [5].

Vitiligo

These depigmented macules or patches occur due to loss of pigment on the skin; no secondary changes are evident (no scale, crusts, or erosions). Vitiligo is considered to be a multifactorial disorder; hypotheses on its development include neural, biochemical, and autoimmune mechanisms [9]. The association with autoimmune conditions such as autoimmune thyroiditis, pernicious anemia, diabetes, rheumatoid arthritis, and alopecia areata supports the likely autoimmune etiopathogenesis of vitiligo [9,10]. The association between vitiligo and autoimmune thyroid disease has been suggested due to the presence of thyroid antibodies (antithyroglobulin and anti–thyroid peroxidase antibodies) and abnormalities in thyroid function [11,12]. In a retrospective study of 1436 patients who had vitiligo, atopic/nummular eczema was seen in 20 (1.4%) patients, bronchial asthma in 10 (0.7%), diabetes mellitus in 8 (0.6%) [13], thyroid disease in 7 (0.5%), and alopecia in 6 (0.4%) [14]. These findings stress the importance of a thorough assessment for autoimmune diseases in selected patients who have vitiligo. Vitiligo has also been associated with endocrinopathies (auotimmune polyglandular syndromes) [12], different skin diseases (psoriasis Ref. [15], lichen planus Ref. [16]), and rare syndromes (Vogt-Koyanagi-Harada syndrome Ref. [11]) [9].

Common areas affected are those around orifices (perioral, periorbital) and on areas of frequent trauma. Despite its benign nature, it has devastating implications due to the cosmetic problems it causes, and patients often seek camouflaging agents to conceal the defects. Differential diagnoses for flat hypopigmented lesions are postinflammatory hypopigmentation noted after various inflammatory cutaneous disorders (infections and drug-related eosinophilic and scaling skin syndromes); tinea versicolor that has fine scaling treated with antifungal agents; and pityriasis alba that also may have fine scales and is common in atopic dermatitis.

Heliotrope rash

Dermatomyositis may manifest with a violaceous discoloration of the eyelids, upper cheeks, forehead, and temples called a helioptrope cutaneous eruption, named after the color of the heliotrope flower. The cutaneous eruption can evolve to include underlying edema of the eyelids before, during, or after the development of muscle weakness; however, a subset may lack any evidence of myopathy. Diagnosis is through a skin biopsy to differentiate it from chronic eyelid dermatitis such as contact dermatitis. Pathology may show nonspecific inflammatory changes indistinguishable from lupus erythematosus [17]. There is epidermal atrophy, basement membrane degeneration, vacuolar alteration of basilar keratinocytes, a sparse lymphocytic inflammatory infiltrate around blood vessels, and interstitial mucin deposition [18].

Port-wine stains

Vascular malformations include port-wine stains, salmon patches, and malformations associated with syndromes (Sturge-Weber, Cobb, and Klippel-Trénaunay). Port-wine stains (nevus flammeus) are unilateral and commonly affect the face and other areas. They are present at birth up to 0.3% and range in size from a few millimeters to very large, covering the whole face or limb [19]. They are flat, erythematous to violaceous patches with irregular well-delineated borders and are initially smooth but may become popular, nodular, or cobblestoned. They differ from hemangiomas in that they increase in size proportionate to child growth, then remain stable throughout life but may darken. Port-wine stains over the eyelid in the distribution of the trigeminal nerve (V1) has a risk of being associated with Sturge-Weber syndrome, which is associated with central nervous system findings (angioma of the meninges, hemiparesis contralateral to the skin lesions, epilepsy), mental retardation, renal angioma, coarctation of the aorta, visual impairment, high arched palate, and abnormally developed ears.

Xanthelasmas and plane xanthomas

Xanthelasmas affecting the eyelids, called xanthelasma palpebrum, are a variant of xanthomas, which are bilateral symmetric flat-topped yellowish papules or plaques located typically on the inner or outer canthus of the upper eyelid, rarely involving the lower eyelid or obstructing vision. Female sex and increasing age are predisposing factors. Xanthelasma may be associated with familial hypercholesterolemia but approximately 50% of patients have normal cholesterol levels [20]. Pathology of these lesions shows the presence of xanthoma cells—foamy, lipid-laden histiocytes—in the superficial dermis in perivascular and periadnexal areas [21]. When they appear before the age of 40 years, they may have a higher likelihood of being associated with familial hypercholesterolemia [22]. There may be an associated risk of atherosclerosis and pancreatitis in lesions found to be associated with lipid abnormalities. Hence, it is valuable to screen for lipid abnormalities in these patients. They have also been found to occur more often in diabetics [23].

Seborrheic keratosis

Seborrheic keratoses are very common benign cutaneous growths that may be skin-colored to hyperpigmented and occur anywhere on the body and commonly involve the eyelids. They are more common with increasing age and appear as well-circumscribed, thick, keratotic papules or plaques that have a smooth and flat surface or an irregular and rough surface. They can be brown, tan, or black and have a characteristic stuck-on appearance. Unlike actinic keratoses, they are not related to sun exposure and are benign. A genetic form is common in blacks and is termed dermatosis papulosa nigra. Even young and middle-aged blacks may develop these multiple brown-black, smooth, dome-shaped, or pedunculated 2- to 3-mm papules, usually on the face and neck.

Skin tags

Skin tags or acrochordon are frequently found on the eyelids but may also be found anywhere on the body, especially on the axilla, neck, and inguinal region. They may start as small brown or skin-colored growths with a short stalk and may evolve to larger polyps with longer narrow stalks. There have been several reports suggesting that skin tags may be a marker for the presence of colonic polyps in symptomatic patients [24–26]. In a prospective study of 100 asymptomatic patients, no association was found between skin tags and colonic polyps [25]. A review of the literature and results of a meta-analysis show a significant association between skin tags and colonic polyps in 777 symptomatic patients, but no association in 268 asymptomatic patients [25]. Hence, the mere presence of acrochordons (skin tags) should not be used as an indication for screening colonoscopy.

Warts

Unlike the seborrheic keratoses and skin tags previously reviewed, warts are transient viral infections secondary to human papilloma virus (HPV). HPV infects the skin through breaks that easily occur on thin skin such as eyelids. Recent interest in warts has emerged due to their occurrence in immunocompromised individuals such as those who have HIV infection. Flat warts (verruca plana) are flat-topped and may be found on the face and eyelids and other areas of the body; common warts (verruca vulgaris) are less commonly seen on the face and more common on the extremities. There are many HPV types identified, with various types causing different clinical behavior and location preference [26]. Flat warts are often seen on the face and eyelids and may be present in large numbers as flat-topped papules that are skin-colored to tan to pinkish, whereas the more hyperkeratotic common warts do not normally occur on the eyelids.

Comedones

Comedones are commonly called blackheads when they are open comedones and white heads when they are closed comedones. These represent a stage in acne vulgaris and are caused by plugging of the hair follicle due to increased stickiness of keratinocytes. Comedones are common in adolescents on the face, nose, and chin. Senile comedones, which are larger, occur in the elderly around the eyes and temples and may be attributed to excessive sun exposure [27]. The sun damage causes the pilosebaceous duct to become distended and more easily filled with keratinocytes.

Syringoma

Syringomas are small, firm, flesh-colored, flat-topped or dome-shaped papules ranging from 1 to 5 mm commonly found on the lower eyelids and malar area but may also be present on the forehead, chest, and abdomen. They represent benign tumors of the sweat duct and have no malignant potential. They are found at any age but occur more commonly in the third and fourth decades and in women. They usually appear in crops. Palpebral syringomas are a common cutaneous pathology in Down syndrome, more commonly in female patients [28].

Rosacea

Rosacea is often mistaken for acne, but the major difference is the lack of comedones. Rosacea may comprise erythema, edema, papules, pustules, or telangiectasias occurring on the cheeks, forehead, nose, and eyes. Patients look like they have a chronic blush. Rhinophyma is the involvement of the nose and is characterized by a bulbous appearance with chronic inflammation and hypertrophy. The actor W.C. Fields represents an example of rosacea involving the nose. The cause is unknown, but genetic, environmental, vascular, and inflammatory factors and microorganisms such as *Demodex folliculorum* and *Helicobacter pylori* have been considered [29]. The mite *Demodex folliculorum*, a normal resident fauna of hair follicles, has been found in increased numbers in patients who have rosacea [30]. Precipitating factors for this eruption include consumption of alcohol or hot beverages, spices, sun exposure, and stress.

Symptoms of ocular rosacea may range from mild to severe. Nonspecific symptoms may include conjunctivitis, blepharitis, soreness, lacrimation, and grittiness. Aside from involvement of the lid (blepharitis, chalazion), ocular rosacea can involve the conjunctiva (conjunctivitis, keratoconjunctivitis sicca), sclera (scleritis, episcleritis, scleral perforation), iris (iritis, iridocyclitis), and cornea (punctuate keratopathy, scarring, corneal perforation, corneal neovascularization, ulceration, and blindness) [31]. Starr [32] examined the eyes of patients who had rosacea and found ocular complications in 58% and corneal involvement in 33%. Recent articles on the prevalence of ocular rosacea in patients who had acne rosacea suggest that between 6% and 18% of acne rosacea patients have signs or symptoms of ocular rosacea, but few cases are confirmed by an ophthalmologist [33]. Twenty percent of patients who have acne rosacea have ocular symptoms before the skin lesions [34]. Rosacea is found more often in female patients, but ocular rosacea occurs equally in both sexes. In patients who have acne rosacea and ocular complaints, a multidisciplinary approach is recommended, including evaluation by an ophthalmologist.

Lipoid proteinosis

Lipoid proteinosis is a rare genodermatosis characterized by protein infiltration of the skin, oral cavity, and larynx. The first clinical sign is hoarseness caused by infiltration of the vocal cords [35]. Patients are easily recognized due to their husky voice, inability to protrude the tongue and thickened eyelids [36]. The involvement of the eyelids with tiny papules produces the classic string of beads sign appearance [35,36]. Waxy, yellow papules and nodules on the skin or generalized skin thickening may also be seen.

Angioedema

Angioedema refers to the deeper swelling of the skin involving the subcutaneous layer. The overlying epidermis is normal, nonpruritic, and nonpitting. Any part of the body may be affected with angioedema, but the more common areas are the eyelids, lips, and genitalia. Possible causes of acute angioedema include an immunoglobulin (Ig)E-mediated allergic reaction to food or drugs. Although any food can provoke a reaction, relatively few foods are responsible for the most significant food-induced allergic reactions: milk, eggs, peanuts, tree nuts, fish, and shellfish [37]. In food-allergic patients who have atopic dermatitis, the ingestion of the food item can provoke the whole spectrum of IgE-mediated symptoms, from oral allergy syndrome to severe anaphylaxis [38]. Common drugs that cause angioedema are beta-lactam antibiotics (penicillins, penicillin derivatives, cephalosporins), sulfa-based antibiotics such as trimethoprim-sulfamethoxazole, insulin, extracts, heterologous antisera (equine antitoxins and antilymphocyte globulin), murine monoclonal antibodies, protamine, and heparin [39]. Local and systemic angioedema may be caused by hymenoptera stings or fire ant bites [40].

Bradykinin-induced angioedema is another cause of nonallergic angioedema that can be acquired or genetic. Examples are hereditary angioedema and angioedema secondary to use of angiotensin-converting enzyme (ACE) inhibitors. A well-known relationship exists between angioedema and ACE inhibitors (with angioedema occurring in 0.1%–6% of patients taking these drugs), which is thought to be due to defective degradation of bradykinin or substance P [41].

Contact urticaria

Contact urticaria is characterized by urticaria that develops due to contact with certain substances. The eruption commonly appears within 30 minutes to an hour after contact and results in erythema, pruritus, burning, and urticaria. A severe manifestation of contact urticaria of the conjunctiva manifesting with bulging chemotic conjunctiva is commonly seen in severe allergic conjunctivitis, which is typically bilateral. When contact urticaria affects only one eye, it is more commonly caused by the patient bringing the allergen to the eye by way of the fingers due to eye rubbing.

Erysipelas

Erysipelas is a deep infection of the dermis and subcutaneous tissue commonly caused by *Streptococcus pyogenes*. The eyelids may be involved, and erysipelas is characteristically found on one eye with associated erythema, tense edema, and tenderness. Patients may experience high fever, headache, and vomiting. This infection should be differentiated from allergic manifestations that are more commonly painless.

Trichinosis

Pyrexia, eyelid, or facial edema and myalgia represent the principal syndrome of the acute stage of trichinosis [42]. Other systemic symptoms include nausea, diarrhea, and muscle pain. Trichinosis can be complicated by myocarditis, thromboembolic disease, and encephalitis. Diagnosis is through the identification of *Trichinella* on muscle biopsy or by identification of larvae in the blood.

Chalazion

A chalazion is a slow-growing, often recurrent painless nodule on the eyelid caused by blockage of the meibomian gland, which is located on the tarsal plate of the lid about 3 to 4 mm from the margin. The skin over the nodule is freely movable but adherent to the tarsal plate. It may occasionally be associated with irritation of the conjunctiva. If it ruptures into the tarsal plate, granulation could result. More than half of chalazia resolve spontaneously.

Hordeolum

A hordeolum (stye) is an acute, suppurative, painful, localized inflammation of the eyelid margin involving the follicles of the eyelashes, the meibomian glands (sebaceous glands that empty out into the eyelashes), or the glands of Zeis (sebaceous glands that do not empty out into the eyelashes). *Staphylococcus aureus* is found in most cases. Exudation of purulent material may be seen from the hair follicle or on the conjunctiva.

Nevi

Nevi may erupt on the eyelids. In a retrospective analysis of 80 patients who had benign eyelid and conjunctival tumors (86 tumors), the most frequent tumor was intradermal nevus (44.6%), seborrheic keratosis (16.1%), and compound nevus (10.7%) in eyelid tumors, and compound nevus (29.2%) and intradermal nevus (25.0%) in conjunctival tumors.

Sarcoid

Cutaneous involvement in sarcoid occurs in 20% to 35% of patients [43]. Various specific cutaneous lesions occur in sarcoid, including maculopapules, plaques, nodules, lupus pernio, scar infiltration, alopecia, ulcerative lesions, and hypopigmentation. Erythema nodosum is the most common nonspecific dermatologic manifestation of sarcoid. Lesions may occur on the eyelid as nodules, swelling, scars, or lupus pernio. Lupus pernio appears as violaceous, infiltrated nodules that may be found on the eyelids and lid margin and on the external nares, ears, or along the vermillion border of the lips. Histologic analysis of specific lesions shows noncaseating granulomas consistent with sarcoid. Sarcoid is also commonly associated with uveitis and must be differentiated from chronic conjunctivitis by signs and symptoms such as increased photosensitivity, pain, and unilateral involvement.

Hemangioma

Hemangiomas and malformations are congenital vascular lesions. Hemangiomas are classified as strawberry hemangiomas, which occur at birth or during the first year of life and affect more girls than boys. Most of these lesions are small and harmless, proliferating for 8 to 18 months, then regressing over the next 5 to 8 years. They appear as bright red, well-circumscribed masses that may start out flat and telangiectatic and become nodular, protuberant, and compressible. They are benign but may cause difficulty if they compress vital organs or interfere with normal function. Cavernous hemangiomas are similar to strawberry hemangiomas but are collections of dilated vessels deeper in the dermis and subcutaneous tissue. They may appear as skin-colored, pink, red, or blue masses. Hemangiomas may involve the eyelids, and when there is a possibility of encroachment of the orbit, early management is sought. Approximately 30% of hemangiomas resolve by the fourth birthday, 50% by the fifth birthday, and 75% by the seventh birthday, with 95% undergoing complete or partially complete regression [44].

Basal cell carcinoma

Basal cell carcinoma (BCC) is the most common malignancy affecting the periorbital area. It presents more commonly on the lower eyelid and medial canthus [45]. The age-adjusted incidence rates per 100,000 population per year for BCC of the eyelid are 16.9 for men and 12.4 for women [46]. It is slow growing and locally invasive but rarely metastasizes. The most common presentation of BCC is a shiny, waxy, pearly nodule with rolled borders and small visible telangiectasias on the surface. It is painless and immobile. Variants of the nodular type include the nodular-ulcerative form (also called rodent ulcer wherein the nodule ulcerates centrally) and the morpheaform or sclerosing type (characterized by a pale indurated plaque). Effacement of the meibomian gland orifices with loss of adnexal structures provides a further clue to the typical nodular appearance. Lesions may bleed on manipulation due to increased friability.

Squamous cell carcinoma

Squamous cell carcinomas (SCC) are less common, representing about 5% of eyelid cancers. When they occur on the eyelids, they tend to be seen more often on the upper eyelid. Unlike BCC, they metastasize more often. Risk factors include chronic sun exposure, increasing age, and type

I skin types. Other predisposing factors are immunosuppression and exposure to radiation, arsenic, and coal tar. SCC may arise de novo or from premalignant lesions such as actinic keratosis. The typical presentation of SCC is a shallow ulcer that is often crusted over a reddish base with a surrounding ridgelike border. Associated loss of eyelashes and destruction of the surrounding eyelid structure are additional clues. SCC must be differentiated from a keratoacanthoma, which is benign but grows rapidly and has a horny horn arising from a central crater. Due to the higher rate of metastasis (up to 10%) in SCC, a more aggressive approach is optimal.

Sebaceous carcinoma

Sebaceous carcinoma is a rare cancer involving the eyelid (1%–5.5% of all malignancies of the eyelid), but when present, it is an aggressive and threatening condition with a high tendency for recurrence, invasion, and local or distant metastasis. It arises from the sebaceous glands, of which about 75% are located in the periorbital area. In this region, the appearance is variable and may mimic other benign conditions such as a wart, chronic blepharitis, or a chalazion that is recurrent. When in doubt, a biopsy is suggested. There is a rare association with Muir-Torre syndrome, which should be evaluated in a patient who has sebaceous carcinoma [47].

Malignant melanoma

Malignant melanoma involving the eyelid is less common, developing in about 1% of eyelid tumors [48]. About half are of the nodular variant and approximately 40% are the superficially spreading type. When evaluating pigmented lesions that are suspicious, one needs to examine the lesion for ABCDs: asymmetry, irregular border, variegate color (pigmentation), and rapidly increasing diameter. Malignant melanomas metastasize, so early detection, excision, and evaluation for metastatic disease are of vital importance. Tumor thickness is an important predictor of prognosis. Margin control by mapped serial excision or modified Mohs' micrographic surgery is a useful technique to ensure complete excision and minimization of local recurrence [49].

Eyelid dermatitis

Pruritic, erythematous, weeping, scaly, inflamed eyelids are caused by many etiologies. The more common causes include atopic dermatitis, contact dermatitis, contact urticaria, rosacea, seborrhea, and psoriasis [50].

A number of studies have been conducted to determine the frequency of various skin disorders causing eyelid dermatitis. Atopic dermatitis as a cause of eyelid dermatitis was reported in 39% [51], 23% [52], and 14% [53]. Allergic contact dermatitis was the etiology of eyelid dermatitis in 65%

[53] and 46% [52]. Irritant contact dermatitis was the cause of eyelid dermatitis in 24% [51], 16% [53] and 15% [52].

It was noted that elderly patients had a higher tendency for contact dermatitis to be allergic rather than irritant in nature. Women were affected more commonly [54]. Ocular rosacea was noted in 3% to 58% of patients who had cutaneous rosacea, and when there was ocular involvement, the peak age of onset was in the fifth decade [55]. Contact urticaria is less commonly diagnosed. Other dermatitis conditions of the eyelids include SD, psoriasis, dry eyes, dermatomyositis, and overlapping connective tissue disease.

A retrospective study [54] analyzing 1215 patients patch tested over 10 years showed that of the 105 patients who had eyelid dermatitis, 43.8% had allergic contact dermatitis, 36.2% had SD, 11.4% had other dermatitis/dermatosis, 7.6% had irritant contact dermatitis, 3.8% had psoriasis, and 2.9% had atopic dermatitis. With isolated eyelid dermatitis, SD was the most frequent diagnosis (46.3%), followed by allergic contact dermatitis (35.2%).

Guin [56] demonstrated in 2004 that over a 2.5-year study period, 215 patients presented with eyelid dermatitis for the first time. Women were predominantly affected (173 versus 42). Of the 215 patients, 165 had allergic contact dermatitis; another 9 had protein contact dermatitis without relevant positive patch tests; 37 (12%) had atopic dermatitis; 35 (16%) had SD, psoriasis, or both; 5 had rosacea or periorbital dermatitis; 2 had dermatomyositis; and others had infections [56].

Ayala and colleagues [57] studied 447 patients who had eyelid dermatitis and found that 50.2% were diagnosed with allergic contact dermatitis, 20.9% were found to have irritant contact dermatitis, 13.5% were affected by atopic dermatitis, 6.3% had SD, 6.5% were affected by nonspecific xerotic dermatitis, and 2.3% had psoriasis. These investigators noted that the main risk factor for allergic contact dermatitis was four-eyelid involvement, the main risk factor for irritant contact dermatitis was onset of symptoms between 2 to 6 months, and the main risk factor for atopic dermatitis was the onset of symptoms after 6 months along with personal history of atopy [57].

Atopic dermatitis

Atopic dermatitis occurs in patients who have an atopic background, that is, a personal or family history of asthma, allergic rhinitis, or eczema. Criteria for the diagnosis of atopic dermatitis include major and minor criteria [58]. Major criteria include severe pruritus, family/personal history of atopy, and areas of predilection of the rash (cheeks and extensors in infants, antecubital and popliteal areas for older children and adults). Numerous minor criteria include cataracts, cheilitis, conjunctivitis, perifollicular accentuation, facial pallor/erythema, food intolerance, hand dermatitis, ichthyosis, elevated IgE, cutnaeous infections, Dennie-Morgan fold, itching when sweating, keratoconus, keratosis pilaris, nipple dermatitis, orbital darkening, palmar hyperlinearity, pityriasis alba, white dermatographism, wool intolerance, and xerosis. There is a genetic predisposition for the development of T_H2 inflammatory response and elevated IgE in response to allergens. Hence, atopics usually have high levels of total IgE [59]. Patients who have atopic dermatitis have "twitchy skin," whereby their skin is hyperreactive or hyperesthetic. Wahlgren and colleagues [60] described this phenomenon as allokinesis, which refers to the sensation of itch in atopics in response to stimuli that would not cause itch in nonatopics. The major problem is pruritus, which occurs with or without visible eczema. Thus, there is a vicious cycle of itch causing the eczema, which is made worse by further itching.

The eyelids are commonly involved in atopic dermatitis because they are thin, exposed to irritants, and more easily traumatized by scratching. Constant rubbing leads to chronic changes and inflammation of the eyelid. Eyelid dermatitis was due to atopy in 14% of cases as reported by Valsecchi and colleagues [53], in 23% by Nethercott and colleagues [52], and in 39% as reported by Svennson and Moller [51]. The common presentation of atopic dermatitis of the eyelids consists of symmetric, scaly, erythematous, mildly lichenified plaques on the upper eyelids with or without concomitant involvement of the lower eyelids. The more chronic the eruption, the darker and more lichenified the lesions become. Atopics are also more prone to acquiring other types of eyelid dermatitis such as contact dermatitis. The appearance of the typical rash in areas of predilection and other major and minor criteria are helpful to differentiate atopic dermatitis from other eyelid dermatitis. If the possibility of contact dermatitis is considered, patch testing may be performed.

Many eye changes occur in association with atopic dermatitis. Conjunctivitis and keratoconjunctivitis may commonly occur in conjunction with allergic rhinitis and allergic conjunctivitis. "Allergic shiners" are dark circles around the eyes secondary to venous congestion. In addition, there may be loss of eyelashes, lid edema, itching, burning, tearing, chemosis, and mucoid discharge. The presence of an extra fold under the lower eyelids called the Dennie-Morgan fold is a clue to the presence of atopy. Cataracts can develop secondary to chronic severe atopic dermatitis. Keratoconus is a rare manifestation of atopic dermatitis characterized by a conical eyeball. A very rare complication is retinal detachment.

Many triggering factors contributing to the itch are sweat and heat, irritants such as wool clothing, exposure to cigarette smoke, and aeroallergens such as dust mites. Specific allergens may cause flare-ups of the dermatitis and may occur by way of contact, inhalation, ingestion, or injection [61]. Due to defects in innate and acquired immune responses in patients who have atopic dermatitis, patients have an increased susceptibility to bacterial, fungal, and viral infections [62]. Atopics are prone to staphylococcal colonization, which may lead to chronic anterior blepharitis when the colonization occurs on the eyelid. A subset of atopics may be sensitive to allergens expressed by the yeast *Malasezzia furfur* [62]. In addition, atopics are more commonly affected by contact dermatitis [63].

Contact dermatitis

Acute, subacute, and chronic

Contact dermatitis is the most common cutaneous eruption of the eyelids. The eyelid is prone to contact dermatitis because it is thin, pliable, and soft [64]. Contact dermatitis is also categorized according to its evolution into acute, subacute, and chronic forms. Acute contact dermatitis of the eyelid is characterized by itchy, erythematous, vesicular or papular inflammation. The subacute forms are [65] less vesicular and red and start to become more thickened and scaly. Chronic contact dermatitis is dry, thick, lichenified, more scaly, and usually less pruritic.

Epidemiology

Allergic contact dermatitis has been considered the most common of the many dermatologic conditions found with eyelid dermatitis [63]. In a retrospective study of 203 patients who had persistent or recurrent eyelid dermatitis, 74% were found to have relevant contact dermatitis. In a study of 1781 patients diagnosed with contact dermatitis over a 6-year period, 4.2% had allergy to cosmetic products.

Another retrospective analysis studied 1554 patients diagnosed as having conjunctivitis with or without dermatitis on the eyelids. Fifty-six percent [66] had a positive reaction to at least one of the contact allergens tested. The main sources were topical pharmaceutic products (antibiotics, corticosteroids), cosmetics (fragrance components, preservatives, emulsifiers, hair care and nail products), metals (nickel), rubber derivatives, resins (eg, epoxy resin), and plants [67].

In the 2003–2004 data of the North American Contact Dermatitis Group (NACDG) [68], 268 patients were found to have a final diagnosis of allergic contact dermatitis of the eyelids alone. Gold was the most frequently encountered etiology (12.5%).

Irritant versus allergic

Contact dermatitis may be categorized as irritant or allergic. Irritant contact dermatitis is more common and develops secondary to the application of an irritating substance. Irritant contact dermatitis is a more diffuse, less well defined area of inflammation that develops depending on strength and concentration of the substance, duration of contact, condition of the eyelid before contact (eg, the presence of fissures or prior inflammation), and individual susceptibility. Allergic contact dermatitis is secondary to delayed hypersensitivity reaction to the substance that is T-cell mediated and occurs after previous sensitization. Patients who develop allergic contact dermatitis are genetically predisposed with an atopic background. The appearance and distribution of the inflammation correspond to the area of contact (eg, cosmetics used on the eyelids) but may be more diffuse due to rubbing of the eyelids with the material (eg, nail polish) and occur more rapidly within 12 to 24 hours after a period of prior sensitization. Although irritant and allergic contact dermatitis have some characteristics that distinguish one from the other, they are not always readily distinguishable [66].

Etiologies

In general, rhus (poison ivy) and chrysanthemums are the most common causes of allergic contact dermatitis. For the eyelids, a common substance causing allergic contact dermatitis is nail polish coming in contact with the eyelid through scratching. Important sources of contact dermatitis include nickel (from glasses, jewelry, metal eyelash curlers), cosmetics, fragrances, contact lens solutions, and topical medications such as corticosteroids and neomycin, or preservatives such as formaldehyde resin and benzalkonium chloride [54,63]. There is also airborne contact dermatitis, caused by things such as pollen, dust mites, animal dander, and chemicals suspended in the air. The eyelids are particularly predisposed to airborne contact dermatitis because they are exposed and materials may lodge and get deposited on the upper eyelids.

One meta-analysis showed that nickel (14.7% of tested patients), thimerosal (5.0%), cobalt (4.8%), fragrance mix (3.4%), and balsam of Peru (3.0%) are the most prevalent allergens, whereas the five least prevalent allergens are paraben mix (0.5%), black rubber mix (0.6%), quaternium-15 (0.6%), quinoline mix (0.7%), and caine mix (0.7%). NACDG data, however, show that the five most prevalent allergens are nickel (14.3%), fragrance mix (14%), neomycin (11.6%), balsam of Peru (10.4%), and thimerosal (10.4%) [69].

Cosmetics

Cosmetic alteration of a patient's orbital skin is a common reason for professional consultation [70]. The NACDG conducted a study in 13,216 patients and found contact dermatitis related to cosmetics in 5%. These figures are believed to underestimate the total number of cases because most reactions thought to be trivial are not investigated [69].

The most common cause of contact dermatitis of the eyelids is cosmetics applied to the hair, face, or fingernails rather than to those applied to the actual eye area [66]. Hence, nail polish applied to nails and hair dye applied to the hair and scalp are common causes of eyelid contact dermatitis. Ectopic dermatitis occurs when the primary area of application causes the eruption in another area. Other cosmetics that come in contact with the eyes and may cause eczema are facial creams, foundations, and blush. Eye makeup such as mascara, eye shadow, and eyeliner can cause burning and itch in predisposed individuals. Irritation may also develop from propylene glycol and soap emulsifiers or from volatile components such as mineral spirits, isoparaffins, and alcohol [66].

The common ingredients in cosmetics causing contact dermatitis of the eyelid include various pigments, fragrances, resins, additives, nickel, emulsifiers, preservatives, and vehicles. Examples include parabens, phenyl mercuric acetate, imidazolidinyl urea, quaternium-15, potassium sorbate, antioxidants, butylated hydroxyanisole, butylated hydroxytoluene di-tert-butylhydroquinone, colophony, bismuth oxychloride, emollients, lanolin, and propylene glycol [65,71].

p-Phenylenediamine (PPD) is the most frequent sensitizer in hair dyes and semipermanent henna tattooing. It can cause marked edema of the eyelids. Recent reports have shown PPD to cause contact dermatitis secondary to use in permanent eyeliners, or dye in eyelash and eyebrow creams [72,73]. Hair loss developed in one patient secondary to PPD in tinting mascara [74].

Parabens, phenyl mercuric acetate, imidazolidinyl urea, and quaternium-15 are preservatives used to decrease contamination of the cosmetics. Quaternium-15 and imidazolidinyl urea may induce hypersensitivity reactions by the released formaldehyde [75]. To decrease exposure to parabens, potassium sorbate has been used in formulations, but cases of sensitization to sorbic acid have also been reported [76]. Not all individuals who are sensitive to parabens have to avoid it altogether. Some are able to apply parabens-containing products if the underlying skin is intact and devoid of any abnormality or inflammation.

Tetrahydracurcumin derived from extracts of the root of the *Curcuma longa* plant, also known as turmeric, has been found in cosmetics used for skin lightening and protection against UV-B and in antiaging preparations [77]. Sunscreen agents and fragrances can also cause photoallergic dermatitis, in which exposure to the UV light is required for the development of contact dermatitis.

In general, cosmetics are manufactured such that potential irritants are usually weak, especially if they are to be placed in the eye area [66]. The cosmetics industry must ensure that it maintains standards to make products safe for topical application and accidental insertion into the eye [64].

Irritation due to mascara and eye cosmetic preservatives

Mascara is water based or waterproof. Water-based mascara contains emulsifiers such as sodium borate and ammonium stearate, which are irritating to the conjunctiva. Cases of allergic contact dermatitis to shellac in mascara have been reported [78].

Allergic contact dermatitis has been reported after exposure to resin (colophony) [79] and dihydroabietyl alcohol (Abitol) [80,81], which are contained in some mascara products.

In eye shadow makeup, allergies have been reported secondary to ditertiarybutyl hydroquinone, which is an antioxidant; yellow D & C No. 11 dye [82]; and diisopropanolamine, which is used in cosmetic gloss formulas [66]. A special removal product for waterproof eye makeup containing surfactants such as cocamidopropyl betaine has caused allergic contact dermatitis [83]. In these patients, it is recommended that they avoid waterproof products [64].

Fragrance

As per the 2001–2002 report of the NACDG [83], fragrance mix is the fourth most frequent patch-test positive reaction (10.4%) compared with reactions to nickel (16.7%), neomycin (11.6%), balsam of Peru (11.6%), gold (10.2%), and quaternium-15 (9.3%).

Irritation due to conjunctival deposition

The conjunctivae could be irritated by inadvertent deposition of cosmetics such as eyeliner and mascara into the eye. The pigment could cause discoloration of the conjunctiva, discomfort, tearing, and itching or the patient may not be bothered by such deposition of cosmetics and any irritation may go away spontaneously.

Artificial eyelashes may cause irritation secondary to the natural or synthetic fibers or to the adhesive used to attach them to the lids. The adhesive is a mixture of rubber latex, cellulose gums, casein solubilized with alkali or other resins, and water. Although no reports have documented that the rubber latex in the adhesive has caused latex hypersensitivity, there have been reports of latex sensitivity to rubber used in older forms of eyelash curlers [66].

Nail polish

The main allergen responsible for nail polish contact dermatitis is toluene sulfonamide formaldehyde resin (TSFR) [84]. "Hypoallergenic" nail polish has been manufactured, whereby a polyester resin replaces the TSFR. There have been a few cases of contact dermatitis caused by phthalic anhydride/trimellitic anhydride/glycols copolymer, which is not available for patch testing, but contact dermatitis can be diagnosed using patch testing of the varnish itself [85]. One should note that the dermatitis from nail lacquer is not found on the nails and the surrounding nail fold, which are thicker, more resistant areas. Some reactions have occurred with artificial nails containing cyanoacrylate or methacrylates [86].

Metals

Nickel and mercury are well-recognized contact allergens. Nickel is the most common positive patch test. The exposure to nickel is common due to the use of fancy jewelry and accessories. Stainless steel products are recommended in susceptible individuals in whom nickel-plated eyelash curlers and tweezers may cause reactions [66]. Mercury is found in thimerosal, a commonly used antiseptic or preservative in vaccines and topical medications. Mercury is also found in dental amalgam and in thermometers. Gold and palladium have been detected as contactants and have been included in patch-test screening trays. Cobalt is another possible etiologic agent. Cobalt and palladium allergy may be associated with nickel allergy [87].

Aeroallergens

There have been reported cases of contact dermatitis secondary to airborne contactants [66]. Dermatitis can occur from exposure to burning poison ivy. Other contact allergens that are airborne and cause eyelid dermatitis are insecticides, animal dander, and dust mites [63], household sprays, and occupational volatile chemicals. Other reported causes are household products such as oil of lemon peel and dyes of Florida orange skin, and phosphorous sesquisulfide in "strike anywhere" matches used to light wood fireplaces [88,89].

Medications/eyedrops/contact lens solution

Many topical medications have been reported to cause hypersensitivity of the eyelids and conjunctivae. Neomycin sulfate, which is used for treatment of conjunctivitis, is a common contactant [90]. Lack of resolution or worsening of the condition should raise the suspicion of contact dermatitis.

Allergens identified in topical ophthalmics include antibiotics, antivirals, β-blockers, mydriatics, anesthetics, and preservatives such as benzalkonium chloride, thimerosal, and phenylmercuric acetate [88]. Medicated eye drops and contact lens solutions may contain ingredients that have the potential for irritation or sensitization, leading to eyelid dermatitis, conjunctivitis, or both. Benzalkonium chloride and thimerosal (commonly used preservatives in ophthalmic solutions) may lead to dermatitis [91]. Contact allergy to sodium metabisulfite has been reported rarely so far, leading to the increasing use of this agent as a preservative by manufacturers of cosmetics and medications [92]. An alternative preservative is chlorobutanol, which is rarely sensitizing. Patients who are very sensitive could opt to use preservative-free solutions. Topical medications used for glaucoma have been documented to cause contact dermatitis. A prostaglandin F2 alpha analog called latanoprost used to lower intraocular pressure has been described to cause sensitization. It was reported to cause pruritus, erythema, swelling, and erosions of the eyelids, especially in the elderly, and symptoms can appear several months after therapy [93]. Propine, containing epinephrine hydrochloride, also used to treat glaucoma, has caused patch test–proven ocular hypersensitivity [94].

Paper

Perfume, formaldehyde, or benzalkonium chloride found on facial tissues has been found to produce dermatitis in sensitized individuals. In persons sensitized to formaldehyde, dermatitis could be caused by contact with newsprint and carbon paper products [66].

Plants

Sensitizing plants in cosmetics are tea tree oil, arnica, chamomile, yarrow, citrus extracts, common ivy, aloe, lavender, peppermint, and others. The sensitizing potential of these plants varies [95]. Toxicodendron species include poison ivy, poison oak, and poison sumac and are a cause of contact dermatitis affecting millions of Americans each year [96]. When the eyelids are affected, it can produce marked swelling with minimum dermatitis of the face [66]. The dermatitis may also affect other parts of the body that come in contact with the plant.

Histology

Histologically, eczema is generally characterized by the presence of spongiosis. Spongiosis refers to the increased intercellular edema in the epidermis resulting in the pulling away of the keratinocytes from their surrounding desmosomes. Hence, spongiosis is a pathologic nonspecific finding in contact dermatitis.

Diagnosis

Diagnosis is through clinical suspicion. A compatible history and examination is fundamental in the diagnosis and can be supported by patch testing. Patch testing for poison ivy is not necessary because history and clinical appearance are usually diagnostic. When the diagnosis is in question or the causative substance is unknown, patch testing may be used. The thin-layer rapid epicutaneous patch test is a commercially available Food and Drug Administration (FDA)-approved patch test panel and the global standard [69]. It is an easy diagnostic tool, with 24 patches containing 42 unique allergens and four complex mixtures [97]. The patch is applied on noninflamed skin, removed after 48 hours, and read by an experienced practitioner after 48 and 96 hours. Positive results range from 1 to +2 and depend on the presence of erythema, vesiculation, and induration. Irritant reactions caused by a direct toxic effect that occur after 48 hours should disappear by the fifth day, whereas allergic responses worsen.

There are many limitations to routine patch-test panels. Many possible contactants are not found on the FDA-approved panels available in the United States [54]. These panels contain only approximately 1.4% of the more than 3700 known allergens [97]. Comparison with data from the NACDG suggests that clinically important allergens may be missed by the TRUE test [69]. Hence, due to the difficulty in determining the etiology of eyelid dermatitis with routine patch testing, open and closed patch testing can be performed "as is" with eye cosmetics if liquid cosmetics such as mascara and certain eyeliners are allowed to dry before occlusion [64]. Furthermore, the fragrance mix detects only 70% of perfume-allergic patients and causes false-positive and false-negative reactions [98]. A big problem is the relative lack of information on some of the new ingredients that have been used in hundreds of marketed cosmetic formulations [99]. To assist the clinician in making a diagnosis, Cosmetic Industry On Call [100] provides information to assist in contacting manufacturers who may provide the ingredients necessary for patch testing. Reference information on the chemical concentrations and vehicles to use to test cosmetics ingredients is provided by de Groot and colleagues [101].

Herpes simplex

Herpes simplex is a viral infection caused by herpes simplex virus (HSV) 1 and 2. Herpes simplex may be primary or recurrent. The first or primary infection is usually more severe. On resolution of the primary infection, the virus remains in a latent or dormant phase in the sensory ganglia. For the eyelid, this is the trigeminal or superior cervical ganglion. Recurrent disease occurs with reactivation of the virus, which travels back to the skin from the nerve fiber. These recurrences may be triggered by stress, infections, immunosuppression, UV light, trauma, cold wind, or menstruation. Infection of the eye could involve the periorbital skin, the conjunctiva, or cornea. Typical lesions on the eyelid are grouped vesicles on an erythematous base ("dewdrops on a rose petal") associated with itch and burning with or without ocular involvement. Lesions on the cornea or conjunctiva manifest as erosions or superficial ulcers. With recurrent disease, deeper erosions and stromal keratitis can develop. Untreated infection could lead to herpes simplex keratitis, which is regarded as the leading cause of infectious blindness in the United States [102].

A Tzanck test can be performed to make a quick diagnosis of herpes simplex. It entails scraping the floor of an intact vesicle and examining it under the microscope after staining with Wright's or Giemsa stain. The presence of multinucleated giant cells is considered positive for herpes infection. A more accurate tool is the use of viral culture or testing for herpes simplex antibodies in serum.

Herpes lesions typically improve in 7 to 10 days, but recurrences are common. In immunosuppressed individuals, lesions are more severe, more frequent, harder to treat, and may become disseminated.

Herpes zoster

Herpes zoster, also known as shingles, is caused by varicella-zoster virus. It commonly presents initially as pain followed by a unilateral rash in a dermatomal distribution. The rash begins as erythematous papules that become vesicular and sometimes pustular over an erythematous patch. In immune-competent patients, the eruptions last between 2 and 4 weeks; however, postherpetic neuralgia is a common problem, especially in the elderly. Trigeminal neuralgia, which may occur with ophthalmic zoster, can recur months to years after the resolution of the active lesions and can range in intensity from mild to severe and disabling. Atypical lesions, more severe eruption, and bilateral involvement may occur in immunocompromised individuals.

Vesicles found on the tip or side of the nose, called the Hutchinson's sign, is a clue that the eyes will be affected [103]. These early skin lesions should alert the physician to treat aggressively to prevent potential vision loss. In herpes zoster involving the eyes, or herpes zoster ophthalmicus, about half of the patients have ocular involvement such as conjunctivitis or keratitis.

Clinical diagnosis is usually adequate if a typical eruption is discovered. A Tzanck test showing multinucleated giant cells assists in the diagnosis. Serum antibody testing for herpes zoster antibodies or viral culture differentiates it from herpes simplex.

Treatment considerations for the eyelids

Eyelid dermatitis

Whenever appropriate, finding and eliminating an identifiable cause is the main goal of therapy. Prevention is key. For example, for contact dermatitis, avoidance of the contactant is essential. For cases in which cosmetics play a role in the eyelid dermatitis, Draelos [64] recommended that cosmetics for patients who have eyelid dermatitis be formulated with a paucity of ingredients, an absence of sensitizers, a minimum number of irritants, and no cutaneous sensory or vasodilatory stimulants.

Saline compresses and baby shampoo wiped gently on the affected areas are safe and mild remedies used to help alleviate the scaling and crusting of blepharitis. For SD lesions, topical antifungal creams, shampoos, and lotions are used with much improvement [5]. Antidandruff shampoos that have fungistatic ingredients such as selenium sulfide and zinc pyrithione are advised for regular use on active lesions and two to three times a week to prevent eruptions. Systemic antifungals and antibiotics (erythromycin or tetracycline) are reserved for severe infections, superinfection, or persistent inflammation.

Management of eyelid dermatitis (contact dermatitis, atopic dermatitis, SD) includes improvement of inflammation using corticosteroids. This treatment should be used with caution because the eyelids are very thin and become more prone to side effects of topical steroids such as thinning of the skin, visible blood vessels, and more serious ocular side effects such as glaucoma and cataracts with chronic use, especially with high potency. Most inflammatory conditions respond to topical corticosteroids. Possible side effects of steroids used on the eyelids include atrophy, telangiectasias, glaucoma, cataract formation, and risk of infection [104]. The mildest and nonfluorinated steroids should be used and only for a brief period of time [105,106]. The potential for side effects increases with the longer use of higher potency steroids. For severe cases, oral steroids may be warranted.

In light of the side effects of steroids, more physicians now prescribe the newer topical calcineurin inhibitors (TCIs)—pimecrolimus (Elidel) or tacrolimus (Protopic). TCIs cause minimal systemic absorption [107,108] and have a low incidence of side effects such as local burning, stinging, and itching [109,110]. They can be used for longer periods of time. TCIs help decrease the inflammatory features of dermatitis and decrease the need for steroids, which have many side effects when applied chronically and on thin skin such as the eyelids [111,112]. The safety of the TCIs in children younger than 2 years is controversial [8].

Measures to avoid itching are of utmost value to prevent the itch–scratch cycle associated with atopic dermatitis. Cold compresses alleviate the sensation of itch. Because histamine is not the cause of the inflammation or itch, antihistamines are not recommended, apart from the use of sedating antihistamines to help the patient fall asleep. When identified, triggering factors such as irritants, tobacco smoke, and exposure to aeroallergens should be avoided.

Infections

Infections of the eyelids are treated according to the etiology. A culture or eye swab is recommended to confirm the diagnosis. Use topical (eg, mupirocin, polysporin) or oral antibiotics for bacterial infections such as pyodermas. Use antivirals (oral acyclovir, valacyclovir) for viral infections such as herpes simplex and herpes zoster.

Treatment for herpes simplex should be started early, within the first 2 days of the infection. The treatment of choice is systemic antivirals such as acyclovir or valacyclovir. Topical acyclovir (Zovirax) can be used for herpes keratitis, in which the infection is confined to the epithelium [113]. Topical acyclovir, trifluridine, or vidarabine has been found to result in greater proportion of healing within 1 week of treatment compared with idoxuridine [102]. Corticosteroids can be added for herpetic stromal disease and iritis. Ocular HSV disease can be treated with 12 months of acyclovir to reduce the recurrence of ocular and orofacial HSV. This long-term prophylaxis for patients who have a history of HSV stromal keratitis is important to prevent recurrences and visual loss [113].

Herpes zoster is treated with antivirals. Acyclovir should be started as early as possible, preferably within the first 72 hours (164,165). Starting treatment early has been shown to decrease the duration of the illness and decrease the risk of ocular and systemic complications [113]. Giving an oral steroid early in addition to antivirals is an option to improve the early quality of life in herpes zoster patients. Additional measures include symptomatic treatment of pain and prevention of secondary infection. The varicella-zoster virus vaccine is used for prevention of herpes zoster [114].

Warts may be transient infections but may spread, recur, and become difficult to treat. With this in mind, various treatment options have been tried with variable success [115]. Surgical measures include electrodessication, laser, and excision. Destructive modalities include cryotherapy, photodynamic therapy, salicylic acid, and trichloroacetic acid. These modalities have good results in destroying lesions. Other modalities include antiproliferative agents such as 5-fluorouracil, intralesional bleomycin, and podophyllin. Therapies targeting the immune system include interferons, imiquimod, and duct tape occlusion therapy [116].

Molluscum contagiosum may resolve spontaneously and may be left alone, especially in young children. Lesions may last 2 to 4 months, with autoinoculation causing more lesions to erupt. Most lesions resolve by 6 to 9 months, but others persist for longer periods up to few years. Conventional therapy relies on tissue destruction using modalities such as curettage, cryotherapy, carbon dioxide laser, electrodessication, trichloroacetic acid, and cantharidin. More recently, topical immune modulators have been used with some success [117,118].

Inflammation

Acne is treated with keratolytics such as tretinoin to loosen up the impacted keratinocytes. Alternatively, acne surgery using comedone extractors is a quick remedy to extract the contents of the follicle.

Treatment for rosacea was evaluated in a recent meta-analysis; however, the quality of the studies was generally poor [119,120]. There is evidence for the use of topical metronidazole and azelaic acid and some evidence for the use of oral metronidazole and tetracycline. Tetracycline or erythromycin is the primary treatment option for rosacea. The lesions that are thought to respond to this treatment include blepharitis, keratitis, and inflammatory papules and pustules. The efficacies of doxycycline and tetracycline, including treatment effect, optimal dose, duration of therapy, and side effects when used for ocular rosacea, have not been established [121]. Minocycline or doxycycline (100–200 mg/d) may be tried to decrease the blushing. Metronidazole (200 mg two times a day) is another option. Response is hard to predict. Some lesions clear in 2 to 4 weeks, whereas others require chronic suppression. Isotretinoin has been effective in severe refractory cases of rosacea. A newer treatment modality for rosacea is low-dose (40 mg) doxycycline monohydrate (Oracea), which is used as an anti-inflammatory agent, not as an antibiotic. The low dose allows for maintenance, with less chance for development of resistance [122]. It may be used alone or in combination with topical metronidazole [123]. Topical therapy may be used for mild rosacea or for maintenance. Topical metronidazole (Metrogel) 0.75% or

1% is commonly used [124]. It may exert its effect by inhibiting the neutro-phil-induced oxidative injury. Clindamycin is another option for topical application, especially for pustular lesions. Use of 15% azelaic acid showed a clear improvement, as rated by physicians and patients [123]. Sulfur/sulfa-cetamide lotion also controls pustules. These topical creams may be used alone for milder disease or in combination with oral antibiotics. Lack of response to antibiotics may be due to demodex infestation or tinea, which can be confirmed using potassium hydroxide smear and be treated with crotamiton, lindane, sulfur/salicylic acid lotions.

For ocular rosacea, lid hygiene is important. Warm compresses and gentle massage of the tarsal plate help to decrease the lipid secretions from the meibomian glands. For dry eyes that may accompany ocular rosa-cea, artificial tears are effective. Bacterial overgrowth on the lids is treated with topical antibiotics. Inflammatory lesions respond to steroid applica-tions used for short durations to avoid telangiectasias and other local effects of steroids.

Urticaria and angiodema

In the more acute forms in which an identifiable cause is known or sus-pected, avoidance is mainstay of treatment, followed by symptomatic relief of swelling with antihistamines and glucocorticoids. Therapy is more chal-lenging when a cause is not found despite extensive workup. Empiric ther-apy that includes H_1 with or without H_2 blockers may be effective. If the eruption is more chronic, control is sought with use of regular daily H_1 an-tihistamines, followed by the addition of other classes of H_1. Doxepin, a tri-cyclic antidepressant that has both H_1 and H_2 inhibition, has been a rewarding adjunctive therapy. Side effects of antihistamines such as som-nolence in the sedating types should be taken into consideration. Corticoste-roids and immune modulators may be tried in refractory and severe cases.

In the hereditary forms of angioedema, treatment is much different. Pro-phylactic treatment of the condition for long-term management and before surgical procedures includes the use of attenuated androgens (danazol) and antifibrinolytics (aminocaproic acid). Treatment with fresh frozen plasma and plasma-derived C1 inhibitor concentrate (available in Europe and in phase 3 trials in the United States) has been used for acute attacks. Newer treatment modalities that target specific elements of the complement or kinin pathways are being developed. Measures to replace C1 inhibitor with plasma-derived or recombinant C1 inhibitor and to inhibit bradykinin with a highly specific kallekrein inhibitor (ecallantide or DX-88) or a specific bradykinin-B2-receptor antagonist (Icatibant) are in development [125–128]. These treatments may prove effective in acute attacks and are being studied for their potential use as prophylaxis [129]. Rituximab has been tried for treatment of acquired angioedema associated with lymphoproliferative and autoimmune diseases [128].

Benign tumors and growths

Benign growths on the eyelids include milia, syringomas, chalazia, hordeola, moles, skin tags, and xanthelasmas. Milia are benign cysts that can be removed using a comedone extractor after being pricked with a blade tip or lancet. Application of mild pressure will allow extrusion of soft, white material. For those who do not want to undergo extraction, topical retinoids can be tried but have less success and should be used with caution around the eyelids because they are irritating. Patients seek treatment of syringomas for cosmetic purposes. Effective treatment methods include electrodessication and curettage or low-dose electrocoagulation [130]. More recently developed treatments consist of the use of lasers [131]. More than half of chalazia resolve spontaneously. Conservative management is through warm compresses. Some ophthalmologists inject steroids into the lesions that are not infected [42]. Drainage and excision (and cautery and curettage) may be done. These surgical procedures and injections have potential for hypopigmentation, atrophy, and disfigurement. Argon laser treatment is an interesting alternative technique, particularly in cases with cosmetic indications [132]. A hordeolum may be self-limiting and may drain spontaneously. Supportive measures include warm compresses or removal of an eyelash if the hordeolum is external. For more immediate relief of the infection, incision and drainage may be performed. If the infection spreads beyond the immediate area of the nodules, topical and systemic antibiotics are indicated.

Due to the benign nature of moles, no treatment is necessary. Patients seek removal for cosmetic reasons or because of irritation, interruption with normal function (eg, the mole may be in the line of vision), or suspicion that lesions are atypical or malignant. Surgical excision or lasers are used for removal of moles depending on the situation [43,133]. The use of Q-switched lasers has revolutionized the treatment of nevi of Ota [134–136]. Although good results may be achieved with laser ablation of these lesions, laser treatment modalities for congenital melanocytic nevi remains controversial because of the potential for malignancy [134].

Xanthelasmas may be removed with chemicals such as trichloroacetic acid or liquid nitrogen. They may be surgically excised or removed using lasers [21]. Despite successful treatment, lesions often recur.

Skin tags are benign growths commonly removed for cosmetic reasons or when function is impaired (such as lesions obstructing vision if occurring near the eyes). Simple surgical excision can be performed by way of curettage, cautery, snipping (when small or pedunculated), cryotherapy, or lasers. When lesions are atypical or the diagnosis is in doubt, histologic biopsy is recommended to rule out premalignant and malignant lesions such as melanoma.

Malignant tumors

A diagnostic biopsy assists in the proper evaluation. Surgical treatment of carcinomas may have good results. Smaller lesions may be treated with electrodessication and curettage. Larger lesions can be surgically excised or treated with cryosurgery, chemical surgery, radiotherapy. For areas that need more aggressive management such as large areas, those found in difficult locations such as around the medial and lateral canthi, or recurrent lesions, referral to a skilled Mohs' surgeon is recommended.

Despite rare metastasis of BCC, the tendency for local invasion warrants early intervention and removal. The overall cure rate is approximately 95%; however, despite excision, lesions seen arising from the medial canthus have been found to have a high recurrence rate (~60%) [137].

SCC has a higher rate of metastasis (up to 10%) such that a more aggressive approach is optimal. Immediate histologic monitoring of surgical margins with frozen sections or Mohs' micrographic surgery also allows for smaller margins of excision in an area where tissue conservation is important [138]. Mohs' surgery is the treatment of choice to ensure complete removal, especially in difficult-to-manage areas.

As with other cancers of the eyelid, wide local excision or Mohs' surgery is necessary for sebaceous carcinomas [139]. Prognosis is poor, with mortality second only to malignant melanoma. A clinicopathologic study of sebaceous carcinoma revealed the occurrence of death in 9% and mutilating exenteration in 23% of the patients studied [140].

Malignant melanomas metastasize, so early detection, excision, and evaluation for metastatic disease are of vital importance. Tumor thickness is an important predictor of prognosis. Margin control by mapped serial excision or by modified Mohs' micrographic surgery is a useful technique to ensure complete excision and minimization of local recurrence [49].

"Cosmetic" lesions of the eyelids

Vascular lesions

Due to the natural course of hemangiomas, they are usually left alone. Treatment is available when the lesions present cosmetic problems, affect surrounding organs, or interfere with normal functions. When sought, treatment for hemangiomas includes oral steroids, intralesional steroids [141], ultrapotent topical steroids [142], and laser [45,143].

Port-wine stains are cosmetic problems. Treatment is with the use of lasers. Alternatively, camouflage techniques (DermaBlend, CoverMark) may be used to cover the defect.

Vitiligo

Vitiligo involving the eyelids is best treated with cover-up measures. Cosmetic camouflaging agents such as DermaBlend and Covermark are available and can be chosen to match the patient's natural skin color. For localized vitiligo, topical corticosteroids are the preferred drugs. Extensive lesions over the body may be treated with topical or oral psoralens with UV-A light exposure (PUVA). In a recent double-blind randomized control trial, 56 patients who had nonsegmental vitiligo, narrow-band UV-B therapy was found to be superior to oral PUVA therapy [144,145]. Newer therapies include topical immunomodulators (tacrolimus, pimecrolimus), which display comparable effectiveness over steroids with fewer side effects; vitamin D analogs; surgical therapy or transplantation; laser therapy; L-phenylalanine therapy; and pseudocatalase [146].

Others

Dermatomyositis is hard to treat and is often resistant. The mainstay of treatment is corticosteroids that are tapered according to clinical response, creatine kinase levels, and side effect profile [147]. Inadequate response or need for steroid-sparing agents may prompt the use of hydroxychloroquine [148], dapsone [149], or immunomodulators such as methotrexate, azathioprine [150], cyclosporine [151], and mycophenolate mofetil [152].

References

[1] Kanitakis J. Anatomy, histology and immunohistochemistry of normal human skin. Eur J Dermatol 2002;12(4):390–9 [quiz: 400–1].

[2] Ha RY, Nojima K, Adams WP Jr, et al. Analysis of facial skin thickness: defining the relative thickness index. Plast Reconstr Surg 2005;115(6):1769–73.

[3] Fitzpatrick TB, Freedberg IM. Fitzpatrick's dermatology in general medicine. 6th edition. New York: McGraw-Hill; 2003, Medical Pub. Division. xxxi, p. 2594.

[4] Gupta AK, Madzia SE, Batra R. Etiology and management of seborrheic dermatitis. Dermatology 2004;208(2):89–93.

[5] Gupta AK, Batra R, Bluhm R, et al. Skin diseases associated with *Malassezia* species. J Am Acad Dermatol 2004;51(5):785–98.

[6] Gupta AK, Bluhm AR, Cooper EA, et al. Seborrheic dermatitis. Dermatol Clin 2003;21(3): 401–12.

[7] Rigopoulos D, Paparizos V, Katsambas A, et al. Cutaneous markers of HIV infection. Clin Dermatol 2004;22(6):487–98.

[8] Rallis E, Nasiopoulou A, Kouskoukis C, et al. Pimecrolimus cream 1% can be an effective treatment for seborrheic dermatitis of the face and trunk. Drugs Exp Clin Res 2004;30(5–6): 191–5.

[9] Sehgal VN, Srivastava G. Vitiligo: auto-immunity and immune responses. Int J Dermatol 2006;45(5):583–90.

[10] Ongenae K, Van Geel N, Naeyaert JM. Evidence for an autoimmune pathogenesis of vitiligo. Pigment Cell Res 2003;16(2):90–100.

[11] Barnes L. Vitiligo and the Vogt-Koyanagi-Harada syndrome. Dermatol Clin 1988;6(2): 229–39.

[12] Amerio P, Tracanna M, De Remigis P, et al. Vitiligo associated with other autoimmune diseases: polyglandular autoimmune syndrome types 3B+C and 4. Clin Exp Dermatol 2006; 31(5):746–9.

[13] Gould IM, Gray RS, Urbaniak SJ, et al. Vitiligo in diabetes mellitus. Br J Dermatol 1985; 113(2):153–5.

[14] Handa S, Kaur I. Vitiligo: clinical findings in 1436 patients. J Dermatol 1999;26(10): 653–7.

[15] Hwang SM, Ahn SK, Choi EH. Psoriasis occurring in amelanotic lesions. J Dermatol 1998; 25(1):66–7.

[16] Rubisz-Brzezinska J, Buchner SA, Itin P. Vitiligo associated with lichen planus. Is there a pathogenetic relationship? [see comment] Dermatology 1996;192(2):176–8.

[17] Lever WF, Elder DE. Lever's histopathology of the skin. 9th edition. Philadelphia: Lippincott Williams & Wilkins; 2005. xvi, p. 1229.

[18] Janis JF, Winkelmann RK. Histopathology of the skin in dermatomyositis. A histopathologic study of 55 cases. Arch Dermatol 1968;97(6):640–50.

[19] Habif TP. Clinical dermatology: a color guide to diagnosis and therapy. 3rd edition. St. Louis: Mosby; 1996. xii, p. 898.

[20] Bergma R. The pathogenesis and clinical significance of xanthelasma palpebrarum. J Am Acad Dermatol 1994;30(2 Pt 1):236–42.

[21] Rohrich RJ, Janis JE, Pownell PH. Xanthelasma palpebrarum: a review and current management principles. Plast Reconstr Surg 2002;110(5):1310–4.

[22] Scriver CR. The metabolic basis of inherited disease. 6th edition. New York: McGraw-Hill Information Services Co.,; 1989. Health Professions Division. 2 v. (xxviii 3006, 85 p.).

[23] Stawiski MA, Voorhees JJ. Cutaneous signs of diabetes mellitus. Cutis 1976;18(3):415–21.

[24] Varma JR. Skin tags:–a marker for colon polyps? J Am Board Fam Pract 1990;3(3):175–80.

[25] Piette AM, Meduri B, Fritsch J, et al. Do skin tags constitute a marker for colonic polyps? A prospective study of 100 asymptomatic patients and metaanalysis of the literature. Gastroenterology 1988;95(4):1127–9.

[26] Cox JT. Epidemiology and natural history of HPV. J Fam Pract 2006;(Suppl):3–9.

[27] Jackson R. Elderly and sun-affected skin. Distinguishing between changes caused by aging and changes caused by habitual exposure to sun. Can Fam Physician 2001;47:1236–43.

[28] Schepis C, Siragusa M, Palazzo R, et al. Palpebral syringomas and Down's syndrome. Dermatology 1994;189(3):248–50.

[29] Buechner SA. Rosacea: an update. Dermatology 2005;210(2):100–8.

[30] Roihu T, Kariniemi AL. Demodex mites in acne rosacea. J Cutan Pathol 1998;25(10): 550–2.

[31] Mannis MJ, Macsai MS, Huntley AC. Eye and skin disease. Philadelphia: 1996. Lippincott-Raven; xxiii, 705 p.

[32] Starr PA. Oculocutaneous aspects of rosacea. Proc R Soc Med 1969;62(1):9–11.

[33] Stone DU, Chodosh J. Ocular rosacea: an update on pathogenesis and therapy. Curr Opin Ophthalmol 2004;15(6):499–502.

[34] Ghanem VC, Mehra N, Wong S, et al. The prevalence of ocular signs in acne rosacea: comparing patients from ophthalmology and dermatology clinics. Cornea 2003;22(3):230–3.

[35] Bozda KE, Gul Y, Karaman A. Lipoid proteinosis. Int J Dermatol 2000;39(3):203–4.

[36] Thappa DM, Gupta S, Thappa DM, et al. Eyelid beading—a useful diagnostic clue for lipoid proteinosis. Indian Pediatr 2001;38(1):97.

[37] Sicherer SH, Sampson HA, Sicherer SH, et al. 9. Food allergy. J Allergy Clin Immunol 2006;117(2 Suppl Mini-Primer):S470–5.

[38] Wuthrich B, Wuthrich B. Food-induced cutaneous adverse reactions. Allergy 1998;53(46): 131–5.

[39] Executive summary of disease management of drug hypersensitivity: a practice parameter. Joint Task Force on Practice Parameters of the American Academy of Allergy, Asthma and Immunology, the American College of Allergy, Asthma and Immunology and the Joint Council of Allergy, Asthma and Immunology. Ann Allergy Asthma Immunol 1999; 83(6 Pt 3):665–700.

[40] Golden DB, Golden DBK. Stinging insect allergy. Am Fam Physician 2003;67(12):2541–6.

[41] Byrd JB, Adam A, Brown NJ, et al. Angiotensin-converting enzyme inhibitor-associated angioedema. Immunol Allergy Clin North Am 2006;26(4):725–37.

[42] Ben Simon GJ, Huang L, Nakra T, et al. Intralesional triamcinolone acetonide injection for primary and recurrent chalazia: is it really effective? [see comment] Ophthalmology 2005; 112(5):913–7.

[43] Greve B, Raulin C. [Medical dermatologic laser therapy. A review]. Hautarzt 2003;54(7): 594–602 [in German].

[44] van de Kerkhof PC, de Rooij M, Steijlen PM. Spontaneous course of hemangiomas: facts and speculations. Int J Dermatol 1998;37(2):101–2.

[45] Lindgren G, Diffey BL, Larko O. Basal cell carcinoma of the eyelids and solar ultraviolet radiation exposure. Br J Ophthalmol 1998;82(12):1412–5.

[46] Cook BE Jr, Bartley GB. Epidemiologic characteristics and clinical course of patients with malignant eyelid tumors in an incidence cohort in Olmsted County, Minnesota. Ophthalmology 1999;106(4):746–50.

[47] Rishi K, Font RL. Sebaceous gland tumors of the eyelids and conjunctiva in the Muir-Torre syndrome: a clinicopathologic study of five cases and literature review [see comment] [erratum appears in Ophthal Plast Reconstr Surg. 2004 May;11(5):953]. Ophthal Plast Reconstr Surg 2004;20(1):31–6.

[48] Garner A, Koornneef L, Levene A, et al. Malignant melanoma of the eyelid skin: histopathology and behaviour. Br J Ophthalmol 1985;69(3):180–6.

[49] Chan FM, O'Donnell BA, Whitehead K, et al. Treatment and outcomes of malignant melanoma of the eyelid: a review of 29 cases in Australia. Ophthalmology 2007;114(1): 187–92.

[50] Zug KA, Palay DA, Rock B. Dermatologic diagnosis and treatment of itchy red eyelids. Surv Ophthalmol 1996;40(4):293–306.

[51] Svensson A, Moller H. Eyelid dermatitis: the role of atopy and contact allergy. Contact Dermatitis 1986;15(3):178–82.

[52] Nethercott JR, Nield G, Holness DL. A review of 79 cases of eyelid dermatitis. J Am Acad Dermatol 1989;21(2 Pt 1):223–30.

[53] Valsecchi R, Imberti G, Martino D, et al. Eyelid dermatitis: an evaluation of 150 patients. Contact Dermatitis 1992;27(3):143–7.

[54] Amin KA, Belsito DV. The aetiology of eyelid dermatitis: a 10-year retrospective analysis. Contact Dermatitis 2006;55(5):280–5.

[55] Browning DJ, Proia AD. Ocular rosacea. Surv Ophthalmol 1986;31(3):145–58.

[56] Guin JD. Eyelid dermatitis: a report of 215 patients. Contact Dermatitis 2004;50(2): 87–90.

[57] Ayala F, Fabbrocini G, Bacchilega R, et al. Eyelid dermatitis: an evaluation of 447 patients. Am J Contact Dermat 2003;14(2):69–74.

[58] Hanifin JM, Lobitz WC Jr. Newer concepts of atopic dermatitis. Arch Dermatol 1977; 113(5):663–70.

[59] Leung DY. Role of IgE in atopic dermatitis. Curr Opin Immunol 1993;5(6):956–62.

[60] Wahlgren CF, Hagermark O, Bergstrom R. Patients' perception of itch induced by histamine, compound 48/80 and wool fibres in atopic dermatitis. Acta Derm Venereol 1991; 71(6):488–94.

[61] O'Donnell BF, Foulds IS. Contact allergic dermatitis and contact urticaria due to topical ophthalmic preparations. Br J Ophthalmol 1993;77(11):740–1.

[62] Baker BS. The role of microorganisms in atopic dermatitis. Clin Exp Immunol 2006;144(1): 1–9.

[63] Guin JD. Eyelid dermatitis: experience in 203 cases. J Am Acad Dermatol 2002;47(5): 755–65.

[64] Draelos ZD. Special considerations in eye cosmetics. Clin Dermatol 2001;19(4):424–30.

[65] de Groot AC. Contact allergy to cosmetics: causative ingredients. Contact Dermatitis 1987; 17(1):26–34.

[66] Bielory L. Contact dermatitis of the eyelids. Immunol Allergy Clin North Am 1997;17(1): 131–8.

[67] Goossens A. Contact allergic reactions on the eyes and eyelids. Bull Soc Belge Ophtalmol 2004;(292):11–7.

[68] Rietschel RL, Warshaw EM, Sasseville D, et al. Common contact allergens associated with eyelid dermatitis: data from the North American Contact Dermatitis Group 2003–2004 study period. Dermatitis 2007;18(2):78–81.

[69] Krob HA, Fleischer AG Jr, D'Agostino R, et al. Prevalence and relevance of contact dermatitis allergens: a meta-analysis of 15 years of published T.R.U.E. test data. J Am Acad Dermatol 2004;51(3):349–53.

[70] Beltrani VS. Eyelid dermatitis. Curr Allergy Asthma Rep 2001;1(4):380–8.

[71] Groot ACd, Weyland JW, Nater JP. Unwanted effects of cosmetics and drugs used in dermatology. 3rd edition. Amsterdam; New York: Elsevier; 1994. xii 770 p.

[72] Hansson C, Weyland JW, Nater NP, et al. Allergic contact dermatitis from 2-chloro-p-phenylenediamine in a cream dye for eyelashes and eyebrows. Contact Dermatitis 2001;45(4): 235–6.

[73] Teixeira M, de Wachter L, Ronsyn E, et al. Contact allergy to para-phenylenediamine in a permanent eyelash dye. Contact Dermatitis 2006;55(2):92–4.

[74] Wachsmuth R, Wilkinson M. Loss of eyelashes after use of a tinting mascara containing PPD. Contact Dermatitis 2006;54(3):169–70.

[75] Fisher AA. Allergic contact dermatitis from Germall 115, a new cosmetic preservative. Contact Dermatitis 1975;1(2):126.

[76] Fisher AA, Fisher AA. Cutaneous reactions to sorbic acid and potassium sorbate. Cutis 1980;25(4):350.

[77] Thompson DA, Tan BB. Tetrahydracurcumin-related allergic contact dermatitis. Contact Dermatitis 2006;55(4):254–5.

[78] Le Coz CJ, Leclere JM, Arnoult E, et al. Allergic contact dermatitis from shellac in mascara. Contact Dermatitis 2002;46(3):149–52.

[79] Fisher AA, Fisher AA. Allergic contact dermatitis due to rosin (colophony) in eyeshadow and mascara. Cutis 1988;42(6):507–8.

[80] Rapaport MJ, Rapaport MJ. Sensitization to Abitol. Contact Dermatitis 1980;6(2):137.

[81] Dooms-Goossens A, Degreef G, Luytens E, et al. Dihydroabietyl alcohol (Abitol): a sensitizer in mascara. Contact Dermatitis 1979;5(6):350–3.

[82] Calnan CD, Calnan CD. Quinazoline yellow SS in cosmetics. Contact Dermatitis 1976;2(3): 160–6.

[83] Pratt MD, Belsito DV, DeLeo VA, et al. North American Contact Dermatitis Group patch-test results, 2001–2002 study period. Dermatitis 2004;15(4):176–83.

[84] Panati C. Extraordinary origins of everyday things. 1st edition. New York: Harper & Row; 1987. xi 463.

[85] Nassif AS, Le Coz CJ, Collet E. A rare nail polish allergen: phthalic anhydride, trimellitic anhydride and glycols copolymer. Contact Dermatitis 2007;56(3):172–3.

[86] Guin JD, Guin JD. Eyelid dermatitis from methacrylates used for nail enhancement. Contact Dermatitis 1998;39(6):312–3.

[87] Garner LA, Garner LA. Contact dermatitis to metals. Dermatol Ther 2004;17(4):321–7.

[88] Herbst RA, Maibach HI, Herbst RA, et al. Allergic contact dermatitis from ophthalmics: update 1997. Contact Dermatitis 1997;37(5):252–3.

[89] Burge SM, Powell SM, Burge SM, et al. Contact urticaria to phosphorus sesquisulphide. Contact Dermatitis 1983;9(5):424.

[90] Prystowsky SD, Allen AM, Smith RW, et al. Allergic contact hypersensitivity to nickel, neomycin, ethylenediamine, and benzocaine. Relationships between age, sex, history of exposure, and reactivity to standard patch tests and use tests in a general population. Arch Dermatol 1979;115(8):959–62.

[91] van Ketel WG, Melzer-van Riemsdijk FA, van Ketel WG, et al. Conjunctivitis due to soft lens solutions. Contact Dermatitis 1980;6(5):321–4.

[92] Seitz CS, Brocker EB, Trautmannn A, et al. Eyelid dermatitis due to sodium metabisulfite. Contact Dermatitis 2006;55(4):249–50.

[93] Lai CH, Lai IC, Chi CC, et al. Allergic contact dermatitis caused by latanoprost ophthalmic solution. Eur J Ophthalmol 2006;16(4):627–9.

[94] Gaspari AA, Gaspari AA. Contact allergy to ophthalmic dipivalyl epinephrine hydrochloride: demonstration by patch testing. Contact Dermatitis 1993;28(1):35–7.

[95] Schempp CM, Schopf E, Simon JC, et al. [Plant-induced toxic and allergic dermatitis (phytodermatitis)]. Hautarzt 2002;53(2):93–7 [in German].

[96] Gladman AC, Gladman AC. Toxicodendron dermatitis: poison ivy, oak, and sumac. Wilderness Environ Med 2006;17(2):120–8.

[97] Belsito DV, Belsito DV. Patch testing with a standard allergen ("screening") tray: rewards and risks. Dermatol Ther 2004;17(3):231–9.

[98] de Groot AC, Frosch PJ, de Groot AC, et al. Adverse reactions to fragrances. A clinical review. Contact Dermatitis 1997;36(2):57–86.

[99] Barker MO. Newer cosmetic ingredients:–new patch testing problems? Am J Contact Dermat 1998;9(2):130–5.

[100] Cosmetic Toiletry and Fragrance Association. Cosmetic industry on call. Washington, DC: Cosmetic, Toiletry, and Fragrance Association; 1982. p. 38.

[101] de Groot AC, van Ginkel CJ, Weijland JW, et al. [Statement of ingredients of cosmetics]. Ned Tijdschr Geneeskd 1997;141(36):1747–8 [in Dutch].

[102] Pepose JS, Holland GN, Wilhelmus KR. Ocular infection & immunity. St. Louis: Mosby; 1996. xl. 1552 p.

[103] Zaal MJ, Volker-Dieben HJ, D'Amaro J. Prognostic value of Hutchinson's sign in acute herpes zoster ophthalmicus. Graefes Arch Clin Exp Ophthalmol 2003;241(3): 187–91.

[104] Turpeinen M, Salo OP, Leisti S, et al. Effect of percutaneous absorption of hydrocortisone on adrenocortical responsiveness in infants with severe skin disease. Br J Dermatol 1986; 115(4):475–84.

[105] Hoare C, Li Wan Po A, Williams H, et al. Systematic review of treatments for atopic eczema. Health Technol Assess 2000;4(37):1–191.

[106] Del Rosso J, Friedlander SF, Del Rosso J, et al. Corticosteroids: options in the era of steroid-sparing therapy. J Am Acad Dermatol 2005;53(1 Suppl 1):S50–8.

[107] Staab D, Pariser D, Gottlieb AB, et al. Low systemic absorption and good tolerability of pimecrolimus, administered as 1% cream (Elidel) in infants with atopic dermatitis: a multicenter, 3-week, open-label study. Pediatr Dermatol 2005;22(5):465–71.

[108] Harper J, Smith C, Rubins A, et al. A multicenter study of the pharmacokinetics of tacrolimus ointment after first and repeated application to children with atopic dermatitis. J Invest Dermatol 2005;124(4):695–9.

[109] Reitamo S, Rustin M, Ruzicka T, et al. Efficacy and safety of tacrolimus ointment compared with that of hydrocortisone butyrate ointment in adult patients with atopic dermatitis. J Allergy Clin Immunol 2002;109(3):547–55.

[110] Housman TS, Norton AB, Feldman SR, et al. Tacrolimus ointment: utilization patterns in children under age 2 years. Dermatol Online J 2004;10(1):2.

[111] Boguniewicz M, Fiedler VC, Raimer S, et al. A randomized, vehicle-controlled trial of tacrolimus ointment for treatment of atopic dermatitis in children. Pediatric Tacrolimus Study Group [see comment]. J Allergy Clin Immunol 1998;102(4 Pt 1):637–44.

[112] Fonacier L, Spergel J, Charlesworth EN, et al. Report of the Topical Calcineurin Inhibitor Task Force of the American College of Allergy, Asthma and Immunology and the American Academy of Allergy, Asthma and Immunology. J Allergy Clin Immunol 2005;115(6): 1249–53.

[113] Kaufman HE. Treatment of viral diseases of the cornea and external eye. Prog Retin Eye Res 2000;19(1):69–85.

[114] Liesegang TJ, Liesegang TJ. Herpes zoster virus infection. Curr Opin Ophthalmol 2004; 15(6):531–6.

[115] Gibbs S, Harvey I, Gibbs S, et al. Topical treatments for cutaneous warts [update of Cochrane Database Syst Rev 2003;(3):CD001781; PMID: 12917913]. Cochrane Database Syst Rev 2006;3:CD001781.
[116] Snoeck R. Papillomavirus and treatment. Antiviral Res 2006;71(2–3):181–91.
[117] Hanson D, Diven DG. Molluscum contagiosum. Dermatol Online J 2003;9(2):2.
[118] Smith KJ, Skelton H. Molluscum contagiosum: recent advances in pathogenic mechanisms, and new therapies. Am J Clin Dermatol 2002;3(8):535–45.
[119] van Zuuren EJ, Gupta AK, Gover MD, et al. Systematic review of rosacea treatments. J Am Acad Dermatol 2007;56(1):107–15.
[120] van Zuuren EJ, Graber MA, Hollis S, et al. Interventions for rosacea [update of Cochrane Database Syst Rev 2004;(1):CD003262; PMID: 14974010]. Cochrane Database Syst Rev 2005;(3):CD003262.
[121] Stone DU, Chodosh J. Oral tetracyclines for ocular rosacea: an evidence-based review of the literature. Cornea 2004;23(1):106–9.
[122] Berman B, Perez OA, Zell D. Update on rosacea and anti-inflammatory-dose doxycycline. Drugs Today 2007;43(1):27–34.
[123] Fowler JF Jr. Combined effect of anti-inflammatory dose doxycycline (40-mg doxycycline, usp monohydrate controlled-release capsules) and metronidazole topical gel 1% in the treatment of rosacea. J Drugs Dermatol 2007;6(6):641–5.
[124] Yoo J, Reid DC, Kimball AB. Metronidazole in the treatment of rosacea: do formulation, dosing, and concentration matter? J Drugs Dermatol 2006;5(4):317–9.
[125] Levy JH, O'Donnell PS, Levy JH, et al. The therapeutic potential of a kallikrein inhibitor for treating hereditary angioedema. Expert Opin Investig Drugs 2006;15(9):1077–90.
[126] Bas M, Adams V, Suvorava T, et al. Nonallergic angioedema: role of bradykinin. Allergy 2007;62(8):842–56.
[127] Bork K, Frank J, Grundt B, et al. Treatment of acute edema attacks in hereditary angioedema with a bradykinin receptor-2 antagonist (Icatibant). J Allergy Clin Immunol 2007;119(6):1497–503.
[128] Lock RJ, Gompels MM. C1-inhibitor deficiencies (hereditary angioedema): where are we with therapies? Curr Allergy Asthma Rep 2007;7(4):264–9.
[129] Zuraw BL. Current and future therapy for hereditary angioedema. Clin Immunol 2005;114(1):10–6.
[130] Park HJ, Lee DY, Lee JH, et al. The treatment of syringomas by CO(2) laser using a multiple-drilling method. Dermatol Surg 2007;33(3):310–3.
[131] Wang JI, Roenigk HH Jr. Treatment of multiple facial syringomas with the carbon dioxide (CO2) laser. Dermatol Surg 1999;25(2):136–9.
[132] Ruban JM. [Treatment of benign eyelid conditions with argon laser]. J Fr Ophtalmol 2003;26(1):88–91 [in French].
[133] Raulin C, Schonermark MP, Greve B, et al. Q-switched ruby laser treatment of tattoos and benign pigmented skin lesions: a critical review. Ann Plast Surg 1998;41(5):555–65.
[134] Ferguson REH Jr, Vasconez HC. Laser treatment of congenital nevi. J Craniofac Surg 2005;16(5):908–14.
[135] Chan HHL, Kono T. Nevus of Ota: clinical aspects and management. Skinmed 2003;2(2):89–96 [quiz: 97–8].
[136] Ee HL, Goh CL, Khoo LS, et al. Treatment of acquired bilateral nevus of Ota-like macules (Hori's nevus) with a combination of the 532 nm Q-switched Nd:YAG laser followed by the 1,064 nm Q-switched Nd:YAG is more effective: prospective study. Dermatol Surg 2006;32(1):34–40.
[137] Pieh S, Kuchar A, Novak P, et al. Long-term results after surgical basal cell carcinoma excision in the eyelid region. Br J Ophthalmol 1999;83(1):85–8.
[138] Limawararut V, Leibovitch I, Sullivan T, et al. Periocular squamous cell carcinoma [see comment]. Clin Experiment Ophthalmol 2007;35(2):174–85.

[139] Spencer JM, Nossa R, Tse DT, et al. Sebaceous carcinoma of the eyelid treated with Mohs micrographic surgery. J Am Acad Dermatol 2001;44(6):1004–9.

[140] Zurcher M, Hintschich CR, Garner A, et al. Sebaceous carcinoma of the eyelid: a clinico-pathological study. Br J Ophthalmol 1998;82(9):1049–55.

[141] O'Keefe M, Lanigan B, Byrne SA. Capillary haemangioma of the eyelids and orbit: a clinical review of the safety and efficacy of intralesional steroid. Acta Ophthalmologica Scandinavica 2003;81(3):294–8.

[142] Garzon MC, Lucky AW, Hawrot A, et al. Ultrapotent topical corticosteroid treatment of hemangiomas of infancy. J Am Acad Dermatol 2005;52(2):281–6.

[143] Railan D, Parlette EC, Uebelhoer NS, et al. Laser treatment of vascular lesions. Clin Dermatol 2006;24(1):8–15.

[144] Yones SS, Palmer RA, Garibaldinos TM, et al. Randomized double-blind trial of treatment of vitiligo: efficacy of psoralen-UV-A therapy vs narrowband-UV-B therapy [see comment]. Arch Dermatol 2007;143(5):578–84.

[145] Bhatnagar A, Kanwar AJ, Parsad D, et al. Comparison of systemic PUVA and NB-UVB in the treatment of vitiligo: an open prospective study. J Eur Acad Dermatol Venereol 2007; 21(5):638–42.

[146] Forschner T, Buchholtz S, Stockfleth E. Current state of vitiligo therapy: evidence-based analysis of the literature. J Dtsch Dermatol Ges 2007;5(6):467–75.

[147] Choy EHS, Isenberg DA. Treatment of dermatomyositis and polymyositis. Rheumatology 2002;41(1):7–13.

[148] Wallace DJ. The use of chloroquine and hydroxychloroquine for non-infectious conditions other than rheumatoid arthritis or lupus: a critical review. Lupus 1996;(5 Suppl 1):S59–64.

[149] Cohen JB. Cutaneous involvement of dermatomyositis can respond to dapsone therapy. Int J Dermatol 2002;41(3):182–4.

[150] Brasington RD Jr, Kahl LE Jr, Ranganathan P, et al. 14. Immunologic rheumatic disorders. J Allergy Clin Immunol 2003;111(Suppl 2):S593–601.

[151] Reiff A, Rawlings DJ, Shaham B, et al. Preliminary evidence for cyclosporin A as an alternative in the treatment of recalcitrant juvenile rheumatoid arthritis and juvenile dermatomyositis. J Rheumatol 1997;24(12):2436–43.

[152] Gelber AC, Nousari HC, Wigley FM. Mycophenolate mofetil in the treatment of severe skin manifestations of dermatomyositis: a series of 4 cases. J Rheumatol 2000;27(6):1542–5.

ELSEVIER
SAUNDERS

Immunol Allergy Clin N Am
28 (2008) 169–188

IMMUNOLOGY
AND ALLERGY
CLINICS
OF NORTH AMERICA

Pediatric Ocular Inflammation

Rudolph S. Wagner, MD[a],*, Marcella Aquino, MD[b]

[a]Institute of Ophthalmology and Visual Sciences, UMDNJ–New Jersey Medical School,
Doctors Office Center, Suite 6100, PO Box 1709, Newark, NJ 07101-1709, USA
[b]Department of Medicine, Division of Allergy, Immunology, and Rheumatology,
UMDNJ–New Jersey Medical School, 90 Bergen Street, Newark, NJ 07103, USA

Pediatric conjunctivitis often has a benign etiology and a self-limited course [1]. It is common in childhood and may be infectious or noninfectious in nature and acute or chronic in presentation [2]. Infectious causes include bacterial and viral conjunctivitis [1]. Bacterial conjunctivitis is caused by organisms such *Haemophilus influenzae*, *Branhamella catarrhalis*, and *Streptococcus pneumoniae* [3] and presents with mucopurulent (unilateral or bilateral) discharge with normal visual acuity. Treatment is generally with topical antibiotics, but parenteral ceftriaxone is indicated for pathogens such as *Neisseria gonorrhea* [4] or *H influenzae*. Pathogens in viral conjunctivitis include adenoviruses, enteric cytopathic human orphan (ECHO) virus, and human coxsackieviruses. Viral conjunctivitis is generally characterized by a watery discharge. Treatment is supportive. Viral conjunctivitis is commonly associated with childhood exanthems, particularly measles. Allergic conjunctivitis should be considered in any child who presents with watery itchy injected eyes.

Conjunctivitis usually spares the limbal area of the eyes [5]. When perilimbal involvement is present, one must consider other disease states such as keratitis (inflammation of the cornea) or uveitis (inflammation of the anterior segment) [5]. Pain, photophobia, and blurry vision are not usually presenting complaints of conjunctivitis; when present, uveitis, keratitis, and glaucoma should be considered [2]. A serous discharge may be seen with allergic or viral causes [5], whereas a mucoid discharge is highly characteristic of allergy or dry eyes [2]. Allergic conjunctivitis is usually accompanied by other atopic conditions such as asthma, allergic rhinitis, and eczema and usually involves both eyes [1]. If present, preauricular adenopathy suggests a viral etiology [6]. Adenoviral conjunctivitis may be accompanied by

---

* Corresponding author.
E-mail address: wagdoc@comcast.net (R.S. Wagner).

0889-8561/08/$ - see front matter © 2008 Elsevier Inc. All rights reserved.
doi:10.1016/j.iac.2007.12.003

pharyngitis and fever—termed pharyngoconunctival fever [6]. Adenoviral serotypes 8, 19, and 37 are responsible for epidemic keratoconjunctivitis, resulting in loss of visual acuity due to corneal subepithelial infiltrates [7]. Otitis media with conjunctivitis is most often caused by nontypeable *H influenzae*. A child who has conjunctivitis, otitis media, fever, and muco-purluent rhinorrhea may have the conjunctivitis-otitis syndrome [8]. This particular association with otitis media and conjunctivitis was first described by Coffey [9] in 1966 and was coined the conjunctivitis-otitis syndrome by Bodor [8]. Because one fourth of patients who have conjunctivitis concur-rently have otitis media, it is essential that all patients have their ears checked even in the absence of ear pain [8].

Bacterial conjunctivitis

Bacterial conjunctival infection is more likely to be accompanied by a pu-rulent discharge than its viral or allergic counterparts. Although *H influen-zae*, *Streptococcus pneumoniae*, and *B catarrhalis* are the most common etiologies overall, in the neonatal age group, agents such as *Chlamydia trachomatis*, *Staphylococcus aureus*, *Staphylococcus epidermidis*, *Viridans streptococci*, and *Neisseria gonorrhea* are other causative organisms [10–12].

The most common pathogens reported in pediatric bacterial conjunctivi-tis are *H influenzae* and *Streptococcus pneumoniae* (Fig. 1) [13,14]. The intro-duction of the *H influenzae* vaccine (HiB) in 1985 has not reduced the number of cases of conjunctivitis caused by this organism because most cases are caused by a nontypeable strain [15]. There are no data to indicate that the introduction of the heptavalent pneumococcal vaccine (Prevnar-Wyeth) has decreased the frequency of conjunctivitis due to *Streptococcus pneumoniae*. In fact, there were two recent epidemics of conjunctivitis caused by nonencapsulated, nontypeable strains of *Streptococcus pneumoniae*. One of these epidemics occurred on a college campus where more than 600 stu-dents were infected [16]. The second epidemic took place in an elementary

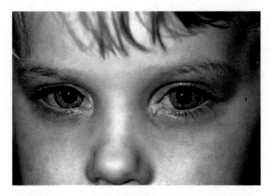

Fig. 1. *Haemophilus influenzae* conjunctivitis with purulent discharge in a 4-year-old child.

school in Maine in December 2002 where 361 students (median age, 6 years) were infected [17]. These data suggest that the incidence of gram-positive bacterial conjunctivitis is increasing, particularly in children and young adults.

Children who have bacterial conjunctivitis usually present with complaints of itching and burning; on examination, purulent or mucopurulent discharge can be appreciated along with eyelid edema, conjunctival erythema, or both (Fig. 2) [3,18]. Although it is clinically difficult to distinguish bacterial from viral etiologies, certain clues, when present, may point toward a bacterial cause. In children younger than 6 years, bacterial causes of conjunctivitis predominant, whereas in children older than 6 years, adenoviruses are the leading pathogen [1]. Time of year is also a helpful clue: bacterial conjunctivitis occurs more frequently during the winter, whereas viral conjunctivitis occurs during the fall [1]. Association of otitis media with conjunctivitis and bilateral conjunctival disease points to a bacterial etiology [19]. Sinusitis and rhinitis can accompany conjunctivitis caused by pneumococci [1].

Viral conjunctivitis/herpes simplex virus infections

Most viral conjunctivitis is caused by Adenoviridae [19]. Overall, 20% of all cases of conjunctivitis are caused by this family of viral pathogens [10,20]. Infection with adenoviruses can manifest as follicular conjunctivitis, pharyngoconjunctival fever, epidemic keratoconjunctivitis, and acute hemorrhagic conjunctivitis [3,5,21]. Pharyngoconjunctival fever is characterized by fever up to 104°F, pharyngitis, and conjunctivitis; it is caused primarily by human adenoviruses 3 and 7, and found in children younger than 10 years [22]. Epidemic keratoconjunctivitis is typically a disease of older children and adults; involvement of the cornea is the predominant finding on physical examination [22]. Adenoviral conjunctivitis is very contagious, with the virus transmitted in schools, workplaces, swimming pools, and medical

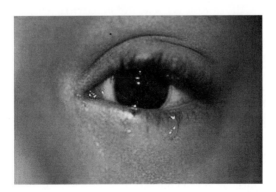

Fig. 2. Conjunctival injection with serous discharge in adenoviral conjunctivitis.

offices [2]. Most cases are spread through direct contact with infected persons or equipment [3]. Health care workers are encouraged to wear gloves, practice good hand washing, and clean instruments after patient contact [3]. Patients should also be encouraged to promote good hand washing and to separate towels of infected and noninfected family members [5]. Treatment is supportive, with symptoms lasting 1 to 3 weeks. Cold compresses, artificial tears, and topical vasoconstrictors may provide some relief [2]. A randomized, double-blind placebo-controlled trial with topical ketorolac versus artificial tears for the treatment of viral conjunctivitis failed to show any statistical difference in patient symptom score (discomfort, itching, foreign-body sensation, tearing, or eyelid swelling) or sign score (conjunctival injection, chemosis, mucous, or eyelid edema) [23]. Topical antibiotics are rarely needed because superinfection with bacterial pathogens is a rare occurrence [2].

Viral etiologies for conjunctivitis other than adenoviruses include ECHO virus, herpesviruses, enteroviruses, Epstein-Barr virus, influenza A virus, human coxsackieviruses, and Kawasaki disease. Patients present with conjunctival injection, watery discharge, conjunctival swelling, a tender preauricular node, and possibly foreign-body sensation [2]. Both eyes may be concurrently infected or the second eye may become involved a few days later; an associated upper respiratory infection may accompany the conjunctivitis [2].

Viral conjunctivitis caused by recurrent herpes simplex virus (HSV) can be vision threatening. Although primary infection usually has a self-limited course, recurrent disease can result in corneal opacification and loss of vision [1]. Primary infection peaks between age 1 and 5 years [3]. Recurrent disease primarily strikes in adulthood [24]. Most ocular infections in children are caused by HSV-1 as opposed to neonatal herpes eye disease, whereby HSV-2 is acquired at delivery [1]. Presentation of eye disease in primary HSV infection may be a nonspecific conjunctivitis (follicular response, serous discharge, and preauricular adenopathy) with or without vesicles of the surrounding skin (Fig. 3) [1]. Without these vesicles present, disease may not be distinguishable from other infectious forms of conjunctivitis. A helpful clue is that most herpetic conjunctivitis (80%) is unilateral [3]. The virus is transmitted from inoculation through direct contact with another individual who is shedding the virus or from autoinoculation of the conjunctiva from a primary infection elsewhere [3]. On examination, involvement of the cornea with the classic dendritic appearance is found in 50% of patients (Fig. 4) [5].

Secondary HSV disease may occur if the trigeminal ganglion is invaded during primary disease. Physical stress may precipitate the second outbreak. These patients now present with a different clinical picture: unilateral red eye with severe pain and sensation of a foreign body but without history of trauma or contact with a foreign body [1]. On examination, a dendritic ulcer on the corneal epithelium is a characteristic feature. Identification can be facilitated by the use of fluorescein dye and by examination with filtered cobalt

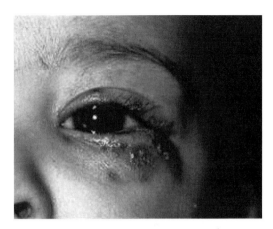

Fig. 3. Periocular vesicles on the eyelids of a child who has primary HSV infection.

blue light [1]. Treatment can be established with topical agents such as trifluridine and vidarabine (limitations include frequent dosing of medication and difficulty administering drops to the pediatric population). Systemic treatment with acyclovir, famciclovir, and valacyclovir may be needed in severe cases or to suppress recurrent lesions [2]. Topical steroids should be avoided because they lead to virus replication.

Treatment of infectious conjunctivitis

Viral conjunctivitis is largely a self-limited disease and not responsive to topical antibiotics. Topical antibiotics are used to treat bacterial conjunctivitis and as prophylaxis for ophthalmia neonatorum (discussed later) and nasolacrimal duct obstruction with purulent discharge (also discussed later) [25]. The efficacy of topical therapy was tested by Gigliotti and colleagues [26] who compared placebo to topical polymyxin-bacitracin ointment in

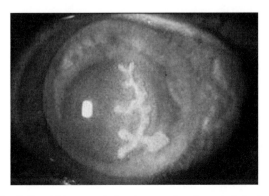

Fig. 4. Dendritic corneal ulcer in secondary herpetic infection.

Table 1
Treatment of bacterial conjunctivitis

Medication	Class	Dosage	Adverse effects	Approximate cost
Trimethoprim-polymixin B (Polytrim)	Combination	Age >2 mo: 1 drop q 3 h × 7–10 d	Burning, stinging, itching, eyelid edema, superinfection	10 mL = $33.99
Sodium sulfacetamide 10% (Bleph-10)	Sulfonamide	Age >2 mo: 1–2 drops q 2–3 h during the day × 7–10 d	Local irritation, stinging, burning, superinfection, sensitization Severe: Stevens-Johnson syndrome	5 mL = $20.99
Ciprofloxacin 0.3% solution (Ciloxan)	Quinolone	Age >1 y: 1–2 drops q 2 h while awake × 2 d, then bid for the next 5 d	Burning, lid margin crusting, scales, foreign-body sensation, pruritus, conjunctival hyperemia	5 mL = $54.42
Ofloxacin solution (Ocuflox)	Quinolone	Age >1 y: 1–2 drops q 2 h while awake × 2 d, then qid for the next 5 d	Superinfection, photophobia, lacrimation, burning, stinging, redness, itching, dry eye Rare: anaphylaxis and Stevens-Johnson syndrome	5 mL = $50.19
Tobramycin 0.3% (Tobrex)	Aminoglycoside	1–2 drops q 4 h for mild to moderate infections	Superinfection, itching, swelling, erythema Rare: thrombocytopenia and bronchospasm	5 mL = $49.05

Drug	Class	Dosing	Side effects	Cost
Erythromycin 0.5% ointment	Macrolide	1-cm ribbon to lower conjunctival sac up to 6 × per day × 7–10 d	Ocular irritation, erythema, hypersensitivity reactions	3.5 g = $7.99
Moxifloxacin 0.5% solution (Vigamox)	Fluoroquinolone	Age >1 yr: 1 drop tid × 7 d	Conjunctival irritation, dry eye, visual acuity changes, ocular pain/pruritus/redness; Serious: hypersensitivity reaction, superinfection, subconjunctival hemorrhage	3 mL = $68.58
Gatifloxacin 0.3% solution (Zymar)	Fluoroquinolone	Age >1 yr: 1 drop q 2 h while awake × 2 d, then qid for 5 d	Conjunctival irritation, lacrimation, dry eye, ocular discharge/pain/redness; Serious: hypersensitivity reaction, superinfection, subconjunctival hemorrhage	5 mL = $62.88

children aged 1 month to 18 years. By day 8, both groups were cured (no significant *P* value). Treatments with topical antibiotics led to a faster cure and a greater likelihood of clearing the organism.

As previously stated, most causes of bacterial conjunctivitis are caused by gram-positive and gram-negative organisms, and treatment should be tailored accordingly. Options include trimethoprim-polymixin B (Polytrim), which has broad-spectrum antibiotic coverage, is inexpensive, and has minimal side effects (ocular irritation) (Table 1) [25]. Sodium sulfacetamide 10% (Bleph-10) is also an inexpensive option covering gram-positive organisms but causes significant stinging on application [25]. Topical fluoroquinolones such as ciprofloxacin 0.3% (Ciloxan) and ofloxacin (Ocuflox) have broad-spectrum coverage against gram-positive and gram-negative organisms but are more expensive choices [1]. Aminoglycosides are frequently prescribed for bacterial conjunctivitis; gentamicin and tobramycin have good gram-negative coverage but do not cover organisms such as *Chlamydia*, and corneal epithelial toxicity may be seen with extensive use [25]. Erythromycin is another inexpensive option with good gram-positive and *Chlamydia* coverage; however, it has poor activity against *Haemophilus* species, *B catarrhalis*, gram-negative organisms, and staphylococcal species [25]. Administration may be by drops or with ointment. Ointments tend to blur vision, which may be a consideration in school-aged children [1]. Overall, the side effects of topical agents, including hypersensitivity, are local in nature, with systemic effects being rare [25]. Neomycin preparations should be avoided because there is a higher likelihood of cell-mediated sensitivity to these agents [6].

Recently, fourth-generation topical fluoroquinolones have been introduced for the treatment of bacterial conjunctivitis. These agents, including gatifloxacin 0.3% and moxifloxacin 0.5%, have increased efficacy against gram-positive organisms and reduced the potential for bacterial resistance [27]. Moxifloxacin is the only fluoroquinolone that can be administered in the less frequent, three-times-daily dosing schedule. The relatively low minimum inhibitory concentration of moxifloxacin for isolates of the common pathogens that cause pediatric conjunctivitis in addition to the high conjunctival tissue levels reached compared with other topical antibiotics make it ideal for eradicating the organism quickly and for subsequent rapid clinical cures [28]. A recent study demonstrated the need to exclude children with infectious conjunctivitis from school until clinical signs and symptoms are resolved. Treatment of bacterial conjunctivitis with the fourth-generation fluoroquinolones may provide the opportunity to get children back to school the next day following initiation of treatment [29].

Combination therapies of antibiotics and corticosteroids are available. These therapies are not generally recommended unless a firm diagnosis is obtained because they are able to increase intraocular pressure with prolonged use and cause aggravation of ocular HSV infections (causing the virus to proliferate) [1].

Nasolacrimal duct obstruction

Congenital nasolacrimal obstruction is a common disorder in infants and results in persistent tearing and may lead to infections such as dacryocystitis, orbital cellulitis, and bacterial conjunctivitis [30]. It occurs when a membranous fold obstructs the lower end of the nasolacrimal duct [1]. The condition is usually apparent when the infant is 3 to 12 weeks old [1]. The true incidence of this disorder in healthy newborns remains controversial. The most frequently quoted number of 6% comes from a study of 200 consecutive live births in the 1940s in which nasolacrimal patency was assessed by the presence or absence of discharge on compression of the lacrimal sac [31]. The incidence of the disorder, however, is considered higher in children who have craniofacial disorders and Down syndrome [32].

Epiphora (persistent, overflow tearing) is the most common but least specific presenting sign. The conjunctiva is usually clear, with only one eye typically being affected [1]. Blepharitis with matting of the lids and lashes is part of the clinical presentation (Fig. 5) [1]. It is essential to determine whether the epiphora is due to overproduction of tears (trichiasis, foreign body, corneal abrasion, or abnormal eyelid position) or obstruction of outflow tract [30]. The patency of the lacrimal outflow system can be assessed using the modified fluorescein disappearance test. Fluorescein mixed with topical anesthetic is placed into the lower conjunctival fornix of each eye and excess solution and tears are blotted with a tissue. After 5 minutes, the child is examined. Light passed through a cobalt blue filter helps to identify residual fluorescein, which should not be present [33,34]. MacEwen and Young [34] found this test to be 90% sensitive and 100% specific for the presence of nasolacrimal obstruction in their prospective study of 80 patients.

The natural course of the disease appears to be spontaneous remission. In MacEwen and Young's [35] study of 4792 infants in Scotland, they saw spontaneous remission throughout the first year of life, with 96% of the cases resolving before the age of 1 year and 350 cases resolving within the

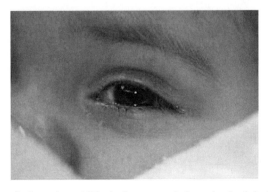

Fig. 5. Watery discharge in a child who has congenital nasolacrimal duct obstruction.

first month alone. Conservative treatment consists of topical antibiotics and lacrimal sac massage. A topical antibiotic ointment may aid the inflammation at the lid margin [1,36]. Lacrimal sac massage, first described by Crigler [36], is the technique of placing one finger over the common canaliculus to block upward flow and then stroking downward along the lacrimal sac to increase hydrostatic pressure and attempt to break a membrane at the opening of the nasolacrimal duct into the nose (Fig. 6). Although studies quote varying degrees of success for lacrimal sac massage, it is not harmful.

Most investigators recommend probing and irrigation as the next intervention after conservative management. The procedure to probe and irrigate the nasolacrimal duct canal is performed under general anesthesia [1]. Early intervention occurs when the procedure is performed on a child younger than 1 year. Advantages to early probing are earlier relief of symptoms, the avoidance of complications of nasolacrimal obstruction (the development of acute dacryocystitis, conjunctivitis, and cellulitis), and decreasing the chance of fibrosis and scarring of the nasolacrimal system that would make further treatment difficult [30]. The main disadvantages to early probing are that it requires surgical intervention in patients who might have complete resolution of symptoms with conservative management and places the infant at risk for complications such as the creation of false passages and the morbidity from general anesthesia [30]. After the age 1 year, the success rate of probing decreases with increasing age. The addition of balloon catheter dilatation of the lacrimal sac (Lacri-Cath) at the time of probing may result in improved success rates. When probing is not successful, a silicone tube may be placed into the nasolacrimal canal.

Allergic conjunctivitis

Children are subject to the same ocular allergies as their adult counterparts. Allergic conjunctivitis can be divided into acute and chronic

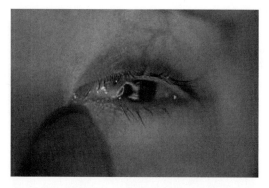

Fig. 6. Mucous expressed from the lacrimal puncta with digital pressure over the lacrimal sac is diagnostic of congenital nasolacrimal duct obstruction.

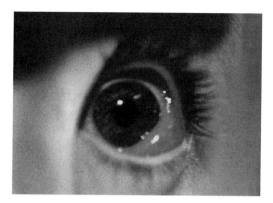

Fig. 7. Acute conjunctival chemosis (edema) in allergic conjunctivitis.

disorders. Seasonal allergic conjunctivitis and perennial allergic conjunctivitis can be placed into the acute disorder category, whereas chronic allergic diseases are made up of vernal keratoconjunctivitis, atopic keratoconjunctivitis, and giant papillary conjunctivitis. The inflammation encountered on the ocular surface results in itching, tearing, and lid/conjunctival edema (Fig. 7).

The allergic response in conjunctivitis is typically elicited by ocular exposure to allergens that causes cross-linkage of membrane-bound immunoglobulin (Ig)E, which triggers mast cell degranulation, releasing a cascade of allergic and inflammatory mediators [37]. Allergens may be seasonal culprits (pollen, weeds, molds, grasses) or perennial ones (animal dander, dust mites, cockroaches) [1]. Vernal conjunctivitis occurs in two forms: limbal vernal, with the infiltration of eosinophils at the superior limbus; and a form with large papules forming on the palpebral conjunctiva. Both forms are particularly difficult to treat and may require a topical steroid in addition to a combination antihistamine–mast cell stabilizer (Fig. 8).

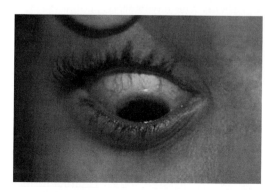

Fig. 8. Eosinophilic infiltrate on superior limbus in limbal vernal conjunctivitis.

Treatment with cold compresses, eyewashes with artificial tears, and avoidance of allergens (dust mite covers) are nonspecific measures to counsel the allergic patient. The use of topical therapy allows for direct and local application while avoiding the ocular drying effects evident with the use of systemic oral antihistamines [38]. Combinations of antihistamines and topical vasoconstrictors provide relief from itch but are not recommended for long-term use because they may cause a reduction in body temperature, central nervous system depression, headache, cardiac arrhythmias, and papillary dilation [25]. Naphcon-A, which contains naphazoline hydrochloride and pheniramine maleate, is presently available over-the-counter for children older than 6 years (Table 2) [1].

H_1 receptor antagonists such as levocabastine hydrochloride (Livostin 0.05%) are available for use in patients 12 years and older, with a suggested application regimen of four times daily to relieve ocular pruritus [1]. Azelastine (Optivar) is a second-generation H_1 receptor antagonist with the added component of being an inhibitor of histamine–mast cell release. It can be prescribed in children older than 3 years and applied twice daily for relief. Comparisons of the two agents show a similar profile of tolerability and symptomatic relief [39].

Combination antihistamine–mast cell stabilizers have the advantage of rapid symptomatic relief given by immediate histamine receptor antagonism along with the long-term disease-modifying benefit of mast cell stabilizers. It should be noted that not all medications of this class are equivalent [37]. Olopatadine, ketotifen, and epinastine ophthalmic solutions have indications for the treatment of allergic conjunctivitis in patients age 3 years and older.

Another class of medications includes corticosteroids; however, caution is advised considering the potential side effects (cataracts, increased intraocular pressure, and corneal melts). The use of corticosteroids is typically reserved for patients not responsive to the previously mentioned therapies or for severe forms of allergy; namely, vernal keratoconjunctivitis and atopic keratoconjunctivitis [37]. As mentioned previously, the use of topical corticosteroids in patients who have herpetic conjunctival disease can cause rapid proliferation of the virus and corneal scarring. If needed, rimexolone (Vexol), a derivative of prednisolone approved for the treatment of allergic conjunctivitis that becomes inactivated in the anterior chamber of the eye, may be an option [40] because it demonstrates efficacy while decreasing safety concerns (intraocular pressure) [41,42].

Topical nonsteroidal anti-inflammatory drugs (NSAIDs) are effective for use in allergic conjunctivitis through their interruption of prostaglandin synthesis. Ketorolac (Acular) has been shown to diminish the ocular itching and conjunctival hyperemia associated with allergic conjunctivitis [43]. The advantage of this class of agents over corticosteroids is that NSAIDs do not increase intraocular pressure, induce cataract formation, or interfere with wound healing. Ocular irritation, however, is commonly associated

Table 2
Treatment of allergic conjunctivitis

Medication	Class	Dosage	Adverse effects	Approximate cost
Naphazoline-pheniramine (Naphcon-A)	Antihistamine/decongestant (over-the-counter)	Age >6 y: 1–2 drops each eye q 3–4 h prn	Mydriasis, irritation, redness, blurred vision, headache Serious: central nervous system depression, increased intraocular pressure	15 mL = $12.00
Ketorolac 0.5% (Acular)	Nonsteroidal anti-inflammatory drug	Age >12 y: 1 drop each eye qid × 1 wk	Burning, stinging, hyperemia, corneal infiltrate Serious: corneal ulcer, erosion or perforation, keratitis	10 mL = $150.00
Azelastine 0.05% (Optivar)	H$_1$ receptor antagonist	Age >3 y: 1 drop each eye bid	Burning, stinging, bitter taste, ocular pain	6 mL = $78.03
Olopatadine 0.2% (Pataday)	H$_1$ receptor antagonist/ mast cell stabilizer	Age >3 y: 1 drop each eye qd	Headache, burning, dry eye, hyperemia, foreign-body sensation	2.5 mL in a 4 mL bottle = $80.00
Epinastine 0.05% solution (Elestat)	H$_1$ receptor antagonist/ mast cell stabilizer	Age >3 y: 1 drop each eye bid	Ocular burning, hyperemia, pruritus, upper respiratory infection, headache, cough, folliculosis	5 mL = $83.28
Rimexolone 1% (Vexol)	Corticosteriod	Adult dosing: 1–2 drops each eye qid × 2 wk	Blurred vision, burning, redness Serious: cataract, loss of vision, superinfection	5 mL = $28.99

with the use of these agents, especially in contact lens wearers. Use of topical NSAIDs is limited to age 12 years and older.

Immunotherapy, which involves administration of selected allergens to which the patient is allergic by way of a subcutaneous, gastrointestinal, mucosal, or sublingual route, has aided greatly in the treatment of allergic rhinitis symptoms [40]. Some clinical studies have focused on the improvement in ocular symptoms with immunotherapy [44,45]. Benefits of this modality must be weighed against the time commitment, risk of systemic reactions, and difficulty in administering injections to the pediatric population.

Neonatal conjunctivitis

Conjunctivitis in the first month of life (ophthalmia neonatorum) is the most common infection in the neonatal period [10,11,46]. It occurs in 1.6% to 12% of newborns [20]. The etiologies include chemical, bacterial, and viral [46]. The most common cause is from chemical irritation followed by *C trachomatis* infection [20]. Chemical conjunctivitis is commonly induced by the use of eye drop prophylaxis, especially silver nitrate but also erythromycin and tetracycline ointments [46]. It typically appears within 6 to 8 hours of application and remits spontaneously in 1 to 2 days. No treatment is necessary and Gram stain shows no organisms [46].

Regarding infectious etiology, the most common infectious cause is due to *C trachomatis* acquired during delivery from mother to child: a vaginally born infant to a mother who has an active chlamydial infection has a 50% chance of acquiring the organism [46]. Of these infants, roughly one fourth to one half develop conjunctivitis [4]. Symptoms typically begin at age 5 to 14 days (it can be seen earlier if amniotic membranes rupture prematurely) [47] and vary widely, from conjunctival injection to severe edema with mucopurulent discharge. The inflammatory reaction consists mostly of polymorphonuclear leukocytes, and pseudomembrane formation may occur as the exudate adheres to the conjunctiva [47]. The pseudomembranes may be appreciated by everting the eyelid. The cornea is usually spared, and systemic treatment with erythromycin (oral erythromycin base or ethylsuccinate, 50 mg/kg/d in four divided doses for 14 days) usually results in healing without complications (Fig. 9) [47]. Sometimes a second course of erythromycin is needed because the efficacy of erythromycin is approximately 80% [4]. Untreated infection may persist and carries the risk of corneal and conjunctival scarring [47]. The preferred method for diagnosis is culture of the conjunctiva (from the everted eyelid) and pharynx. Nonculture tests that are acceptable to the Food and Drug Administration for use with conjunctival specimens include (1) an enzyme immunoassay that uses enzyme-labeled chlamydial-specific antibodies to detect chlamydial lipopolysaccharide and (2) direct fluorescent antibody assays that use

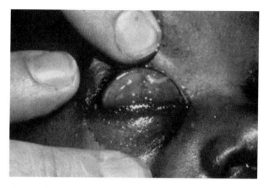

Fig. 9. Pseudomembrane formation on the palpebral conjunctiva in neonatal chlamydial conjuctivitis.

fluorescein-conjugated monoclonal antibodies to stain antigens in smears [47]. Appropriate treatment must also be obtained for the mother and her partner [4].

Neonatal conjunctivitis from *C trachomatis* must be distinguished from other bacterial causes, especially *Neisseria gonorrhoeae*. Some clinical features may aid in this distinction. First, gonococcal ophthalmia usually occurs at an earlier age, around age 2 to 5 days, although overlap can occur [47]. Second, gonococcal disease usually has a more rapidly progressive course than that caused by *C trachomatis* [47]. The disease in gonococcal ophthalmia neonatorum is usually bilateral, with prominent eyelid edema with chemosis [48]. Discharge from the eyes may initially appear watery but quickly develops into a mucopurulent discharge (Fig. 10) [48]. In severe cases, corneal ulceration or perforation may occur [1]. It usually has a benign outcome with treatment (ceftriaxone, 25–50 mg/kg, administered intravenously or intramuscularly [IV or IM] with a maximum of 125 mg for one

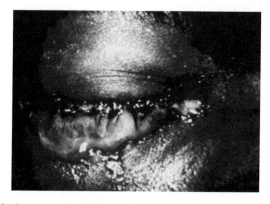

Fig. 10. Acute purulent discharge in gonococcal neonatal conjunctivitis.

dose or cefotaxime, 100 mg/kg, administered IV or IM for one dose) [4] and with aggressive irrigation several times a day until the purulence subsides [4,46]. The patient should also be evaluated for disseminated infection such as arthritis, meningitis, or sepsis because the conjunctivae serve as portals of entry [48]. Isolation of *Neisseria gonorrhoeae* by culture performed on conjunctival exudates, blood, synovial fluid, or cerebrospinal fluid is standard for diagnosis [48]. The mother and her sexual contacts should also be treated for gonorrhea [46].

Other potential microbes for neonatal conjunctivitis are *H influenzae, Streptococcus pneumoniae, Staphylococcus aureus, Neisseria cineria, Pseudomonas* sp, *Proteus* sp, *Klebisella pneumoniae*, enterococci, HSV, and adenoviruses [48]. Infections with most of these other organisms may be treated with topical antibiotics except for *Pseudomonas aeruginosa* [46]. This infection presents with edema, erythema, purulent discharge, or endophthalmitis [46,49] and can cause corneal perforations, blindness, and death [46]. Presumptive diagnosis is made when gram-negative rods are seen on Gram stain of exudates, with growth in culture confirming the diagnosis [46]. Treatment with topical and systemic aminoglycosides is necessary [49].

Congenital glaucoma

The primary clinical manifestations of congenital glaucoma are tearing, photophobia, corneal clouding and edema, redness, and enlargement of the eye [1]. Some of these symptoms (tearing, redness, edema) may prompt physicians to think of conjunctivitis. The abnormality of congenital glaucoma is a defect in the iridocorneal angle of the anterior chamber that obstructs the outflow of aqueous fluid [1]. The consequent rise in intraocular pressure leads to corneal edema and enlargement. Surgery is necessary to reduce this rise in intraocular pressure [1]. Glaucoma classification is vast, and this disease has associations with systemic abnormalities such as Sturge-Weber syndrome, neurofibromatosis type 1, Marfan syndrome, trisomy 13 syndrome, trisomy 21 syndrome, and Rubinstein-Taybi syndrome [50].

Uveitis

Uveitis includes inflammation of the iris (iritis), ciliary body (cyclitis), and choroid (choroiditis) [6]. It can be classified anatomically into the following categories: anterior, intermediate, posterior, and diffuse [1]. Patients complain of decreased or hazy vision, pain, and photophobia, with a sensation of black floating spots [1]. Typical presentation for anterior uveitis is conjunctival injection with a miotic pupil and ciliary flush (Fig. 11) [6]. Due to its primary presentation with tearing and red eye, uveitis may be confused with conjunctivitis.

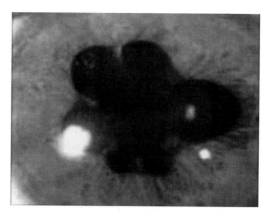

Fig. 11. Irregularly shaped pupil secondary to synechia formation in recurrent anterior uveitis.

Children represent 5% to 10% of patients seen at tertiary referral centers for uveitis, with slightly more cases seen in female patients [51]. A retrospective, multicenter observational study in England of patients younger than 16 years who had uveitis found a prevalence of 4.9 in 100,000 [52]. Anterior and posterior uveitis account for most cases (30%–40% and 40%–50%, respectively), with intermediate uveitis accounting for 10% to 20% and diffuse uveitis accounting for 5% to 10% of cases [51]. In children, the most common cause of anterior uveitis is juvenile rheumatoid arthritis [51]. Toxoplasmic retinochoroiditis is the most frequent type of posterior uveitis [51]. Intermediate uveitis and diffuse uveitis are mostly bilateral, chronic, and of idiopathic etiology [51]. Cunningham [51] described the most common complications in children to be cataract formation, band keratopathy, glaucoma, and cystoid macular edema, with one fourth to one third of uveitis patients being left with severe vision loss.

Anterior uveitis may be granulomatous or nongranulomatous [6]. Granulomatous causes include sarcoidosis, tuberculosis, syphilis, and toxoplasmosis [6]. Nongranulomatous anterior uveitis is associated with ankylosing spondylitis, sacroiliitis, Reiter syndrome, psoriasis, Behçet's syndrome, and infections (HSV, varicella-zoster virus) [6]. The sequelae of anterior uveitis are formation of synechia (adhesions of the posterior iris to the anterior capsule of the lens), angle closure glaucoma, and cataract formation [1].

Posterior uveitis presents with inflammatory cells in the vitreous, retinal vasculitis, and macular edema, which threaten visual acuity [1]. Causes of posterior uveitis include congenitally transmitted toxoplamosis, toxocariasis, tuberculosis, syphilis, Lyme disease, cat-scratch disease, rubella retinitis, HSV, and cytomegalovirus [51]. Panuveitis involves all three portions of the uveal track and, in one Israeli study, it was linked to a systemic autoimmune disease in over 95% of cases [53].

References

[1] Wagner RS. Ocular allergy: pediatric concerns of ocular inflammation. Immunol Allergy Clin North Am 1997;17:161–77.
[2] Morrow GL, Abbott RL. Conjunctivitis [see comment]. Am Fam Physician 1998;57(4):735–46.
[3] Weiss A. Acute conjunctivitis in childhood. Curr Probl Pediatr 1994;24(1):4–11.
[4] American Academy of Pediatrics. Committee on Infectious Diseases. Red book: report of the Committee on Infectious Diseases. 25th edition. Elk Grove Village (IL): American Academy of Pediatrics; 2000.
[5] Steinkuller PG, Edmond J, Chen R. Ocular infections. In: Feigin RD, Cherry JD, editors. Textbook of pediatric infectious diseases. 4th edition. Philadelphia: WB Saunders; 1998.
[6] Hara JH. The red eye: diagnosis and treatment. Am Fam Physician 1996;54(8):2423–30.
[7] Riordan-Eva P, Vaughan D. Eye. Current medical diagnosis & treatment. Stamford (CT): Appleton & Lange; 1996. p. 156–80.
[8] Bodor FF. Conjunctivitis-otitis syndrome. Pediatrics 1982;69(6):695–8.
[9] Coffey JD Jr. Otitis media in the practice of pediatrics. Bacteriological and clinical observations. Pediatrics 1966;38(1):25–32.
[10] Fransen L, Van den Berghe P, Mertens A, et al. Incidence and bacterial aetiology of neonatal conjunctivitis. Eur J Pediatr 1987;146(2):152–5.
[11] Sandstrom I. Etiology and diagnosis of neonatal conjunctivitis. Acta Paediatr Scand 1987;76(2):221–7.
[12] Sandstrom KI, Bell TA, Chandler JW, et al. Microbial causes of neonatal conjunctivitis. J Pediatr 1984;105(5):706–11.
[13] Gigliotti F, Williams WT, Hayden FG, et al. Etiology of acute conjunctivitis in children. J Pediatr 1981;98(4):531–6.
[14] Weiss A, Brinser JH, Nazar-Stewart V. Acute conjunctivitis in childhood. J Pediatr 1993;122(1):10–4.
[15] Alrawi AM, Chern KC, Cevallos V, et al. Biotypes and serotypes of *Haemophilus influenzae* ocular isolates. Br J Ophthalmol 2002;86(3):276–7.
[16] Martin M, Turco JH, Zegans ME, et al. An outbreak of conjunctivitis due to atypical *Streptococcus pneumoniae* [see comment]. N Engl J Med 2003;348(12):1112–21.
[17] Pneumococcal conjunctivitis at an elementary school–Maine, September 20–December 6, 2002. MMWR Morb Mortal Wkly Rep 2003;52(4):64–6.
[18] Gigliotti F. Acute conjunctivitis of childhood. Pediatr Ann 1993;22(6):353–6.
[19] Teoh DL, Reynolds S. Diagnosis and management of pediatric conjunctivitis. Pediatr Emerg Care 2003;19(1):48–55.
[20] Gigliotti F. Acute conjunctivitis. Pediatr Rev 1995;16(6):203–7, quiz 208.
[21] Weber CM, Eichenbaum JW. Acute red eye. Differentiating viral conjunctivitis from other, less common causes [see comment]. Postgrad Med 1997;101(5):185–6, 195–6.
[22] Dawson C, Sheppard J. Follicular conjunctivitis. In: Tasman W, Jaeger E, editors. Duane's clinical opthalmology. Philadelphia: JB Lippincott; 1991.
[23] Shiuey Y, Ambati BK, Adamis AP. A randomized, double-masked trial of topical ketorolac versus artificial tears for treatment of viral conjunctivitis. Ophthalmology 2000;107(8):1512–7.
[24] Syed NA, Hyndiuk RA. Infectious conjunctivitis. Infect Dis Clin North Am 1992;6(4):789–805.
[25] Wallace DK, Steinkuller PG. Ocular medications in children. Clin Pediatr 1998;37(11):645–52.
[26] Gigliotti F, Hendley JO, Morgan J, et al. Efficacy of topical antibiotic therapy in acute conjunctivitis in children. J Pediatr 1984;104(4):623–6.

[27] Lichtenstein SJ, Dorfman M, Kennedy R, et al. Controlling contagious bacterial conjunctivitis [see comment]. J Pediatr Ophthalmol Strabismus 2006;43(1):19–26.

[28] Wagner RS, Abelson MB, Shapiro A, et al. Evaluation of moxifloxacin, ciprofloxacin, gatifloxacin, ofloxacin, and levofloxacin concentrations in human conjunctival tissue. Arch Ophthalmol 2005;123(9):1282–3.

[29] Ohnsman CM. Exclusion of students with conjunctivitis from school: policies of state departments of health [see comment]. J Pediatr Ophthalmol Strabismus 2007;44(2): 101–5.

[30] Kapadia MK, Freitag SK, Woog JJ. Evaluation and management of congenital nasolacrimal duct obstruction. Otolaryngol Clin North Am 2006;39(5):959–77.

[31] Guerry D, Kendig EL. Congenital impatency on the naso-lacrimal duct. Arch Ophthalmol 1948;39:193–204.

[32] Berk AT, Saatci AO, Ercal MD, et al. Ocular findings in 55 patients with Down's syndrome. Ophthalmic Genet 1996;17(1):15–9.

[33] Zappia RJ, Milder B. Lacrimal drainage function. 2. The fluorescein dye disappearance test. Am J Ophthalmol 1972;74(1):160–2.

[34] MacEwen CJ, Young JD. The fluorescein disappearance test (FDT): an evaluation of its use in infants. J Pediatr Ophthalmol Strabismus 1991;28(6):302–5.

[35] MacEwen CJ, Young JD. Epiphora during the first year of life. Eye 1991;5(Pt 5): 596–600.

[36] Crigler L. The treatment of congenital dacryocystitis. JAMA 1923;81:21–4.

[37] Ono SJ, Abelson MB. Allergic conjunctivitis: update on pathophysiology and prospects for future treatment. J Allergy Clin Immunol 2005;115(1):118–22.

[38] Welch D, Ousler GW III, Nally LA, et al. Ocular drying associated with oral antihistamines (loratadine) in the normal population—an evaluation of exaggerated dose effect. Adv Exp Med Biol 2002;506(Pt B):1051–5.

[39] Giede C, Metzenauer P, Petzold U, et al. Comparison of azelastine eye drops with levocabastine eye drops in the treatment of seasonal allergic conjunctivitis. Curr Med Res Opin 2000; 16(3):153–63.

[40] Bielory L. Ocular allergy guidelines: a practical treatment algorithm. Drugs 2002;62(11): 1611–34.

[41] Hirneiss C, Neubauer AS, Kampik A, et al. Comparison of prednisolone 1%, rimexolone 1% and ketorolac tromethamine 0.5% after cataract extraction: a prospective, randomized, double-masked study. Graefes Arch Clin Exp Ophthalmol 2005;243(8):768–73.

[42] Biswas J, Ganeshbabu TM, Raghavendran SR, et al. Efficacy and safety of 1% rimexolone versus 1% prednisolone acetate in the treatment of anterior uveitis—a randomized triple masked study. Int Ophthalmol 2004;25(3):147–53.

[43] Flach AJ, Jaffe NS, Akers WA. The effect of ketorolac tromethamine in reducing postoperative inflammation: double-mask parallel comparison with dexamethasone. Ann Ophthalmol 1989;21(11):407–11.

[44] Juniper EF, Kline PA, Ramsdale EH, et al. Comparison of the efficacy and side effects of aqueous steroid nasal spray (budesonide) and allergen-injection therapy (Pollinex-R) in the treatment of seasonal allergic rhinoconjunctivitis. J Allergy Clin Immunol 1990;85(3): 606–11.

[45] Del Prete A, Loffredo C, Carderopoli A, et al. Local specific immunotherapy in allergic conjunctivitis. Acta Ophthalmol (Copenh) 1994;72(5):631–4.

[46] O'Hara MA. Ophthalmia neonatorum. Pediatr Clin North Am 1993;40(4):715–25.

[47] Darville T. Chlamydia trachomatis infections in neonates and young children. Semin Pediatr Infect Dis 2005;16(4):235–44.

[48] Woods CR. Gonococcal infections in neonates and young children. Semin Pediatr Infect Dis 2005;16(4):258–70.

[49] Olitsky S, Nelson L. Disorders of the conjunctiva. 16th edition. Philadelphia: W.B. Saunders Co.; 2000.

[50] Ho CL, Walton DS. Management of childhood glaucoma. Curr Opin Ophthalmol 2004; 15(5):460–4.
[51] Cunningham ET Jr. Uveitis in children. Ocul Immunol Inflamm 2000;8(4):251–61.
[52] Edelsten C, Reddy MA, Stanford MR, et al. Visual loss associated with pediatric uveitis in English primary and referral centers. Am J Ophthalmol 2003;135(5):676–80.
[53] Weiner A, BenEzra D. Clinical patterns and associated conditions in chronic uveitis. Am J Ophthalmol 1991;112(2):151–8.

ELSEVIER
SAUNDERS

Immunol Allergy Clin N Am
28 (2008) 189–224

IMMUNOLOGY
AND ALLERGY
CLINICS
OF NORTH AMERICA

Ocular Allergy Treatment

Leonard Bielory, MD

*UMDNJ–New Jersey Medical School, 90 Bergen Street, DOC Suite 4700,
Newark, NJ 07103, USA*

Nonpharmacologic interventions are commonly used as first-line treatment of ocular allergy and include avoidance, cold compresses, lubrication, and the use of disposable daily contact lenses. Pharmacologic management of ocular allergy has increased exponentially over the past decade.

Clinically available agents are being expanded to specifically address the various signs and symptoms of inflammation associated with ocular allergy. The increased focus on drug development for treating ocular allergy correlates with the increased awareness of its prevalence in the industrialized countries of the United States and in the European Union. Increasing recognition of the prevalence of ocular allergy has also resulted in an upsurge of research into the pathophysiology and immunology defining the various forms of inflammation and identifying the specific roles of the various mediators of inflammation. This focus has become the basis for the development of novel pharmacologic targets for treating the ocular allergy inflammatory cascade, which include those that target the mast cells, the IgE antibody, and the release of early and late phase mediators (eg, histamine, prostaglandins, leukotrienes, cytokines). The search for of more effective medications for ocular allergy required the development of a standardized model, such as the conjunctival allergen challenge (CAC), also known as the *conjunctival provocation test*. This model allowed more efficient assessment of the efficacy of new agents in treating the allergy signs and symptoms of erythema (redness), pruritus (itching), epiphora (tearing), lid swelling, and conjunctival swelling (chemosis). Many newer agents that have been tested in this model for their impact on the subjective and objective signs have also started to measure the objective efficacy through the presence of cytologic biomarkers, further advancing the understanding of the conjunctival-associated lymphoid tissue allergic response (Fig. 1).

E-mail address: bielory@umdnj.edu

doi:10.1016/j.iac.2007.12.001   *immunology.theclinics.com*

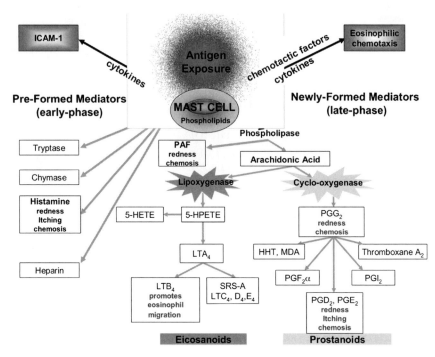

Fig. 1. Effects of the inflammatory cascade in treating allergic conjunctivitis: central role of the mast cell. Antihistamines induce rapid relief from H_1-receptor–mediated itching and inhibit redness through H_2-receptor blockade; mast cell stabilizers stabilize the mast cell membrane, blocking the release of histamine, cytokines, and chemotactic factors; nonsteroidal anti-inflammatory drugs block cyclooxygenase, preventing release of prostanoids; multiple-action agents (antihistamines and mast cell stabilizers) block histamine activity and release, expression of chemokines and intercellular adhesion molecule-1, and leukocyte infiltration; and corticosteroids block all mediators through phospholipase inhibition, increased synthesis of histidine decarboxylase, decreased synthesis of histaminase, and cell membrane stabilization. HETE, hydroxyeicosatetraenoic acid; HHT, heptadecatrienoic; HPETE, hydroperoxyeicosatetraenoic acid; ICAM-1, intercellular adhesion molecule-1; LT, leukotriene; MDA, malonyldialdehyde; PAF, platelet activating factor; PG, prostaglandin; SRS-A, slow reacting substance of anaphylaxis.

Historically, multiple agents have been used to manage allergic conjunctivitis. The classes of agents have included vasoconstrictors, oral and topical antihistamines, mast cell stabilizers, multiple-action agents, nonsteroidal anti-inflammatory agents (NSAIDs), and corticosteroids. Vasoconstrictors are widely available as over-the-counter agents but are not recommended because they are nonspecific and not pharmacologically active in the cascade of events that leads to the overall allergic biphasic reaction. Although they have a rapid onset of action, their reduction of redness is short-lived because of tolerance and they cause rebound hyperemia (ie, the development of conjunctivitis medicamentosa).

Oral antihistamines interfere with systemic allergic events that involve the eye but were clearly inferior compared with topical antihistamines, showing slower onset [1]. Oral antihistamines have as much as a 1- to 2-hour delay from systemic antihistamine administration to delivery to ocular tissues through the tears, whereas topical application provides immediate relief. In addition, oral antihistamines have also been associated with excessive drying, leading to more clinical problems with tear film dysfunction in many patients.

Overall, mast cell stabilizers have a slower onset of action than antihistamines, require multiple daily applications to truly achieve mast cell membrane stabilization, and require initiation before mast cell activation to prevent the initial trigger of the allergic cascade. They have been most useful in seasonal management of chronic ocular allergy disorders, such as vernal keratoconjunctivitis (VKC) and chronic giant papillary conjunctivitis, and have been shown to improve healing time of corneal involvement.

The newer multiple-action agents that were previously referred as *dual-action agents* (ie, having histamine blocking and mast cell stabilizing effects) have been the cornerstone of treatment because they incorporate multiple actions, including binding to H_1 and H_2 receptors, mast cell stabilization, and down-regulation of various inflammatory markers, including eosinophils, neutrophils, adhesion molecules, interleukins, and other cytokines that impact the early and late phases of the conjunctival allergic response. Thus, some of these agents are also approved for prophylactic (ie, prevention) treatment of seasonal allergy conjunctivitis (SAC) in countries other than the United States, and for its acute and long-term treatment of this condition.

NSAIDs specifically inhibit prostaglandins and leukotrienes, theoretically impacting mucus secretion, cellular infiltration, erythema, and chemosis. However, they have only been approved for affecting pruritus and do so weakly compared with the new multiple-action agents. Corticosteroids still remain a cornerstone of treatment for severe and chronic ocular allergy because they exert their anti-inflammatory effects at multiple levels, such as stabilizing intracellular and extracellular membranes; down-regulating inflammation through increasing synthesis of anti-inflammatory lipocortins that block phospholipase A2; inhibiting histamine synthesis in mast cells through blocking histidine decarboxylase; increasing histaminase enzyme and thereby reducing levels of unbound histamine; and modulating transcription factors within mast cell nucleus leading to decreased production of multiple late-phase mediators, which perpetuate the persistent and chronic forms of ocular allergy. However, topical corticosteroids have the potential to induce serious side effects, such as cataracts, elevated intraocular pressure (IOP), and infection, and therefore are best used over short periods (up to 2 weeks). For use beyond 2 weeks, IOP and lens clarity should be monitored with an ophthalmologist or other eye care specialist.

Allergen desensitization involves desensitizing a patient against a specific allergen and is most useful in the management of atopic disorders, including SAC, perennial allergic conjunctivitis (PAC), allergic rhinitis, and certain forms of asthma. Allergen desensitization is not indicated for VKC or atopic keratoconjunctivitis (AKC). Although highly effective in selected patients who have SAC and PAC, allergen desensitization should be carefully monitored for its overall risk-to-benefit ratio by specialists highly experienced in allergen immunotherapy who have facilities for treating anaphylaxis. Topical immunosuppressive agents, such as cyclosporine A, are alternative therapies for VKC and AKC. Topical cyclosporine A is an immunomodulator that is approved by the U.S. Food and Drug Administration (FDA) for dry eye but not allergic conjunctivitis.

Comparative clinical trials, which include known therapies and placebos, are essential in constructing a solid basis from which to launch any new drug. This approach especially applies to eye drops for treating SAC, for which the symptomatology, already dependent on the vagaries of the natural pollen challenge season, is further influenced by a positive washing action of the placebo eye drops [2]. Prophylactic treatment can be achieved in various models with a variety of agents, especially those considered mast cell–stabilizing or those having multiple actions, such as antihistamines with antieosinophilic or mast cell–stabilizing properties.

The availability of newer mildly sedating and nonsedating second-generation oral antihistamines has provided patients with a myriad of options, especially for ocular allergy treatment. Many of the selective H_1-receptor antagonists have also shown some anti-inflammatory activity that provides additional impact on the ocular late-phase reaction. Topically applied agents still provide faster relief of ocular symptoms compared with oral (within hours) or intranasal agents (within days). Although their duration of action may not be as long as oral systemic agents, health care providers should be aware of the anticholinergic effects of all first- and second-generation antihistamines, because these may exacerbate a concomitant dry eye condition in a patient who has allergies.

Treatment of ocular allergies is largely based on how much these allergies interfere with patient quality of life [3] (ie, severity of symptoms) [4]. Improvement of these quality of life parameters has been shown to take up to 2.5 weeks under treatment. The easiest and most direct therapeutic method is applying a topical agent to the affected tissue. Several topical agents are available for treatment and, to some degree, prophylaxis of ocular allergies, including vasoconstrictors, antihistamines, mast cell stabilizers, and anti-inflammatory agents. Efficacy of these agents varies among patients, and choice of agent depends on the underlying health of the eye and other variables, such as drug cost, contact lens wear, and potential for compliance.

Allergic conjunctivitis is commonly managed with different topical ocular agents. Tools for assessing the efficacy and effectiveness of these agents often includes the conjunctival provocation test or "a day in the park" models.

In addition, more chronic and severe forms of ocular allergy may require a multidisciplinary approach in consultation with an ophthalmologist. Recommendations for ophthalmologic consultation include persistence use of oral or topical steroids, ocular pain, or persistent "red eye."

Ocular allergy treatment algorithm

The treatment of ocular allergic disorders may follow a stepwise approach based on severity and chronicity that ranges from mildly intermittent to severe persistent forms of conjunctival inflammation. The development of effective therapeutic agents for ocular inflammation was largely ignored until the early 1990s (see Fig. 1). Current treatment is primarily aimed at restoring patient quality of life and may require at least 2 weeks of therapy. Nonpharmacologic therapy consists of minimizing contact with environmental allergens or avoidance, applying cool compresses to the eye, wearing contact lenses, and using preservative-free lubricants [5,6].

Advisory nonprescription interventions

Environmental control

Avoiding allergens remains the first step in managing any ocular disorder; this primary involves using environmental interventions, from removing the offending allergen source to changing occupational venue.

Cold compresses

Cold compresses provide considerable symptomatic relief, especially from ocular pruritus. In general, all refrigerated ocular medications provide additional subjective relief when applied immediately.

Lubrication

Tear substitutes consisting of saline combined with a wetting and viscosity agent, such as methylcellulose or polyvinyl alcohol ("artificial tears"), can be applied topically 2 to 6 times a day as necessary. This substance primarily helps directly remove and dilute allergens that may come in contact with the ocular surface. If tear substitutes are inadequate, ointments or time-released tear replacements (eg, Lacriserts) are commonly used at night to provide moisture to the ocular surface during sleep. The primary concern with chronic lubrication is possible development of a sensitivity to the preservatives found in the multiple-dose bottles. Therefore, patients who require frequent dosing may benefit from use of a preservative-free product to avoid toxic or allergic reactions to preservatives. Unit-dose packaging is generally preservative-free but has increased cost of use. One multidose bottled product, GenTeal (available as a drop or gel), is preserved with sodium perborate, which is chemically converted to water and oxygen within 1 minute of contact with catalase contained in tear film. Rapid degeneration of the preservative allegedly reduces the risk for preservative toxicity or allergy. Ocular lubricants also vary by class, osmolarity, and electrolyte composition. No product has emerged as a clear favorite.

Patients should offered one or two brands from each class of lubricant to try until a suitable product or combination of products is found. A newer form of lubricant, Systane, which contains polyethylene glycol 400 and propylene glycol demulcents with hydroxypropyl-guar as a gelling agent, has been shown to be more effective at reducing the signs and symptoms of dry eye compared with carboxymethylcellulose-containing lubricants [7].

Although the primary pharmacotherapeutic intervention recommended to patients who use specific medication or prescriptions may be to use contact lenses as a "band-aid," the overall goal of medication is to intervene in the various inflammatory mediators leading ocular allergy symptoms.

Contact lenses

Overall patients who have seasonal allergy are commonly recommended to avoid contact lens use during seasonal flare-ups. The need for clean lenses with minimal deposit buildup must be stressed, and the use of daily-wear lenses with rigid disinfecting and cleaning techniques is recommended. Alternatively, daily disposable lenses should be used [8]. However, when these individuals wear contact lenses, they have an increased risk for developing ocular infection. The risk is greatest if the lenses are soft and therefore provide for little tear exchange beneath their surface. Under these circumstances, limited tear flow allows for a greater buildup of lens deposits and metabolic wastes, while permitting increased tear evaporation from the lens surface [9].

A primary treatment of any inflammatory response is the use of a mechanical barrier, such as a bandage. This method is commonly used to treat corneal abrasions, with a bandage covering the eye, allowing the eyelid to act as a bandage to promote faster healing of the damaged cornea. In a study evaluating the impact of daily disposable lenses versus standard chronic wear lenses, 67% of patients reported that the 1-day disposable lenses provided improved comfort compared with 18% who preferred a new pair of habitual lenses, suggesting that the use of 1-day disposable lenses may be an effective strategy for managing patients who have allergies who wear contact lenses [10]. Overall, the newer soft silicone with increased gas permeability provide greater comfort (56%) than rigid gas-permeable lens (14%), whereas 63% of nonatopic and only 47% of atopic subjects described their lenses as very comfortable to wear [11,12].

Decongestants

Topical decongestants primarily act as vasoconstrictors, which are highly effective in reducing erythema and are widely used in combination with topical antihistamines [13]. Topical decongestants are applied two to four times a day as necessary. Few studies have compared the commercially ocular decongestants. Oxymetazoline (Ocuclear) is believed to have a faster onset of action, longer duration of action, and better decongestant effect than naphazoline (Vasocon) and tetrahydrozoline (Visine). Oxymetazoline 0.025% solution has been shown in earlier studies to significantly improve the symptoms of allergic conjunctivitis when given twice a day [14]. Vasocon-strictors that are commonly used in combination with topical antihistamines are either phenylephrine or naphazoline. All ocular medications containing naphazoline in combination with an antihistamine, except Vasocon-A, have been removed from clinical use because of an evaluation by the FDA in 1992 [15]. Vasocon-A, an antihistamine/decongestant combination, has been proven to effectively treat the signs and symptoms (itch and redness) of allergic conjunctivitis. Visine-A (formerly Ocuhist; Pfizer) contains phenir-amine maleate 0.3% and naphazoline 0.025%. The usual dose is one to two drops per eye every 2 hours, up to four times a day. The primary contraindi-cation is for narrow-angle glaucoma. One of the earliest studies comparing the relative efficacies of combination vasoconstrictors in the treatment of allergic conjunctivitis used naphazoline hydrochloride as the vasoconstrictor and antazoline phosphate or pheniramine maleate as the antihistamine in varying concentrations. Patients were specifically queried about their ocular signs (lid swelling, bulbar conjunctival inflammation, and palpebral conjunctival inflammation) and symptoms (itching, tearing, and discomfort) over the course of 1 week. The compounds resulted in different levels of patient com-fort and acceptability but were comparable in ameliorating the signs and symptoms [16].

Vasoconstrictors, such as phenylephrine and tetrahydrozoline, are sym-pathomimetic agents that decrease vascular congestion and eyelid edema though α-receptor stimulation; they do not diminish allergic response. An early study in normal volunteers (n = 11) evaluated two commercial prepa-rations of topical ophthalmic vasoconstrictors (0.02% naphazoline HCI and 0.05% tetrahydrozoline HCI) for whitening ability, duration of action, tolerance, and rebound vasodilation. Both significantly reduced baseline redness after a single use (naphazoline > tetrahydrozoline), but naphazoline maintained its whitening ability without tachyphylaxis after 10 days [17]. Although no evidence of "rebound" was reported after 10 days, conjuncti-vitis from the use of nonprescription (over-the-counter) decongestants that include naphazoline, tetrahydrozoline, or phenylephrine is well-known. In a study of these over-the-counter preparations (N = 70; 137 eyes), three clinical patterns of conjunctivitis were reported: conjunctival hyperemia (n = 50), follicular conjunctivitis (n = 17), and eczematoid blepharoconjunc-tivitis (n = 3). Decongestants were used daily for a median of 3 years (range, 8 hours to 20 years) before presentation and then simply halted. The median time to resolution of symptoms and signs was 4 weeks (range, 1–24 weeks), and patients remained asymptomatic for a median follow-up of 6 months (range, 0–12 years) [18]. Most cases were associated with conjunctival hyper-emia, which was similar to the effect of chronic decongestant use on the nasal mucosa (rhinitis medicamentosa) and thus was designated in a case report as *conjunctivitis medicamentosa* [19].

The follicular and eczematoid forms of decongestant-induced conjunctivitis seem to show a T-cell hyperresponsiveness that has been reported with phenylephrine [20]. Although the chronic use of decongestants is associated with conjunctivitis, some experts believe that chronic use of these agents can produce dry-eye symptoms in some patients, which interfere with tear-film adequacy through decreasing mucin-secreting goblet cells. An animal model chronically treated with vasoconstrictors or artificial tears for varying periods showed no significant difference in the number of goblet cells per light microscopic field compared with controls [21].

Antihistamines

Initially, oral antihistamines were used extensively to systemically control the symptoms of allergic rhinitis, which also included allergic conjunctivitis, but with an obvious delayed onset of action on the ocular domain [22]. However, they can clearly have a longer-lasting effect, exemplified in the study comparing the immediate effect of topical agents (olopatadine) with oral antihistamines (loratadine) [23,24]. Therefore, focus on the development of topical antihistamine agents has increased since 1990.

In a human study, chlorpheniramine, dexbrompheniramine, pyrilamine, and pheniramine significantly reduced the classic histamine-induced conjunctival injection [25,26]. However, the newer second-generation H_1 receptor antagonists have less sedative or anticholinergic effects than earlier compounds [27]. In the human conjunctiva, H_1 stimulation principally mediates the symptom of pruritus, whereas the H_2 receptor seems to be clinically involved in vasodilation [28,29]. The improved effect with H_1 and H_2 blockade was also noted in an animal model using pyrilamine and cimetidine. This study showed histamine-induced ocular surface erythema being virtually abolished by a combination of cimetidine (H_2-receptor antagonist) and pyrilamine (H_1-receptor antagonist), whereas either antagonist administered alone produced no significant reduction [30]. However, the potency of the blockade of the various histamine receptors with the newer topical agents has not been well defined. Although topical antihistamines can be used alone to treat allergic conjunctivitis, they have been shown to have a synergistic effect when used in combination with a vasoconstrictor, similar to the addition of a decongestant in the oral formulations for treating allergic rhinitis [13].

Oral antihistamines

Although studies commonly link oral antihistamine use in the treatment of allergic conjunctivitis to its effect on allergic rhinitis, many show conflicting results regarding their impact on the ocular domain of allergy. For example, in one double-bind, placebo-controlled trial evaluating the efficacy of once-daily cetirizine on various symptoms of rhinitis, including nasal congestion, postnasal discharge, sneezing, rhinorrhea, and nasal itching, and ocular symptoms, including lacrimation and epiphora, showed that all nasal symptoms were positively affected, whereas the ocular symptoms were not [31]. However, in a conjunctival provocation model, cetirizine showed efficacy against symptoms of allergic conjunctivitis [32,33]. In a double-blind conjunctival provocation study, cetirizine administered orally (10 mg twice daily for 4 days) increased the threshold of grass allergen compared with placebo ($P<.004$) by inhibiting redness and itching of the eye [32]. Other studies of oral antihistamines have shown loratadine to have a protective effect in conjunctival provocation tests [34], and desloratadine [35] and fexofenadine [36,37] to significantly reduce ocular symptoms of seasonal allergy rhinitis in placebo-controlled studies. In another study, loratadine was found to increase the allergen threshold in conjunctival provocation tests to 3 to 10 times the baseline level in 60% (6/10) of patients [34]. Other antiallergic drugs under investigation show promising results in the treatment of allergic conjunctivitis; including emedastine, a selective blocker of the H_1 histamine receptor [38].

In other human studies, chlorpheniramine, dexbrompheniramine, pyrilamine, and pheniramine significantly reduced histamine-induced and conjunctival injection [25,26]. Second-generation antihistamines can, however, induce ocular drying [39,40], which may impair the protective barrier provided by the ocular tear film and thus actually worsen allergic symptoms. Similarly, the antimuscarinic binding of topical agents may induce a drying effect after chronic use, but recent animal studies show conflicting results regarding whether chronic treatment with topical agents would have a significant clinical effect in patients [41,42]. Therefore, some experts have suggested that the concomitant use of eye drops may treat ocular allergic symptoms more effectively [43]; ketotifen plus desloratadine [44] and olopatadine plus loratadine [45] have been shown to be more effective than either antihistamine alone.

Topical antihistamines

In general, the earlier topical antihistamines were irritating when administered to the eye. Prolonged use of topical antihistamines is associated with the risk for developing sensitivity reactions that can further aggravate ocular allergies. For antihistamines that are nonselective and block muscarinic receptors in addition to H_1 receptors, ciliary muscle paralysis, mydriasis, and photophobia may result. This effect is more pronounced in patients who have lighter irides. Also related to muscarinic receptor blockade is the risk for angle-closure glaucoma, especially in patients who have a history of narrow-angle glaucoma and those who have narrow angles. The mydriatic effect causes the anterior chamber to become shallower, and decreased aqueous humor outflow leads to increased IOP. The classic signs of acute angle–closure glaucoma include headache, blurry vision, nausea, vomiting, and changes in corneal opacity. Histamine-stimulated phosphatidylinositol turnover and cytokine secretion by human conjunctival epithelial cells are attenuated by compounds with H_1-antagonist activity. However, antihistaminic potency alone does not predict anti-inflammatory potential [46]. The newer topical antihistamines are more effective and have fewer adverse effects.

Topical antihistamines

Levocabastine

Levocabastine was identified from a series of cyclohexylpiperidine derivatives as a potent antiallergic agent having rapid and long-lasting activity. It was approved in 1994 for the treatment of allergic conjunctivitis. Levocabastine is a cyclohexyl-3-methylpiperidine derivative that has rapid onset and prolonged activity. Absorption of levocabastine after ocular instillation of single doses is incomplete, with the absolute bioavailability estimated to range from 30% to 60% in patients who have SAC and healthy subjects, respectively. On repeated ocular administration, steady-state plasma concentrations were virtually attained within 7 days of dosing in healthy subjects. After active doses are administered, only low levels of levocabastine are found systemically; plasma concentrations of the drug typically do not exceed 1 to 2 ng/mL [47]. The drug does not seem to cause central nervous system depression, sedation, or effects on psychomotor performance, probably because the systemic absorption of levocabastine is low after ocular instillation [48]. The elimination half-life of levocabastine ranges from 35 to 40 hours after ocular or oral administration and is similar for single and repeated doses. In vitro studies indicated the high selective binding affinity of levocabastine for H_1 receptors along with its exceptionally slow rate of dissociation from these receptors [49]. Levocabastine (dissociation constant, 52.6 nmol/L) exhibited greater functional activity (50% inhibitory concentration, 8–25 nmol/L) than either antazoline or pheniramine [50].

In an ocular provocation study, 10 of 11 patients treated with levocabastine required a 10-fold increase in allergen to reproduce the same symptoms, although pretreatment with an antihistamine caused an increase in late-phase symptoms in 3 of the 11 patients [51].

Emedastine

Emedastine is a selective H_1 antagonist with no apparent effect on adrenergic, dopaminergic, or serotonin receptors [38]. It was the most potent in ligand binding, phosphatidylinositol turnover, and interleukin (IL)-6 secretion, with dissociation constant and 50% inhibitory concentrations of 1 to 3 nmol/L [52]. In human volunteers dosed bilaterally twice daily for 15 days with 0.05% emedastine fumarate ophthalmic solution, plasma concentrations of the parent compound were generally below the limit of the assay. Relief of the signs and symptoms of allergic conjunctivitis have been shown in patients treated for 6 weeks with emedastine in an environmental study, as has reduction in ocular itching when patients were challenged with antigen at either 10 minutes or 4 hours after dosing with 0.005%/0.05% and 0.05% solutions, respectively. Antazoline hydrochloride, emedastine difumarate, levocabastine hydrochloride, olopatadine hydrochloride, and pheniramine maleate attenuated histamine-stimulated phosphatidylinositol turnover and IL-6 and IL-8 secretion [50]. In another study on conjunctival fibroblasts stimulated with histamine, emedastine significantly reduced production of IL-1, IL-6, and IL-8, whereas azelastine reduced only IL-1 [53]. Clinically, emedastine was similar to ketotifen in a conjunctival provocation model effect on ocular itching [54].

Mast cell–stabilizing agents

Cromoglycate

The prototypic mast cell mediator, cromolyn sodium, has been on the market intermittently in the United States. Its efficacy seems to be concentration-dependent, with a 1% solution having no effect, a 2% solution having a possible effect, and a 4% solution having a probable effect [55]. After many years of clinical use, the possible mechanisms for cromolyn are still not clearly defined. Initially, cromolyn was believed to affect phosphodiesterase or cyclic AMP and B lymphocytes switching from mu (IgM) to epsilon (IgE) heavy chains, which would be a novel potential mechanism for the prevention of mast cell–mediated disorders [56,57]. Sodium cromoglycate was originally approved for more severe forms of conjunctivitis (GPC, AKC, VKC), but many physicians had extended its use to the treatment of allergic conjunctivitis with an excellent safety record, although the original studies reflecting its clinical efficacy showed marginal benefit for allergic conjunctivitis when compared with placebo [58,59].

However, in a study using an opiate conjunctival provocation, prior treatment with cromolyn inhibited ocular mast cell activation, but not necessarily clinical symptoms [60]. A study using topical cromolyn during ragweed season found that the diary eye symptoms were similar among patients using cromolyn on a routine basis (four times daily) and those using cromolyn as needed [61]. However, the regular treatment group had better quality of life with topical cromolyn, whereas the as-needed group showed a trend toward more oral terfenadine use for uncontrolled eye symptoms. Cromolyn effects are not present until 2 to 5 days after the initiation of therapy, with maximum improvement of ocular symptoms noted 15 days after initiation of therapy. Topical cromolyn sodium is equivalent to placebo during the first days of treatment.

In multicenter studies of chronic forms of ocular allergy, vernal conjunctivitis topical cromolyn showed effectiveness in relieving discharge, photophobia, hyperemia, and edema of the eyelids. Itching and changes in visual acuity improvement were equivocal in some studies. However, most studies have shown a lack of efficacy in the major problem associated with vernal conjunctivitis: papillary hypertrophy of the upper tarsal conjunctiva. In the treatment of giant papillary conjunctivitis, patients experienced symptomatic improvement, but little if any change in ocular signs. In AKC, significant improvement was seen after 4 weeks of treatment with ocular cromolyn in the clinical scores for photophobia, discharge, papillary hypertrophy, limbal changes, and corneal changes and the overall clinical assessments of patients. Another study comparing the effects of topical cromolyn with other immunomodulatory agents (cyclosporine and dexamethasone) showed that cromolyn was ineffective after 14 days of treatment with regard to symptoms or the tear levels of eosinophil cationic protein [62].

Cromolyn has also been used in comparison studies and shown to have similar effect to azelastine, with more than 80% improvement compared with the placebo effect of 50% [63]. A comparison study with olopatadine also showed equivalent results between the agents [64].

Cromolyn sodium 4% ophthalmic solution should be applied four to six times daily, with the dosage decreased incrementally to twice daily as symptoms permit. The major adverse effect is burning and stinging, which has been reported in 13% to 77% of patients. This agent is commonly initiated in patients who have moderate symptoms soon after ocular decongestants are administered for immediate relief [59]. Acute chemotic reactions have been reported with cromolyn [65]. The nasal solution of cromolyn sodium is composed in the exact formulation as the ocular solution, except for the additional sterilization procedure required for ophthalmic preparations. Many physicians have used the nasal solution in the eye, making a concerted effort to keep the medication refrigerated and discard it after 4 weeks to decrease the possibility of bacterial contamination. An allergic reaction to topical disodium cromoglycate was reported, which was proven with skin prick tests, conjunctival provocation tests, and circulating IgE-specific antibodies to disodium cromoglycate [66].

Lodoxamide

Lodoxamide is a mast cell stabilizer that has been shown to be approximately 2500 times more potent than cromolyn in preventing histamine release in several animal models [67,68]. Lodoxamide reduced tryptase levels and decreased the recruitment of inflammatory cells in the tear fluid after allergen challenge [69], and has been shown deliver greater and earlier relief in patients who have more chronic forms of conjunctivitis (eg, VKC, AKC, GPC) than cromolyn [70,71]. However, in a study of allergic conjunctivitis, it was only perceived to be clinically better by the patient, and not the physician. Lodoxamide was more effective than placebo [72] and as effective as levocabastine [73]. In patients who have allergic conjunctivitis, its clinical efficacy vis-à-vis cromolyn remains unclear. It has recently been approved for the treatment of all forms of vernal conjunctivitis at a concentration of 0.1% four times daily. Lodoxamide may be used continuously for 3 months. It has been labeled as a schedule B drug for use in pregnancy. It can be used in children from 2 years of age. Tear eosinophil cationic protein (ECP) has also been shown to be a marker for eosinophil activation in ocular allergic disorders and has been used to evaluate the efficacy of lodoxamide and sodium cromoglycate in the treatment of VKC. ECP levels were significantly correlated with signs, symptoms, corneal involvement, and number of eosinophils in tears. Sodium cromoglycate did not prevent tear ECP from increasing, whereas lodoxamide therapy significantly reduced ECP tear levels and thus eosinophil activation, and was more effective than disodium chromoglycate in reducing clinical signs and symptoms [74]. In patients who had VKC, median tear leukotriene B4 and C4 decreased after treatment with disodium cromoglycate 2%, lodoxamide 0.1%, and fluorometholone 0.1% [75]. In the treatment of various forms of VKC, the lodoxamide group experienced a 67% improvement compared with those using topical cyclosporin A [76].

Pemirolast

Pemirolast potassium was originally marketed as a tablet in Japan in 1991 for treating bronchial asthma and allergic rhinitis, and was subsequently developed and registered in Japan as an ophthalmic formulation for the treatment of seasonal allergic and vernal conjunctivitis. It has been studied in children as young as 2 years of age, with no reports of serious adverse events. Antiallergic pharmacology studies have shown that pemirolast is a specific inhibitor of mast cell degranulation inhibiting the release of chemical mediators, such as histamine. In vitro and in vivo studies have shown that the dose-dependent inhibition of antigen-induced chemical mediators is achieved through interference with mediator release, perhaps from the inhibition of phospholipid byproducts involved in intracellular transduction. Ocular antiallergic pharmacology testing has shown that ocular instillation of pemirolast seems to have a potent inhibitor effect on the rat conjunctival IgE–mast cell allergy model. Its potency is more than 100 times that of cromoglycate. In a placebo-controlled study evaluating pemirolast 0.1% four times daily, beginning approximately 1 to 2 weeks before the onset of ragweed season and continuing until after the first killing frost (12–17 weeks duration), patients recorded their daily evaluations of ocular itching in a diary. After the allergy season, patients underwent a second CAC. Evaluable patients (n = 265) recorded a total of 21,491 patient-days of ocular itching data during allergy season. In every 7- or 14-day period, patients treated with pemirolast potassium 0.1% reported more days without any ocular itching compared with patients receiving placebo. Differences favoring pemirolast potassium 0.1% were statistically significant in 63% (10/16) of all 7-day periods ($P < .046$) and 88% (7/8) of all 14-day periods ($P < .016$). After the allergy season, pemirolast potassium 0.1% was significantly superior to placebo in relieving CAC-induced ocular itching, with relief occurring as early as 3 minutes after allergen challenge ($P \leq .034$) [77].

In the specific evaluation of histamine release from the conjunctiva, the simultaneous use of levocabastine and pemirolast significantly decreased histamine content compared with either levocabastine and pemirolast alone. These findings suggest levocabastine not only had antihistaminic activity but also inhibited histamine release [78]. In a pharmaceutical-sponsored study, cromolyn and pemirolast (100 nM–1 mM) failed to significantly inhibit histamine release from human conjunctival mast cells using exposure times of 1 and 15 minutes before challenge, whereas olopatadine did [79]. This finding suggests discordances between in vitro and in vivo studies even while using the human model, and that some antiallergy agents may have more than one mechanism of action.

Nonsteroidal antiinflammatory agents

Ketorolac

Ketorolac tromethamine (Acular), approved in November 1992, is one of the earliest prescription products for treating itch associated with allergic conjunctivitis. Ketorolac, which is a pyrazolone, is a nonsteroidal antiinflammatory agent. Its primary mechanism of action is on the arachidonic acid cascade, where it binds cyclooxygenase to block the production of prostaglandins, but it does not inhibit lipoxygenase or the formation of leukotrienes. Prostaglandins, particularly PGE_2 and PGI_2, are extremely pruritogenic to the conjunctival mucosa [80–82]. Clinical studies have shown that topical NSAIDs significantly diminish the ocular itching and conjunctival hyperemia associated with seasonal antigen-induced allergic conjunctivitis [83] and VKC [84]. Unlike topical corticosteroids, these agents do not mask ocular infections, affect wound healing, increase IOP, or contribute to cataract formation. In a recent study on measles conjunctivitis, it helped decrease the amount of hyperemia and was not associated with any viral spread [85,86].

Although topical ketorolac is currently the only topical NSAID approved by the FDA for use in acute SAC, topical diclofenac may have similar features in the treatment of seasonal allergic conjunctivitis [87]. Ketorolac has been studied in comparison with topical antihistamines, with better outcomes in some cases [87–90]. In a recent study compared topical ketorolac with levocabastine in which the medications were instilled in each eye four times daily for 6 weeks, ketorolac produced the greatest improvements in most efficacy variables, followed by levocabastine and vehicle. Ketorolac was significantly more effective than vehicle in reducing mean itching scores, palpebral hyperemia, bulbar hyperemia, and edema [88]. An experimental model of contact lens–induced conjunctivitis showed that treatment may take up to 2 weeks to have an affect [91]. NSAID-induced asthma does not seem to be a problem, except in patients who have the triad of asthma, nasal polyposis, and aspirin sensitivity [92].

The most frequent adverse events reported with the use of ketorolac ophthalmic solutions (occurring in 40% of patients participating in clinical trials) have been transient stinging and burning on instillation. Other adverse events occurring approximately 1% to 10% of the time during treatment with ketorolac ophthalmic solutions included allergic reactions, corneal edema, iritis, ocular inflammation, ocular irritation, superficial keratitis, and superficial ocular infections. Adverse events reported rarely with the use of ketorolac ophthalmic solutions included corneal infiltrates, corneal ulcer, eye dryness, headaches, and blurred vision. It has been reformulated and is now used to reduce ocular pain after cataract and refractive surgery [93].

Multiple action agents

Olopatadine

Olopatadine (Patanol, Pataday) seems to possess a dual form of action with limited mast cell stabilizing effects and H_1-receptor binding [52,79,94]. Compared with the first-generation antihistamines (antazoline and pheniramine), olopatadine was also noted to inhibit cytokine secretion [52], including tumor necrosis factor (TNF)-α mediator release from human conjunctival mast cells [95–97]. Olopatadine was approximately 10-fold more potent as an inhibitor of cytokine secretion (50% inhibitory concentration, 1.7–5.5 nmol/L) than predicted from binding data, whereas antazoline and pheniramine were far less potent (20- to 140-fold) in functional assays [49]. It has been shown to be significantly more effective than placebo in relieving itching and redness for up to 8 hours [98,99]. Olopatadine also binds to S100 family of calcium-binding proteins similar to amlexanox [100]. In a comparison study with another multiple-action agent, ketotifen, olopatadine showed only slightly better results over 2 weeks of treatment [101]. In one of the few head-to-head studies using the conjunctival provocation model, olopatadine and azelastine treatments were significantly more effective than placebo at reducing itching postchallenge. Subjects gave itching assessments (scale, 0 = no itching to 4 = severe itching) every 30 seconds for 20 minutes (Olopatadine was significantly more effective than azelastine in reducing itching at 3.5 minutes through 20 minutes postchallenge [102].

Ketotifen

Ketotifen (Zaditor), a benzocycloheptathiophene agent, has been used as an orally active prophylactic agent to manage bronchial asthma and allergic disorders. Ketotifen has shown pronounced antihistaminic and antianaphylactic properties, resulting in moderate to marked symptom improvement in most patients who have atopic dermatitis, seasonal or perennial rhinitis, allergic conjunctivitis, chronic or acute urticaria, or food allergy [103]. It recently became generic and is available over-the-counter for treating allergic conjunctivitis. Ketotifen is distinguished from the cromones, sodium cromoglycate and nedocromil, by a conjoint mast cell stabilizing effect; several antimediator properties, including strong H_1-receptor antagonism [104,105]; and inhibition of leukotriene formation [86,106]. A possible effect of ketotifen on the constitutive eosinophil apoptosis and IL-5–mediated eosinophil survival has been postulated to be more induction of primary necrosis than apoptosis [107]. In the guinea pig model, ketotifen was more effective than olopatadine and levocabastine in reducing conjunctival edema and vascular permeability as measured by Evans blue dye leakage in eyelids and eyeballs [108].

In an experimental model for allergic conjunctivitis, chlorpheniramine, ketotifen, and levocabastine were effective in inhibiting cedar pollen-induced conjunctivitis [109]. In the standard CAC model comparing ketotifen with placebo, ketotifen showed up to a 30% decrease in signs and symptom associated with allergic conjunctivitis and a lack of tachyphylaxis over the course of 4 weeks [110]. In another rare head-to-head study of two topical agents (without a placebo control), levocabastine hydrochloride ophthalmic suspension and ketotifen fumarate ophthalmic solution were respectively instilled in the left and right eyes, which were then challenged with the allergen. Pollen allergen–induced ocular symptoms were itching and hyperemia of the palpebral conjunctiva, and itching lasted for more than 5 hours. Moreover, preadministration of antihistamine eye drops suppressed the increases in the ocular symptom scores, eliminating itching within 1 hour. Allergen provoked not only ocular symptoms but also nasal symptoms in 78% of patients [111]. However, ketotifen was not better than a topical cromolyn–chlorpheniramine combination at preventing itching and redness in the CAC model [112].

One study randomly assigned patients who had SAC to one of three groups: two drops per eye twice daily for 30 days of either topical ketotifen 0.025% ophthalmic solution, olopatadine 0.1% ophthalmic solution, or placebo. Clinical scores (itching, tearing, redness, eyelid, swelling, and chemosis) and conjunctival impression cytology specimens were performed on day 0 of the study (baseline), day 15, and day 30. The percentages of cells expressing intercellular adhesion molecule 1, vascular cell adhesion molecule (CAM)-1, human leukocyte antigen (HLA)-DR, and beta 1 integrin (CD29) from conjunctival impression cytology specimens were determined using flow cytometry. Both active-treatment groups noted significant improvements in clinical scores (tearing and itching) and reduction in the expression rates of CAMs and inflammatory markers in conjunctival surface cells within a month [113]. However, in a double-blinded preference study, olopatadine was chosen more than ketotifen [114], perhaps because several studies have reported that ketotifen has a mild stinging affect on the conjunctival surface [104].

Nedocromil

Nedocromil is a pyranoquinoline dicarboxylic acid that was originally believed to be just a mast cell stabilizing agent but is now appreciated to have multiple actions [115], including as an H_1 antagonist with inhibitory effects on various allergic inflammatory cells, mast cells, and eosinophils [116], but with conflicting results on the inhibition of neutrophil migration [117,118]. Nedocromil seems able to stabilize mast cells and inhibit histamine release more than cromolyn [116]. Various studies have suggested that nedocromil may have its effect on B lymphocytes switching from μ (IgM) to ε (IgE) heavy chains, similar to studies for its chemistry-related cousin, cromolyn [56,57,119]. In an animal model, nedocromil was shown to suppress early- and late-phase conjunctival hyperemia, conjunctival edema, eyelid edema, and eosinophil infiltration [120]. Topical nedocromil treatment has been shown in an ocular allergen challenge model to reduce tear concentrations of histamine and prostaglandin D_2 and the number of 3H4-positive mast cells (purportedly the secreted form of IL-4) [121] while increasing the conjunctival tolerance to the allergen [122]. In cultures, nedocromil was shown to abolish the expression of HLA-DR and reduce intracellular adhesion molecule (ICAM)-1 expression [123].

Compared with placebo, nedocromil showed improved control of ocular pruritus and irritation associated with SAC [124–130] and vernal conjunctivitis [131]. In a study involving patients who had PAC, nedocromil eye drops were clinically effective in controlling symptoms that persisted despite previous treatment with cromoglycate [132]. The results of several placebo-controlled studies have shown that nedocromil is effective in alleviating the signs and symptoms of SAC and provide relief in 80% of patients [133,134]. Its safety profile is similar to that of sodium cromoglycate, but it seems to be more potent in treating chronic ocular allergic conditions, such as VKC. In a comparative study, nedocromil sodium 2% eye drops were more efficacious than sodium cromoglycate for treating hyperemia, keratitis, papillae, and pannus and had a quicker effect on itching, grittiness, hyperemia, and keratitis [133]. Nedocromil can be given just twice daily [132] and is associated with stinging or burning of the eyes on application of the drops and a distinctive taste in 5% of the population [135].

Azelastine

Azelastine, which has a half-life of approximately 22 hours, is a second-generation H_1-receptor antagonist that is primarily administered intranasally, although an oral formulation is used in some countries for effective relief of symptoms of allergic rhinitis after oral or intranasal administration [136,137] with a secondary entry in the topical treatment of allergic conjunctivitis [105,138].

Azelastine has been reported to inhibit early allergic response [139,140] and histamine release from rat mast cells after antigen and nonantigen stimuli [140–142], and seems to inhibit IgE secretion from IgE-producing hybridoma FE-3 cells through preventing C-epsilon mRNA expression [143]. The additional prophylactic antiallergic properties are probably partially caused by the inhibition of a broad array of other inflammatory mediators and important receptors for the allergic response, inhibition of superoxide generation by neutrophils and eosinophils [144], inhibition of leukotriene synthesis [145–150], inhibition of TNF-α secretion from rat basophil leukemia cells [151,152] and IL-6 from human leukemic mast cells [96,153], and down-regulation of ICAM-1 in the human conjunctiva [154]. Normal human umbilical cord blood–derived cultured mast cell stimulation with anti-IgE leads to substantial secretion of IL-6, TNF-α, and IL-8, whereas preincubation for 5 minutes resulted in almost maximal inhibition of TNF-α (80%) with 6 μM azelastine, of IL-6 (83%) with 24 μM, and of IL-8 (99%) with 60 μM [155]. When compared with another multiple-action agent in a similar designed experimental model, results with 24 μM azelastine were similar to those with 133 μM of olopatadine (a fivefold difference). At this concentration, these drugs inhibited IL-6 release by 83% and 74%, tryptase release by 55% and 79%, and histamine release by 41% and 45%, respectively [156]. Apart from the ability to inhibit histamine release from mast cells and prevent the activation of inflammatory cells, the antiallergic potency of azelastine is probably partially caused by down-regulation of ICAM1 expression during early- and late-phase response that likely leads to reduced inflammatory cell adhesion to epithelial cells, confirming the prophylactic properties of azelastine [154].

These and various other studies have reflected an extensive array of anti-inflammatory mechanisms of azelastine in the control of allergies and asthma, and it is the only nasal antihistamine spray in the United States that is also approved for treating allergic conjunctivitis [157]. In one study [152], azelastine was instilled into the eyes of patients who had rhinoconjunctivitis sensitive to *Parietaria judaica* both before and after antigen-specific conjunctival challenge (ASCC). When applied 30 minutes after ASCC, a statistically significant reduction in total symptom score (conjunctival hyperemia, lacrimation, itching/burning, eyelid swelling) was observed in azelastine-treated eyes compared with those receiving placebo eye drops, beginning 10 minutes after administration and lasting through the final evaluation 20 minutes later. Total symptom scores were also significantly reduced for up to 6 hours in patients treated twice daily with topical azelastine as opposed to placebo for 1 week before ASCC, accompanied by a significant reduction in conjunctival inflammatory cell infiltration. In a pediatric SAC study comparing the effects of azelastine with levocabastine eye drops, the response rate in the group receiving azelastine eye drops was significantly higher (74%) than that in the placebo group (39%) and comparable with that in the levocabastine group (69%) [158].

In a European study, azelastine significantly improved itching and conjunctival redness compared with placebo ($P < .001$). Tolerability was rated good or better by 97% of patients, with a noticeable bitter taste and some application site stinging. On day 7, ocular symptoms score improved by 1.5 ± 0.9 (compared with 0.5 ± 0.8 for placebo) using a six-point scale with score improvement more than or two in 55% treated with azelastine (versus 14% treated with placebo). Itching and redness further improved at day 42 (score improvement more than two in 95% treated with azelastine versus 33% treated with placebo) and completely resolved for 47% patients treated wit azelastine (versus 10% treated with placebo) [159].

Epinastine

Epinastine (Elestat) is a potent histamine H_1- and H_2-receptor antagonist with mast cell–stabilizing properties. It inhibits histamine release and has other anti-inflammatory activities, and was recently approved in the United States to prevent itching associated with allergic conjunctivitis (olopatadine once-daily formulation was also recently approved for this purpose). It does not significantly penetrate the blood–brain barrier and its safety and tolerability profiles seem to be equal to those of most other topical antihistamines. It is considered a multiple-action agent. Pretreatment with epinastine significantly reduced histamine and TNF-α, whereas IL-5, IL-8, IL-10, and TNF-β profiles were differentially decreased. In vivo, pretreatment with epinastine and olopatadine significantly reduced the clinical scores and eosinophil numbers (n = 6; $P < .05$), whereas epinastine also reduced neutrophils ($P < .02$), reflecting the existence of different patterns of inflammation inhibition [160]. The role of H_1-, H_2-, and H_3-receptor affinities in actual treatment is unclear, but past clinical experience indicates that the presence of multiple binding may be beneficial. In an animal model of histamine-induced vascular leakage, epinastine, azelastine, and ketotifen had a shorter duration of effect than olopatadine [161]. In a recent review, ketotifen, pyrilamine, and epinastine seemed to have the strongest H_1 and H_2 affinities, although a specific study to determine clinical relevance has not been performed [104].

In a major clinical trial, ophthalmologists performed conjunctival provocations to confirm the diagnosis of SAC. The primary end point was ocular itching, and secondary end points included ocular hyperemia, chemosis, ocular mucous discharge (all assessed on a five-point scale), eyelid swelling (assessed on a four-point scale), and tearing. present or absent). Ocular itching was clearly reduced with epinastine compared with placebo ($P = .045$), but ocular itching and hyperemia scores were similar in the epinastine and levocabastine groups [162]. In the human CAC model, multiple signs and symptoms of allergic conjunctivitis were significantly reduced by instillation of epinastine compared with vehicle. Epinastine showed prompt onset (3 minutes) and long duration of action (≥ 8 hours). Mean severity scores were significantly lower with epinastine compared with vehicle at all time points after onset and duration challenges, including ocular itching ($P < .001$); eyelid swelling ($P < .001$); conjunctival ($P < .001$), episcleral ($P < .001$), and ciliary hyperemia ($P < .001$); and chemosis ($P \leq .009$) [163].

A concern also exists about the impact of many antihistamines, and that multiple-action agents with antihistaminic activity may also show anticholinergic activity. In a study comparing loratadine and epinastine, anticholinergic activity was noted to affect the eyes after 4 days of treatment, and loratadine was associated with clinical signs of ocular dryness, including decreased tear volume and tear flow, in contrast with topical epinastine [164]. In a longer (1 month) head-to-head comparison of olopatadine and epinastine in a botulinum toxin B–induced murine model for dry eye, no difference was noted [41], whereas another animal model found epinastine to be superior [42].

Mizolastine

Mizolastine, a benzimidazole derivative, is a second-generation antihistamine that has been shown in experimental studies to possess 5-lipoxygenase inhibitory properties in addition to its H_1-receptor antagonistic activity [165,166]. It has been shown to interrupt intermediate signaling events that regulate cell function, such as through exerting an inhibitory effect on protein kinase C (PKC) activation in a dose-dependent manner [167]. Mizolastine has a terminal beta half-life of approximately 1 hour and a duration of action of at least 2 hours. The compound did not show any anticholinergic effects in a standard animal model using carbachol [168]. Mizolastine has a pronounced effect on nasal blockade that is believed to be linked to its anti-inflammatory properties. European approval for the treatment of perennial allergic rhinoconjunctivitis has shown some beneficial effects on ocular and total nasal scores after 6 months of treatment [165].

In an evaluation of mizolastine's effect on ocular allergy inflammation, it decreased the mean ocular symptom score (which included itching, tearing, and erythema) as reported by patients and physicians by 40% compared with 7% in the placebo group [169]. The decrease was noted within the first 2 weeks and continued for the remainder of the 4-week study. In a 2-week study, mizolastine reduced total symptom scores, nasal scores, and ocular scores at the end of the first week [170]. In perennial allergic rhinitis, mizolastine significantly improved symptoms of nasal obstruction compared with placebo and also significantly reduced nasal membrane color, nasal secretions, and mucosal swelling as shown with rhinoscopy. These effects were maintained over a 5-month treatment period [171]. Mizolastine was shown to have an effect within 1 hour in 50% of patients, and 78% of patients reported a positive effect after the first intake [172]. In another study, mizolastine showed more symptom relief with the first 3 days than cetirizine [173].

Picumast

Picumast dihydrochloride (3,4-dimethyl-7-[4-(4-chlorobenzyl) piperazine-1-yl] propoxycoumarin dihydrochloride) is a compound that seems to have prophylactically active antiallergic properties, which combines inhibition of mediator release and action on H_1-antagonism (and that of its metabolites on M2 and M1 receptors). It was originally believed to have potential in the treatment of bronchial and allergic rhinitis but was found to have limited effect [174,175]. Because the activity profile of picumast differs clearly from that of known prophylactic antiallergic drugs such as cromolyn and ketotifen, as reflected in the systemic administration of picumast in the inhibition of the allergen-induced conjunctivitis model when compared with mepyramine and ketotifen, an ocular formulation was further evaluated [176]. Examination of any specific long-term effects on the lens did not show any opacifications after 1 year of study comparing ketotifen with picumast [177].

Amlexanox

Amlexanox, an azoxanthone derivative that was developed as an ocular antiallergic drug, has shown limited antihistamine properties in guinea pig models of allergic conjunctivitis [109,178–180]. One target is believed to be a heat shock protein because it binds directly to wild-type Hsp90 through the *N*- and *C*-terminal domains [181] and to the S100 family of calcium-binding proteins, a multigenic family of low-molecular-weight Ca(2+)-binding proteins comprising 19 members [100]. It was recently found to inhibit the formation of the fibroblast growth factor (FGF-1), which led to its present position in investigational research in the treatment of aphthous ulcers [182] and is now available as Aphthasol. Although a high concentration was needed, tranilast and amlexanox showed significant inhibition of cedar pollen–induced conjunctivitis (Table 1) [109].

Table 1
Effects of the inflammatory cascade in treating allergic conjunctivitis: several of the more commonly used multiple-action agents

	Azelastine HCl 0.05% (Optivar)	Epinastine HCl 0.05% (Elestat)	Ketotifen fumarate 0.25% (Zaditor)[a]	Olopatadine HCl 0.2% (Pataday)
Indication	Relief of itching associated with allergic conjunctivitis	Relief of itching associated with allergic conjunctivitis	Temporary prevention of itching of the eye caused by allergies	Relief of itching associated with allergic conjunctivitis
Dosage	One drop bid each affected eye	One drop bid each affected eye (≥3 years of age)	One drop q8–12h each affected eye	One drop qd each affected eye
Adverse effects	Transient sting (∼30%) headache (∼15%) bitter taste (∼10%)	Cold symptoms (∼10%) upper respiratory infection (∼10%)	Headache (∼10%–25%) conjunctival injection (∼10%–25%) rhinitis (∼10%–25%)	Cold syndrome (∼10%) pharyngitis (∼10%)

[a] Ketotifen (Zaditor) is now available over-the-counter in the United States.

Topical antihistamines and dry eye

Because all topical antihistamines are also known to have muscarinic binding abilities and may theoretically cause dry eye syndrome complaints with chronic use, an animal model was used to compare the effects of topical olopatadine, epinastine, and lubricant eye drops on dry eye ocular surface disease in the botulinum toxin B–induced mouse model of keratoconjunctivitis sicca. In this model, no statistically significant differences were seen in aqueous tear production among the three different medication groups at all time points throughout the 4-week experimental period. In addition, changes in corneal fluorescein staining of the olopatadine group versus the epinastine group did not show a statistically significant difference. In this botulinum model, the additional placement of topical olopatadine and epinastine does not seem to cause significantly additional damage to the compromised ocular surface secondary to dry eye after continuous 4-week, twice-daily application [41]. However, on examining other animal models, epinastine-treated mice after 2 days showed greater mean tear volumes than olopatadine-treated mice at 15, 45, 90, and 240 minutes, with statistical significance at 15 and 45 minutes ($P<.001$). Olopatadine significantly reduced tear volume compared with untreated controls at 15 and 45 minutes ($P<.001$). After 4 days, tear volumes with epinastine treatment exceeded those with olopatadine treatment at all time points, with statistical significance at 45 minutes ($P<.05$) [42]. Therefore, which of these models has clinical relevance in patients who have ocular allergies remains to be determined.

Steroids

Ophthalmic steroids

Topical corticosteroids are appropriate for treating severe allergic conjunctivitis because of their potent antiinflammatory effect. Corticosteroids block most inflammatory pathways in the allergic reaction, especially the late-phase mediators that perpetuate the persistent and chronic forms of ocular allergy [5,6].

Corticosteroids are divided into ketone and ester corticosteroids and are most commonly used for treating ocular inflammation. Conventional corticosteroids, such as prednisolone and dexamethasone, have a ketone group at the C-20 position that is associated with cataract formation. Substitution of the C-20 group with a chloromethyl ester moiety led to development of loteprednol etabonate (Alrex), currently the only ester corticosteroid approved for treating the signs and symptoms of SAC [183]. Loteprednol etabonate has several potential advantages over ketone corticosteroids. First, loteprednol etabonate has high lipophilicity compared with ketone corticosteroids, which may increase its efficacy by enhancing penetration into target inflammatory cells [184]. Second, loteprednol etabonate's potential for inducing ocular hypertension is minimized by its rapid conversion to inactive metabolites after achieving its therapeutic role [185]. Third, low levels of loteprednol etabonate are detected in plasma, which reduces systemic side effects.

Data from clinical trials in patients who have allergic conjunctivitis show that topical loteprednol etabonate is a safe treatment option. In a placebo-controlled study of giant papillary conjunctivitis, no significant change in IOP was seen after 4 weeks of loteprednol etabonate 0.5% compared with baseline [186]. Data from two 6-week placebo-controlled studies of patients who had SAC showed more effective reduction of symptoms in the group treated with loteprednol etabonate compared with the placebo group [187–189]. A unique feature of loteprednol is the claim that it is a *site-specific* steroid, meaning that the active drug resides at the target tissue long enough to render a therapeutic effect but not long enough to cause the secondary harmful effects of, for example, increased IOP [190,191].

Topical corticosteroids have the potential to induce serious side effects, such as cataracts, elevated IOP, and infection. Therefore, topical corticosteroids are best used over short periods (up to 2 weeks); IOP and lens clarity should be monitored in use beyond 2 weeks. They should not be used in conjunction with a topical antibiotic because if infection is a concern, it may be viral and topical steroids would be contraindicated unless an eye care specialist examines the infection with a biomicroscope.

Intranasal steroids

Increasing evidence supports the effect of intranasal corticosteroids on reducing ocular symptoms associated with allergic rhinitis. Initial evidence for this therapeutic benefit surfaced during placebo-controlled clinical trials studying the effects of intranasal corticosteroids on a spectrum of allergic rhinitis symptoms [192–194]. More recently, studies designed specifically to investigate effects on ocular symptoms have reinforced those observations [195,196]. In a pooled analysis of data from seven randomized placebo-controlled clinical trials of intranasal fluticasone propionate in seasonal allergy rhinitis, both subject and physician ratings of ocular symptom severity on study days 7 and 14 also favored intranasal fluticasone [196].

Not only have intranasal corticosteroids been shown to be superior to placebo in reducing ocular symptoms of allergic rhinitis but also accumulating data suggest that they are comparable to or possibly more effective than oral antihistamines. A meta-analysis of 11 randomized controlled trials found no significant difference in improvement of eye symptoms between intranasal corticosteroids and oral antihistamines [197]. A similar meta-analysis of 10 randomized clinical trials failed to identify any significant difference in ocular symptom relief between intranasal corticosteroids and nonsedating antihistamines [198], suggesting that intranasal corticosteroids are equivalent to oral antihistamines in their effect on the eye or that antihistamines do not work on ocular allergy. However, more recent studies have shown that

intranasal steroids may be a class effect on ocular allergy, because triamcinolone [199], beclomethasone [200], budesonide [201], fluticasone propionate
[195], fluticasone furoate [202] and mometasone furoate have shown this
activity [203].

Immunomodulatory agents

Cyclosporine

Although cyclosporine (CsA) has been available for more than 20 years in
various areas of organ transplantation, its lipophilicity presented a unique
challenge for generating a solution or suspension to be delivered to ocular
surface [204]. In an animal model, CsA 0.1% and 0.5% eye drops significantly
inhibited eosinophilic infiltration into the conjunctiva in mice actively immu-
nized with ragweed compared with vehicle-treated mice, and the inhibition was
similar to that induced with 0.1% betamethasone [205]. Patients who had severe VKC treated with topical 2% cyclosporine A in preservative-free artificial
tears showed improved signs and symptoms, and experienced no side effects
during the 14-week study [206]. In a lower dose regimen, 0.05% cyclosporine
A for steroid-dependent AKC and VKC showed no benefit over placebo as
a steroid-sparing agent [207]. Compared with a 0.5% solution of ketorolac,
CsA 0.5% had a slower onset of improvement over 2 to 4 weeks, with a significant difference in subjective ($P < .005$) and objective ($P < .001$) scores seen between the eyes treated with CsA or placebo at 2 weeks. At 4 weeks, scores for
signs ($P < .001$) and symptoms ($P = .01$) were reduced in the placebo-treated
eyes, with no further improvement in the CsA-treated eyes [208].

Immunotherapy

Immunotherapy was used for the primary treatment of allergies, or spring
"catarrh," before antihistamines and other pharmacologic agents were discovered. In the original report, allergen immunotherapy "measured the
patient's resistance during experiments of pollen extracts to excite a *conjunctival* reaction" [209]. The eye, and not the skin, was the target organ.
The efficacy of allergen immunotherapy is well established, although
allergic rhinitis seems to respond better to treatment compared with allergic
conjunctivitis. In patients who experienced allergic asthma and rhinoconjunctivitis when exposed to specific animal dander (Fel d I allergen), one
study showed that immunotherapy improved overall symptoms of rhinoconjunctivitis, decreased antiallergy medications, and required a 1-log
(10-fold) increase in the dose of allergen to induce a positive ocular challenge test reaction after 1 year of immunotherapy with the cat allergen
[210]. This finding was also noted in an immunotherapy study over 12
months with a purified and standardized preparation of *Dermatophagoides
farinae*, in which patients receiving immunotherapy injections experienced

significant improvement in their subjective symptoms ($P<.028$) and objective cutaneous ($P<.0001$) and conjunctival ($P<.001$) sensitivities. Subjective improvements also correlated well with changes in conjunctival ($P<.01$), and especially skin sensitivity ($P<.005$), subjective improvement [211]. However, whether ocular or nasal symptoms are more responsive is unclear, because the studies were not designed with well-defined patient groups; nor is the natural history of nasal and ocular allergy known. As shown in patients sensitive to ragweed treated for at least 2 years with specific ragweed immunotherapy, symptom assessment postchallenge revealed that nasal symptoms responded more than ocular symptoms when compared with controls [212]. Although initial studies of allergen immunotherapy did not specifically address ocular symptoms in a separate manner [213], more-recent clinical studies have begun to identify improvement in ocular signs and symptoms in a separate category [214–216], including the standard use of subcutaneous immunotherapy [217] and the investigational forms of sublingual immunotherapy [218–220]. In a more recent study, the clinical effect on rhinitis and conjunctivitis achieved during specific subcutaneous immunotherapy even persisted for years after termination of treatment (5-year follow-up). The visual analog scale reflected an two- to threefold improvement for ocular ($P<.001$) and nasal scores ($P<.01$), whereas the conjunctival sensitivity measured with provocation tests were significantly reduced by more than 2-logs of allergen from years 2 to 5 ($P<.001$) [221].

Summary

Pharmacologic treatment of allergic conjunctivitis consists of agents designed to block various pathways in the IgE–mast cell mediated inflammatory cascade. Oral and topical antihistamines target histamine receptors, preventing histamine-mediated symptoms of allergic conjunctivitis, such as itching, watery eyes, chemosis, and periorbital swelling. Antihistamines may have a minimal effect on inflammatory mediators and tend to induce ocular drying, which may limit use. Although topical mast cell stabilizers block the release of histamine, prostaglandins, and leukotrienes through stabilizing mast cell membranes, they are more useful as prophylaxis because they have no effect on already-synthesized inflammatory mediators. Topical multiple-action agents with mast-cell–stabilizing activity have more diverse inhibitory effects on the inflammatory cascade, and will inhibit pre-existing inflammatory mediators and block synthesis of more inflammatory mediators. Because of their ability to block the generation of most inflammatory mediators through inhibition of mast cell phospholipase A2, topical corticosteroids are the most effective treatment for persistent and chronic forms of allergic conjunctivitis. However, corticosteroids are less likely to be prescribed because of their increased risk for cataract formation and elevated IOP, and their restriction to short-term use. According to current treatment recommendations, allergic conjunctivitis is managed in a stepwise

214 BIELORY

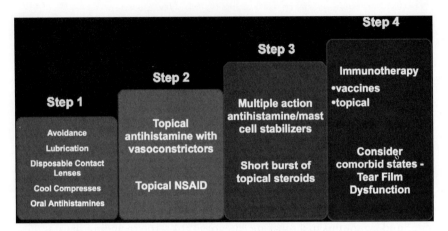

Fig. 2. Stepwise treatment. NSAID, nonsteroidal anti-inflammatory drug.

approach (Fig. 2). Lubricants are initially recommended for disease prevention. In patients who do not experience response, pharmacotherapy is prescribed in the following sequence until acceptable relief of symptoms is achieved: (1) topical antihistamines, alone or in combination with nonsteroidal antiinflammatory drugs; (2) topical antihistamines combined with vasoconstrictors; and (3) multiple-action agents with a short course of corticosteroids.

References

[1] Lanier BQ, Gross RD, Marks BB, et al. Olopatadine ophthalmic solution adjunctive to loratadine compared with loratadine alone in patients with active seasonal allergic conjunctivitis symptoms. Ann Allergy Asthma Immunol 2001;86:641–8.
[2] Pflugfelder SC, Stern ME. Future directions in therapeutic interventions for conjunctival inflammatory disorders. Curr Opin Allergy Clin Immunol 2007;7:450–3.
[3] Friedlaender MH. Epinastine in the management of ocular allergic disease. Int Ophthalmol Clin 2006;46(4):85–6.
[4] Ellis AK, Day JH, Lundie MJ, et al. Impact on quality of life during an allergen challenge research trial. Ann Allergy Asthma Immunol 1999;83(1):33–9.
[5] Bielory L. Ocular allergy guidelines: a practical treatment algorithm. Drugs 2002;62(11): 1611–34.
[6] Bielory L. Update on ocular allergy treatment. Expert Opin Pharmacother 2002;3(5):541–53.
[7] Christensen MT, Cohen S, Rinehart J, et al. Clinical evaluation of an HP-guar gellable lubricant eye drop for the relief of dryness of the eye. Curr Eye Res 2004;28(1):55–62.
[8] Lemp MA. Contact lenses and associated anterior segment disorders: dry eye, blepharitis, and allergy. Ophthalmol Clin North Am 2003;16(3):463–9.
[9] Lemp MA. Is the dry eye contact lens wearer at risk? Yes. Cornea 1990;9(Suppl 1):S48–50 [discussion: S54].
[10] Hayes VY, Schnider CM, Veys J. An evaluation of 1-day disposable contact lens wear in a population of allergy sufferers. Cont Lens Anterior Eye 2003;26(2):85–93.
[11] Kari O, Haahtela T. Is atopy a risk factor for the use of contact lenses? Allergy 1992;47(4 Pt 1): 295–8.

[12] Kari O, Teir H, Huuskonen R, et al. Tolerance to different kinds of contact lenses in young atopic and non-atopic wearers. CLAO J 2001;27(3):151–4.

[13] Abelson MB, Paradis A, George MA, et al. Effects of Vasocon-A in the allergen challenge model of acute allergic conjunctivitis. Arch Ophthalmol 1990;108(4):520–4.

[14] Duzman E, Warman A, Warman R. Efficacy and safety of topical oxymetazoline in treating allergic and environmental conjunctivitis. Ann Ophthalmol 1986;18(1):28–31.

[15] Antazoline in fixed combination with naphazoline for human ophthalmic use: drug efficacy study implementation; Final evaluation. Federal Register 1992;45391–2.

[16] Lanier BQ, Tremblay N, Smith JP, et al. A double-masked comparison of ocular deconges-tants as therapy for allergic conjunctivitis. Ann Allergy 1983;50(3):174–7.

[17] Abelson MB, Butrus SI, Weston JH, et al. Tolerance and absence of rebound vasodilation following topical ocular decongestant usage. Ophthalmology 1984;91(11):1364–7.

[18] Soparkar CN, Wilhelmus KR, Koch DD, et al. Acute and chronic conjunctivitis due to over-the-counter ophthalmic decongestants. Arch Ophthalmol 1997;115(1):34–8.

[19] Spector SL, Raizman MB. Conjunctivitis medicamentosa. J Allergy Clin Immunol 1994; 94(1):134–6.

[20] Thomas P, Rueff F, Przybilla B, et al. Severe allergic contact blepharoconjunctivitis from phenylephrine in eyedrops, with corresponding T-cell hyper-responsiveness in vitro. Con-tact Derm 1998;38(1):41–3.

[21] Shellans S, Rich LF, Louiselle I. Conjunctival goblet cell response to vasoconstrictor use. J Ocul Pharmacol 1989;5(3):217–20.

[22] Alexander M, Rosen LJ, Yang WH. Comparison of topical nedocromil sodium and oral ter-fenadine for the treatment of seasonal allergic conjunctivitis. Clin Ther 1999;21(11):1900–7.

[23] Abelson MB, Lanier RQ. The added benefit of local Patanol therapy when combined with systemic Claritin for the inhibition of ocular itching in the conjunctival antigen challenge model. Acta Ophthalmol Scand Suppl 1999;(228):53–6.

[24] Abelson MB, Welch DL. An evaluation of onset and duration of action of patanol(r) (olopatadine hydrochloride ophthalmic solution 0.1%) compared to claritin(r) (loratadine 10 mg) tablets in acute allergic conjunctivitis in the conjunctival allergen challenge model. Acta Ophthalmol Scand 2000;78(Suppl 230):60–3.

[25] Berdy GJ, Abelson MB, George MA, et al. Allergic conjunctivitis: a survey of new antihis-tamines. J Ocul Pharmacol 1991;7(4):313–24.

[26] Koeffler BH, Lemp MA. The effect of antihistamine (chlorpheniramine maleate) on tear production in humans. Am J Ophthalmol 1980;12:217–9.

[27] Hingorani M, Lightman S. Therapeutic options in ocular allergic disease. Drugs 1995;50(2): 208–21.

[28] Abelson MB, Udell IJ. H2-receptors in the human ocular surface. Arch Ophthalmol 1981; 99(2):302–4.

[29] Udell IJ, Abelson MB. Animal and human ocular surface response to a topical nonimmune mast-cell degranulating agent (compound 48/80). Am J Ophthalmol 1981;91(2):226–30.

[30] Woodward DF, Johnson L, Spada C, et al. Effect of cimetidine and pyrilamine on hista-mine-induced ocular surface hyperemia. J Ocul Pharmacol 1986;2(3):275–8.

[31] Mansmann HC Jr, Altman RA, Berman BA, et al. Efficacy and safety of cetirizine therapy in perennial allergic rhinitis. Ann Allergy 1992;68(4):348–53.

[32] Schoeneich M, Pecoud AR. Effect of cetirizine in a conjunctival provocation test with aller-gens. Clin Exp Allergy 1990;20(2):171–4.

[33] Tosca M, Ciprandi G, Passalacqua G, et al. Cetirizine reduces conjunctival nonspecific hy-perreactivity in children with mite allergy. J Investig Allergol Clin Immunol 1998;8(1):23–6.

[34] Ciprandi G, Buscaglia S, Pesce GP, et al. Protective effect of loratadine on specific conjunc-tival provocation test. Int Arch Allergy Appl Immunol 1991;96(4):344–7.

[35] Meltzer EO, Prenner BM, Nayak A, et al. Efficacy and tolerability of once-daily 5 mg desloratadine, an H1-receptor antagonist, in patients with seasonal allergic rhinitis: assess-ment during the spring and fall allergy seasons. Clin Drug Investig 2001;21(1):25–32.

[36] Casale TB, Andrade C, Qu R, et al. Safety and efficacy of once-daily fexofenadine HCl in the treatment of autumn seasonal allergic rhinitis. Allergy Asthma Proc 1999;20(3):193–8.

[37] Wahn U, Meltzer EO, Finn AF Jr, et al. Fexofenadine is efficacious and safe in children (aged 6-11 years) with seasonal allergic rhinitis. J Allergy Clin Immunol 2003;111(4):763–9.

[38] Sharif NA, Xu S, Yanni J. Emedastine: Pharmacological profile of a novel antihistamine for use in allergic conjunctivitis. Invest Ophthalmol Vis Sci 1995;36:s135.

[39] Nevius JM, Abelson MB, Welch D. The ocular drying effect of oral antihistamines (Loratadine) in the normal population—An evaluation. Invest Ophthalmol Vis Sci 1999;40(4):S549.

[40] Welch D, Ousler GW III, Nally LA, et al. Ocular drying associated with oral antihistamines (loratadine) in the normal population-an evaluation of exaggerated dose effect. Adv Exp Med Biol 2002;506(Pt B):1051–5.

[41] Lekhanont K, Park CY, Combs JC, et al. Effect of topical olopatadine and epinastine in the botulinum toxin B-induced mouse model of dry eye. J Ocul Pharmacol Ther 2007;23(1): 83–8.

[42] Villareal AL, Farley W, Pflugfelder SC, et al. Effect of topical ophthalmic epinastine and olopatadine on tear volume in mice. Eye Contact Lens 2006;32(6):272–6.

[43] Butrus S, Portela R. Ocular allergy: diagnosis and treatment. Ophthalmol Clin North Am 2005;18(4):485–92, v.

[44] Crampton HJ. Comparison of ketotifen fumarate ophthalmic solution alone, desloratadine alone, and their combination for inhibition of the signs and symptoms of seasonal allergic rhinoconjunctivitis in the conjunctival allergen challenge model: a double-masked, placebo- and active-controlled trial. Clin Ther 2003;25(7):1975–87.

[45] Lanier BQ, Gross RD, Marks BB, et al. Olopatadine ophthalmic solution adjunctive to loratadine compared with loratadine alone in patients with active seasonal allergic conjunctivitis symptoms. Ann Allergy Asthma Immunol 2001;86(6):641–8.

[46] Bielory L. Ocular histamine and muscarinic receptor binding. In: Characteristiscs ARB. Newark (NJ): Microsoft Word; 2005.

[47] Yanni JM, Stephens DJ, Parnell DW, et al. Preclinical efficacy of emedastine, a potent, selective histamine H1 antagonist for topical ocular use. J Ocul Pharmacol 1994;10:665–75.

[48] Arriaga F, Rombaut N. Absence of central effects with levocabastine eye drops. Allergy 1990;45(7):552–4.

[49] Leysen JE, Gommeren W. Drug receptor dissociation time, new tool for drug research: receptor binding affinity and drug receptor dissociation profiles of serotonin S2, dopamine D2, histamine H1 antagonists and opiates. Drug Dev Res 1986;8:119–31.

[50] Yanni JM, Sharif NA, Gamache DA, et al. A current appreciation of sites for pharmacological intervention in allergic conjunctivitis: effects of new topical ocular drugs. Acta Ophthalmol Scand Suppl 1999;(228):33–7.

[51] Zuber P, Pecoud A. Effect of levocabastine, a new H1 antagonist, in a conjunctival provocation test with allergens. J Allergy Clin Immunol 1988;82(4):590–4.

[52] Yanni JM, Weimer LK, Sharif NA, et al. Inhibition of histamine-induced human conjunctival epithelial cell responses by ocular allergy drugs. Arch Ophthalmol 1999;117(5):643–7.

[53] Leonardi A, DeFranchis G, De Paoli M, et al. Histamine-induced cytokine production and ICAM-1 expression in human conjunctival fibroblasts. Curr Eye Res 2002;25(3):189–96.

[54] D'Arienzo PA, Leonardi A, Bensch G. Randomized, double-masked, placebo-controlled comparison of the efficacy of emedastine difumarate 0.05% ophthalmic solution and ketotifen fumarate 0.025% ophthalmic solution in the human conjunctival allergen challenge model. Clin Ther 2002;24(3):409–16.

[55] Hyams SW, Bialik M, Neumann E. Clinical trials of disodium cromoglycate in vernal conjunctivitis. J Pediatr Ophthalmol 1976;12:116.

[56] Kimata H, Yoshida A, Ishioka C, et al. Disodium cromoglycate (DSCG) selectively inhibits IgE production and enhances IgG4 production by human B cell in vitro. Clin Exp Immunol 1991;84(3):395–9.

[57] Loh RK, Jabara HH, Geha RS. Disodium cromoglycate inhibits S mu→S epsilon deletional switch recombination and IgE synthesis in human B cells. J Exp Med 1994; 180(2):663–71.
[58] Friday GA, Biglan AW, Hiles DA, et al. Treatment of ragweed allergic conjunctivitis with cromolyn sodium 4% ophthalmic solution. Am J Ophthalmol 1983;95(2):169–74.
[59] Sorkin EM, Ward A. Ocular sodium cromoglycate. An overview of its therapeutic efficacy in allergic eye disease. Drugs 1986;31(2):131–48.
[60] Campbell AM, Demoly P, Michael FB, et al. Conjunctival provocation tests with codeine phosphate. Effect of disodium cromoglycate. Ann Allergy 1993;71(1):51–5.
[61] Juniper EF, Guyatt GH, Ferrie PJ, et al. Sodium cromoglycate eye drops: regular versus "as needed" use in the treatment of seasonal allergic conjunctivitis. J Allergy Clin Immunol 1994;94(1):36–43.
[62] Leonardi A, Borghesan F, Faggian D, et al. Eosinophil cationic protein in tears of normal subjects and patients affected by vernal keratoconjunctivitis. Allergy 1995;50(7):610–3.
[63] James IG, Campbell LM, Harrsion JM, et al. Comparison of the efficacy and tolerability of topically administered azelastine, sodium cromoglycate and placebo in the treatment of seasonal allergic conjunctivitis and rhino-conjunctivitis. Curr Med Res Opin 2003;19(4):313–20.
[64] Katelaris CH, Ciprandi G, Missotten L, et al. A comparison of the efficacy and tolerability of olopatadine hydrochloride 0.1% ophthalmic solution and cromolyn sodium 2% ophthalmic solution in seasonal allergic conjunctivitis. Clin Ther 2002;24(10):1561–75.
[65] Ostler HB. Acute chemotic reaction to cromolyn. Arch Ophthalmol 1982;100(3):412–3.
[66] Valdivieso R, Subiza J, Varela-Losada S, et al. Severe allergic conjunctivitis and chemosis caused by disodium cromoglycate. J Investig Allergol Clin Immunol 1998;8(1):58–60.
[67] Johnson HG, VanHout CA, Wright JB. Inhibition of allergic reactions by cromoglycate and by a new anti-allergy drug U-42,585E.I. Activity in rats. Int Arch Allergy Appl Immunol 1978;56(5):416–23.
[68] Johnson HG, VanHout CA, Wright JB. Inhibition of allergic reactions by cromoglycate and by a new antiallergy drug U-42,585E. II. Activity in primates against aerosolized Ascaris suum antigen. Int Arch Allergy Appl Immunol 1978;56(6):481–7.
[69] Bonini S, Schiavone M, Magrini L, et al. Efficacy of lodoxamide eye drops on mast cells and eosinophils after allergen challenge in allergic conjunctivitis. Ophthalmology 1997;104(5):849–53.
[70] Bloch-Michel E. Evaluation de l'efficacite therapeutique d'un collyre anti-allergique par test photographique. Rev Fr Allergol 1990;30:163–5.
[71] Fahy GT, Easty DL, Collum LM, et al. Randomised double-masked trial of lodoxamide and sodium cromoglycate in allergic eye disease. A multicentre study. Eur J Ophthalmol 1992;2(3):144–9.
[72] Cerqueti PM, Ricca V, Tosca MA, et al. Lodoxamide treatment of allergic conjunctivitis. Int Arch Allergy Immunol 1994;105(2):185–9.
[73] Richard C, Trinquand C, Bloch-Michel E. Comparison of topical 0.05% levocabastine and 0.1% lodoxamide in patients with allergic conjunctivitis. Study Group. Eur J Ophthalmol 1998;8(4):207–16.
[74] Leonardi A, Borghesan F, Avarello A, et al. Effect of lodoxamide and disodium cromoglycate on tear eosinophil cationic protein in vernal keratoconjunctivitis. Br J Ophthalmol 1997;81(1):23–6.
[75] Akman A, Irkec M, Orhan M, et al. Effect of lodoxamide on tear leukotriene levels in giant papillary conjunctivitis associated with ocular prosthesis. Ocul Immunol Inflamm 1998; 6(3):179–84.
[76] Kosrirukvongs P, Vichyanond P, Wongsawad W. Vernal keratoconjunctivitis in Thailand. Asian Pac J Allergy Immunol 2003;21(1):25–30.
[77] Abelson MB, Berdy GJ, Mundorf T, et al. Pemirolast potassium 0.1% ophthalmic solution is an effective treatment for allergic conjunctivitis: a pooled analysis of two prospective,

randomized, double-masked, placebo-controlled, phase III studies. J Ocul Pharmacol Ther 2002;18(5):475–88.

[78] Minami K, Hossen MA, Kamei C. Increasing effect by simultaneous use of levocabastine and pemirolast on experimental allergic conjunctivitis in rats. Biol Pharm Bull 2005;28(3):473–6.

[79] Yanni JM, Miller ST, Gamache DA, et al. Comparative effects of topical ocular anti-allergy drugs on human conjunctival mast cells. Ann Allergy Asthma Immunol 1997;79(6):541–5.

[80] Woodward DF, Nieves AL, William LS, et al. Characterization of receptor subtypes involved in prostanoid-induced conjunctival pruritus and their role in mediating allergic conjunctival itching. J Pharmacol Exp Ther 1996;279(1):137–42.

[81] Woodward DF, Nieves AL, Hawley SB, et al. The pruritogenic and inflammatory effects of prostanoids in the conjunctiva. J Ocul Pharmacol Ther 1995;11(3):339–47.

[82] Woodward DF, Nieves AL, Friedlaender M, et al. Interactive effects of peptidoleukotrienes and histamine on microvascular permeability and their involvement in experimental cutaneous and conjunctival immediate hypersensitivity. Eur J Pharmacol 1989;164(2):323–33.

[83] Ballas Z, Blumenthal M, Tinkelman DG, et al. Clinical evaluation of ketorolac tromethamine 0.5% ophthalmic solution for the treatment of seasonal allergic conjunctivitis. Surv Ophthalmol 1993;38(Suppl):141–8.

[84] Sharma A, Gupta R, Ram J, et al. Topical ketorolac 0.5% solution for the treatment of vernal keratoconjunctivitis. Indian J Ophthalmol 1997;45(3):177–80.

[85] Toker MI, Erdem H, Erdogan H, et al. The effects of topical ketorolac and indomethacin on measles conjunctivitis: randomized controlled trial. Am J Ophthalmol 2006;141(5):902–5.

[86] Tomioka H, Yoshida S, Tanaka M, et al. Inhibition of chemical mediator release from human leukocytes by a new antiasthma drug, HC 20-511 (ketotifen). Monogr Allergy 1979;14: 313–7.

[87] Tauber J, Raizman MB, Ostrov CS, et al. A multicenter comparison of the ocular efficacy and safety of diclofenac 0.1% solution with that of ketorolac 0.5% solution in patients with acute seasonal allergic conjunctivitis. J Ocul Pharmacol Ther 1998;14(2):137–45.

[88] Donshik PC, Pearlman D, Pinnas J, et al. Efficacy and safety of ketorolac tromethamine 0.5% and levocabastine 0.05%: a multicenter comparison in patients with seasonal allergic conjunctivitis. Adv Ther 2000;17(2):94–102.

[89] Khosravi E, Elena PP, Hariton C. Allergic conjunctivitis and uveitis models: reappraisal with some marketed drugs. Inflamm Res 1995;44(1):47–54.

[90] Tinkelman DG, Rupp G, Kaufman H, et al. Double-masked, paired-comparison clinical study of ketorolac tromethamine 0.5% ophthalmic solution compared with placebo eyedrops in the treatment of seasonal allergic conjunctivitis. Surv Ophthalmol 1993;38(Suppl):133–40.

[91] Friedlaender MH. Contact lens induced conjunctivitis: a model of human ocular inflammation. CLAO J 1996;22(3):205–8.

[92] Sitenga GL, Ing EB, Van Dellen RG, et al. Asthma caused by topical application of ketorolac. Ophthalmology 1996;103(6):890–2.

[93] Perry HD, Donnenfeld ED. An update on the use of ophthalmic ketorolac tromethamine 0.4%. Expert Opin Pharmacother 2006;7(1):99–107.

[94] Sharif NA, Xu SX, Yanni JM, et al. Olopatadine (AL-4943A): ligand binding and functional studies on a novel, long acting H1-selective histamine antagonist and anti-allergic agent for use in allergic conjunctivitis. J Ocul Pharmacol Ther 1996;12(4):401–7.

[95] Cook EB, Stahl JL, Barney NP, et al. Olopatadine inhibits TNFalpha release from human conjunctival mast cells. Ann Allergy Asthma Immunol 2000;84(5):504–8.

[96] Lippert U, Moller A, Welker P, et al. Inhibition of cytokine secretion from human leukemic mast cells and basophils by H1- and H2-receptor antagonists. Exp Dermatol 2000;9(2):118–24.

[97] Yanni JM, Stephens DJ, Miller ST, et al. The in vitro and in vivo ocular pharmacology of olopatadine (AL-4943A), an effective anti-allergic/antihistaminic agent. J Ocul Pharmacol Ther 1996;12(4):389–400.

[98] Abelson MB. Evaluation of olopatadine, a new ophthalmic antiallergic agent with dual activity, using the conjunctival allergen challenge model. Ann Allergy Asthma Immunol 1998;81(3):211–8.

[99] Abelson MB, Spitalny L. Combined analysis of two studies using the conjunctival allergen challenge model to evaluate olopatadine hydrochloride, a new ophthalmic antiallergic agent with dual activity. Am J Ophthalmol 1998;125(6):797–804.

[100] Kishimoto K, Kaneko S, Ohmori K, et al. Olopatadine suppresses the migration of THP-1 monocytes induced by S100A12 protein. Mediators Inflamm 2006;2006(1):42726.

[101] Aguilar AJ. Comparative Study of clinical efficacy and tolerance in seasonal allergic conjunctivitis management with 0.1% olopatadine hydrochloride versus 0.05% ketotifen fumarate. Acta Ophthalmol Scand 2000;78(Suppl 230):52–5.

[102] Spangler DL, Bensch G, Berdy GJ. Evaluation of the efficacy of olopatadine hydrochloride 0.1% ophthalmic solution and azelastine hydrochloride 0.05% ophthalmic solution in the conjunctival allergen challenge model. Clin Ther 2001;23(8):1272–80.

[103] Grant SM, Goa KL, Fitton A, et al. Ketotifen. A review of its pharmacodynamic and pharmacokinetic properties, and therapeutic use in asthma and allergic disorders. Drugs 1990; 40(3):412–48.

[104] Bielory L, Ghafoor S. Histamine receptors and the conjunctiva. Curr Opin Allergy Clin Immunol 2005;5(5):437–40.

[105] Bielory L, Lien KW, Bigelsen S. Efficacy and tolerability of newer antihistamines in the treatment of allergic conjunctivitis. Drugs 2005;65(2):215–28.

[106] Nishimura N, Ito K, Tomioka H, et al. Inhibition of chemical mediator release from human leukocytes and lung in vitro by a novel antiallergic agent, KB-2413. Immunopharmacol Immunotoxicol 1987;9(4):511–21.

[107] Hasala H, Malm-Erjefalt M, Erjefalt J, et al. Ketotifen induces primary necrosis of human eosinophils. J Ocul Pharmacol Ther 2005;21(4):318–27.

[108] Schoch C. Effect of ketotifen fumarate, olopatadine, and levocabastine on ocular active anaphylaxis in the guinea pig and ocular immediate hypersensitivity in the albino rat. Ocul Immunol Inflamm 2005;13(1):39–44.

[109] Takada M, Yamada T, Nakahara H, et al. Experimental allergic conjunctivitis in guinea pigs induced by Japanese cedar pollen. Biol Pharm Bull 2000;23(5):566–9.

[110] Greiner JV, Mundorf T, Dubiner H, et al. Efficacy and safety of ketotifen fumarate 0.025% in the conjunctival antigen challenge model of ocular allergic conjunctivitis. Am J Ophthalmol 2003;136(6):1097–105.

[111] Dake Y, Enomoto T, Cheng L, et al. Effect of antihistamine eye drops on the conjunctival provocation test with Japanese cedar pollen allergen. Allergol Int 2006;55(4):373–8.

[112] Leonardi A, Busca F, et al. The anti-allergic effects of a cromolyn sodium-chlorpheniramine combination compared to ketotifen in the conjunctival allergen challenge model. Eur J Ophthalmol 2003;13(2):128–33.

[113] Avunduk AM, Tekelioglu Y, Turk A, et al. Comparison of the effects of ketotifen fumarate 0.025% and olopatadine HCl 0.1% ophthalmic solutions in seasonal allergic conjunctivitis: a 30-day, randomized, double-masked, artificial tear substitute-controlled trial. Clin Ther 2005;27(9):1392–402.

[114] Leonardi A, Zafirakis P. Efficacy and comfort of olopatadine versus ketotifen ophthalmic solutions: a double-masked, environmental study of patient preference. Curr Med Res Opin 2004;20(8):1167–73.

[115] Corin RE. Nedocromil sodium: a review of the evidence for a dual mechanism of action. Clin Exp Allergy 2000;30(4):461–8.

[116] Gonzalez JP, Brogden RN. Nedocromil sodium. A preliminary review of its pharmacodynamic and pharmacokinetic properties, and therapeutic efficacy in the treatment of reversible obstructive airways disease. Drugs 1987;34(5):560–77.

[117] Carolan EJ, Casale TB. Effects of nedocromil sodium and WEB 2086 on chemoattractant-stimulated neutrophil migration through cellular and noncellular barriers. Ann Allergy 1992;69(4):323–8.

[118] Silva PM, Martins MA, Castro-Faria-Neto HC, et al. Nedocromil sodium prevents in vivo generation of the eosinophilotactic substance induced by PAF but fails to antagonize its effects. Br J Pharmacol 1992;105(2):436–40.

[119] Loh RK, Jabara HH, Geha RS. Mechanisms of inhibition of IgE synthesis by nedocromil sodium: nedocromil sodium inhibits deletional switch recombination in human B cells. J Allergy Clin Immunol 1996;97(5):1141–50.

[120] Hoyos L, Norris A, Vargaftig BB. Effects of nedocromil sodium on antigen-induced conjunctivitis in guinea pigs. Adv Ther 2000;17(1):1–6.

[121] Ahluwalia P, Anderson DF, Wilson SJ, et al. Nedocromil sodium and levocabastine reduce the symptoms of conjunctival allergen challenge by different mechanisms. J Allergy Clin Immunol 2001;108(3):449–54.

[122] Hammann C, Kammerer R, Gerber M, et al. Comparison of effects of topical levocabastine and nedocromil sodium on the early response in a conjunctival provocation test with allergen. J Allergy Clin Immunol 1996;98(6 Pt 1):1045–50.

[123] Diebold Y, Calonge M, Carretero V, et al. Expression of ICAM-1 and HLA-DR by human conjunctival epithelial cultured cells and modulation by nedocromil sodium. J Ocul Pharmacol Ther 1998;14(6):517–31.

[124] Blumenthal M, Casale T, Dockhorn R, et al. Efficacy and safety of nedocromil sodium ophthalmic solution in the treatment of seasonal allergic conjunctivitis. Am J Ophthalmol 1992;113(1):56–63.

[125] Leino M. Studies comparing efficacy of nedocromil sodium eye drops with sodium cromoglycate and placebo in seasonal allergic conjunctivitis. Ocul Immunol Inflamm 1993;1:21–3.

[126] Leino M, Carlson C, Jaanio E, et al. Double-blind group comparative study of 2% nedocromil sodium eye drops with placebo eye drops in the treatment of seasonal allergic conjunctivitis. Ann Allergy 1990;64(4):398–402.

[127] Leino M, Ennevaara K, Latvala AL, et al. Double-blind group comparative study of 2% nedocromil sodium eye drops with 2% sodium cromoglycate and placebo eye drops in the treatment of seasonal allergic conjunctivitis. Clin Exp Allergy 1992;22(10):929–32.

[128] Melamed J, Schwartz RH, Hirsch SR, et al. Evaluation of nedocromil sodium 2% ophthalmic solution for the treatment of seasonal allergic conjunctivitis. Ann Allergy 1994;73(1):57–66.

[129] Spraul CW, Lang GK. Allergic and atopic diseases of the lid, conjunctiva, and cornea. Curr Opin Ophthalmol 1995;6(4):21–6.

[130] Stockwell A, Easty DL. Group comparative trial of 2% nedocromil sodium with placebo in the treatment of seasonal allergic conjunctivitis. Eur J Ophthalmol 1994;4(1):19–23.

[131] Bonini S, Barney NP, Schiavone M, et al. Effectiveness of nedocromil sodium 2% eyedrops on clinical symptoms and tear fluid cytology of patients with vernal conjunctivitis. Eye 1992;6(Pt 6):648–52.

[132] van Bijsterveld OP, Moons L, Verdonck M, et al. Nedocromil sodium treats symptoms of perennial allergic conjunctivitis not fully controlled by sodium cromoglycate. Ocular Immunol Inflamm 1994;2:177–86.

[133] Verin PH, Dicker ID, Mortemousque B. Nedocromil sodium eye drops are more effective than sodium cromoglycate eye drops for the long-term management of vernal keratoconjunctivitis. Clin Exp Allergy 1999;29(4):529–36.

[134] Verin P. Treating severe eye allergy. Clin Exp Allergy 1998;28(Suppl 6):44–8.

[135] Kjellman NI, Stevens MT. Clinical experience with Tilavist: an overview of efficacy and safety. Allergy 1995;50(Suppl 21):14–22 [discussion: 34–8].

[136] Bernstein JA. Azelastine hydrochloride: a review of pharmacology, pharmacokinetics, clinical efficacy and tolerability. Curr Med Res Opin 2007;23(10):2441–52.

[137] Lieberman PL, Settipane RA. Azelastine nasal spray: a review of pharmacology and clinical efficacy in allergic and nonallergic rhinitis. Allergy Asthma Proc 2003;24(2):95–105.

[138] Bielory L, Buddiga P, Bigelson S. Ocular allergy treatment comparisons: azelastine and olopatadine. Curr Allergy Asthma Rep 2004;4(4):320–5.

[139] McTavish D, Sorkin EM. Azelastine. A review of its pharmacodynamic and pharmacokinetic properties, and therapeutic potential. Drugs 1989;38(5):778–800.

[140] Shin MH, Baroody F, Proud D, et al. The effect of azelastine on the early allergic response. Clin Exp Allergy 1992;22(2):289–95.

[141] Brockman HL, Momsen MM, Knudtson JR, et al. Interactions of olopatadine and selected antihistamines with model and natural membranes. Ocul Immunol Inflamm 2003;11(4): 247–68.

[142] Chand N, Pillar J, Diamantis W, et al. Inhibition of IgE-mediated allergic histamine release from rat peritoneal mast cells by azelastine and selected antiallergic drugs. Agents Actions 1985;16(5):318–22.

[143] Hanashiro K, Sunagawa M, Tokeshi Y, et al. Antiallergic drugs, azelastine hydrochloride and epinastine hydrochloride, inhibit ongoing IgE secretion of rat IgE-producing hybridoma FE-3 cells. Eur J Pharmacol 2006;547(1–3):174–83.

[144] Busse W, Randlev B, Sedgwick J. The effect of azelastine on neutrophil and eosinophil generation of superoxide. J Allergy Clin Immunol 1989;83(2 Pt 1):400–5.

[145] Chand N, Diamantis W, Sofia RD. Modulation of in vitro anaphylaxis of guinea-pig isolated tracheal segments by azelastine, inhibitors of arachidonic acid metabolism and selected antiallergic drugs. Br J Pharmacol 1986;87(2):443–8.

[146] Chand N, Nolan K, Diamantis W, et al. Inhibition of leukotriene (SRS-A)-mediated acute lung anaphylaxis by azelastine in guinea pigs. Allergy 1986;41(7):473–8.

[147] Chand N, Nolan K, Sofia RD, et al. Changes in aeroallergen-induced pulmonary mechanics in actively sensitized guinea pig: inhibition by azelastine. Ann Allergy 1990;64(2 Pt 1): 151–4.

[148] Chand N, Pillar J, Diamantis W, et al. Effect of azelastine on activation and release stages of allergic histamine secretion in rabbit basophils. Res Commun Chem Pathol Pharmacol 1991;72(1):121–4.

[149] Chand N, Pillar J, Nolan K, et al. Inhibition of allergic and nonallergic leukotriene C4 formation and histamine secretion by azelastine: implication for its mechanism of action. Int Arch Allergy Appl Immunol 1989;90(1):67–70.

[150] Chand N, Sofia RD. Azelastine–a novel in vivo inhibitor of leukotriene biosynthesis: a possible mechanism of action: a mini review. J Asthma 1995;32(3):227–34.

[151] Hide I, Toriu N, Nuibe T, et al. Suppression of TNF-alpha secretion by azelastine in a rat mast (RBL-2H3) cell line: evidence for differential regulation of TNF-alpha release, transcription, and degranulation. J Immunol 1997;159(6):2932–40.

[152] Nakata Y, Hide I. Calcium signaling and protein kinase C for TNF-alpha secretion in a rat mast cell line. Life Sci 1998;62(17–18):1653–7.

[153] Shichijo M, Inagaki N, Nakai N, et al. The effects of anti-asthma drugs on mediator release from cultured human mast cells. Clin Exp Allergy 1998;28:1228–36.

[154] Ciprandi G, Buscaglia S, Catrullo A, et al. Azelastine eye drops reduce and prevent allergic conjunctival reaction and exert anti-allergic activity. Clin Exp Allergy 1997;27(2):182–91.

[155] Kempuraj D, Huang M, Kandere-Grzybowska K, et al. Azelastine inhibits secretion of IL-6, TNF-alpha and IL-8 as well as NF-kappaB activation and intracellular calcium ion levels in normal human mast cells. Int Arch Allergy Immunol 2003;132(3):231–9.

[156] Kempuraj D, Huang M, Kandere K, et al. Azelastine is more potent than olopatadine n inhibiting interleukin-6 and tryptase release from human umbilical cord blood-derived cultured mast cells. Ann Allergy Asthma Immunol 2002;88(5):501–6.

[157] Friedlaender MH, Harris J, LaVallee N, et al. Evaluation of the onset and duration of effect of azelastine eye drops (0.05%) versus placebo in patients with allergic conjunctivitis using an allergen challenge model. Ophthalmology 2000;107(12):2152–7.

[158] Sabbah A, Marzetto M. Azelastine eye drops in the treatment of seasonal allergic conjunctivitis or rhinoconjunctivitis in young children. Curr Med Res Opin 1998;14(3):161–70.

[159] Nazarov O, Petzold U, Haase H, et al. Azelastine eye drops in the treatment of perennial allergic conjunctivitis. Arzneimittelforschung 2003;53(3):167–73.

[160] Galatowicz G, Ajayi Y, Stern ME, et al. Ocular anti-allergic compounds selectively inhibit human mast cell cytokines in vitro and conjunctival cell infiltration in vivo. Clin Exp Allergy 2007;37(11):1648–56.

[161] Beauregard C, Stephens D, Roberts L, et al. Duration of action of topical antiallergy drugs in a Guinea pig model of histamine-induced conjunctival vascular permeability. J Ocul Pharmacol Ther 2007;23(4):315–20.

[162] Whitcup SM, Bradford R, Lue J, et al. Efficacy and tolerability of ophthalmic epinastine: a randomized, double-masked, parallel-group, active- and vehicle-controlled environmental trial in patients with seasonal allergic conjunctivitis. Clin Ther 2004;26(1):29–34.

[163] Abelson MB, Gomes P, Crampton HJ, et al. Efficacy and tolerability of ophthalmic epinastine assessed using the conjunctival antigen challenge model in patients with a history of allergic conjunctivitis. Clin Ther 2004;26(1):35–47.

[164] Ousler GW III, Workman DA, Torkildsen GL. An open-label, investigator-masked, crossover study of the ocular drying effects of two antihistamines, topical epinastine and systemic loratadine, in adult volunteers with seasonal allergic conjunctivitis. Clin Ther 2007;29(4):611–6.

[165] Scadding GK, Tasman AJ, Murrieta-Aguttes M, et al. Mizolastine is effective and well tolerated in long-term treatment of perennial allergic rhinoconjunctivitis. Riperex Study Group. J Int Med Res 1999;27(6):273–85.

[166] Triggiani M, Giannattasio G, Balestrieri B, et al. Differential modulation of mediator release from human basophils and mast cells by mizolastine. Clin Exp Allergy 2004;34(2):241–9.

[167] Xia Q, Zhou WM, Yang S, et al. Influence of mizolastine on antigen-induced activation of signalling pathways in murine mast cells. Clin Exp Dermatol 2006;31(2):260–5.

[168] Danjou P, Molinier P, Berlin I, et al. Assessment of the anticholinergic effect of the new antihistamine mizolastine in healthy subjects. Br J Clin Pharmacol 1992;34(4):328–31.

[169] Bachert C, Brostoff J, Scadding GK, et al. Mizolastine therapy also has an effect on nasal blockade in perennial allergic rhinoconjunctivitis. RIPERAN Study Group. Allergy 1998; 53(10):969–75.

[170] Leynadier F, Bousquet J, Murrieta M, et al. Efficacy and safety of mizolastine in seasonal allergic rhinitis. The Rhinase Study Group. Ann Allergy Asthma Immunol 1996;76(2):163–8.

[171] Horak F. Clinical advantages of dual activity in allergic rhinitis. Allergy 2000;55(Suppl 64): 34–9.

[172] Bachert C, Vovolis V, Margari P, et al. Mizolastine in the treatment of seasonal allergic rhinoconjunctivitis: a European clinical experience with 5408 patients managed in daily practice (PANEOS SAR Study). Allergy 2001;56(7):653–9.

[173] Sabbah A, Daele J, Wade AG, et al. Comparison of the efficacy, safety, and onset of action of mizolastine, cetirizine, and placebo in the management of seasonal allergic rhinoconjunctivitis. MIZOCET Study Group. Ann Allergy Asthma Immunol 1999;83(4):319–25.

[174] Slapke J, Muller S, Boerner D. A one-year double-blind clinical study of the efficacy and tolerability of picumast dihydrochloride versus ketotifen in patients with bronchial asthma. Arzneimittelforschung 1989;39(10A):1368–72.

[175] Wilhelms OH, Roesch A, Schaumann W. Picumast dihydrochloride (Auteral), a new antiallergic inhibitor of mediator release and action. Agents Actions Suppl 1991;34:335–49.

[176] Roesch A, Schaumann W, Wilhelms OH, et al. Antiallergic activity of picumast dihydrochloride in several animal species. Arzneimittelforschung 1989;39(10A):1310–6.

[177] Hockwin O, Muller-Breitenkamp U, Laser H, et al. Lens safety study with Picumast dihydrochloride–a double masked study using the Scheimpflug method. Lens Eye Toxic Res 1990;7(3–4):625–30.

[178] Rankov G, Sasaki K, Fukuda M. Pharmacodynamics of Amlexanox (AA-673) in normal and anaphylactic rat conjunctiva and its effect on histamine concentration. Ophthalmic Res 1990;22:359–64.

[179] Kamei C, Izushi K, Nakamura S. Effects of certain antiallergic drugs on experimental conjunctivitis in guinea pigs. Biol Pharm Bull 1995;18:1518–21.

[180] Kamei C, Izushi K, Tasaka K. Inhibitory effect of levocabastine on experimental allergic conjunctivitis in guinea pigs. J Pharmacobiodyn 1991;14:467–73.

[181] Okada M, Itoh H, Hatakeyama T, et al. Hsp90 is a direct target of the anti-allergic drugs disodium cromoglycate and amlexanox. Biochem J 2003;374:433–41.

[182] Rajalingam D, Kumar TK, Soldi R, et al. Molecular mechanism of inhibition of nonclassical FGF-1 export. Biochemistry 2005;44(47):15472–9.

[183] Bausch, Lomb Pharmaceuticals, I. Alrex (loteprednol etabonate ophthalmic suspension 0.2%). Prescribing Information. Physicians Desk Reference. Florida, USA, 1998.

[184] Howes JF. Loteprednol etabonate: a review of ophthalmic clinical studies. Pharmazie 2000; 55(3):178–83.

[185] Bartlett JD, Horwitz B, Howes JF. Intraocular pressure response to loteprednol etabonate in known steroid responders. J Ocul Pharmacol 1993;9(2):157–65.

[186] Bartlett JD, Howes JF, Ghormley NR, et al. Safety and efficacy of loteprednol etabonate for treatment of papillae in contact lens-associated giant papillary conjunctivitis. Curr Eye Res 1993;12(4):313–21.

[187] Dell SJ, Lowry GM, Northcutt JA, et al. A randomized, double-masked, placebo-controlled parallel study of 0.2% loteprednol etabonate in patients with seasonal allergic conjunctivitis. J Allergy Clin Immunol 1998;102(2):251–5.

[188] Dell SJ, Shulman DG, Lowry GM, et al. A controlled evaluation of the efficacy and safety of loteprednol etabonate in the prophylactic treatment of seasonal allergic conjunctivitis. Loteprednol Allergic Conjunctivitis Study Group. Am J Ophthalmol 1997;123(6):791–7.

[189] Shulman DG, Lothringer LL, Rubin JM, et al. A randomized, double-masked, placebo-controlled parallel study of loteprednol etabonate 0.2% in patients with seasonal allergic conjunctivitis. Ophthalmology 1999;106(2):362–9.

[190] Bielory L. Clinical experience with topical corticosteroids and other therapies. Allergy Clinical Immunology International 2007;19(Suppl 1):19–26.

[191] Bielory L. Update: ocular steroids in the treatment of allergic conjunctivitis. Allergy Clinical Immunology International 2007;19(Suppl 1):9–15.

[192] Settipane G, Korenblat PE, Winder J, et al. Triamcinolone acetonide Aqueous nasal spray in patients with seasonal ragweed allergic rhinitis: a placebo-controlled, double-blind study. Clin Ther 1995;17(2):252–63.

[193] Tinkelman D, Falliers C, Gross G, et al. Multicenter evaluation of triamcinolone acetonide nasal aerosol in the treatment of adult patients with seasonal allergic rhinitis. Ann Allergy 1990;64(2 Pt 2):234–40.

[194] Welsh PW, Stricker WE, Chu CP, et al. Efficacy of beclomethasone nasal solution, flunisolide, and cromolyn in relieving symptoms of ragweed allergy. Mayo Clin Proc 1987;62(2): 125–34.

[195] Bernstein DI, Levy AL, Hampel FC, et al. Treatment with intranasal fluticasone propionate significantly improves ocular symptoms in patients with seasonal allergic rhinitis. Clin Exp Allergy 2004;34(6):952–7.

[196] DeWester J, Philpot EE, Westlund RE, et al. The efficacy of intranasal fluticasone propionate in the relief of ocular symptoms associated with seasonal allergic rhinitis. Allergy Asthma Proc 2003;24(5):331–7.

[197] Weiner JM, Abramson MJ, Puy RM. Intranasal corticosteroids versus oral H1 receptor antagonists in allergic rhinitis: systematic review of randomised controlled trials. BMJ 1998;317(7173):1624–9.

[198] Stempel DA, Thomas M. Treatment of allergic rhinitis: an evidence-based evaluation of nasal corticosteroids versus nonsedating antihistamines. Am J Manag Care 1998;4(1):89–96.

[199] Condemi J, Schulz R, Lim J. Triamcinolone acetonide aqueous nasal spray versus loratadine in seasonal allergic rhinitis: efficacy and quality of life. Ann Allergy Asthma Immunol 2000;84(5):533–8.

[200] Giger R, Pasche P, Cheseaux C, et al. Comparison of once- versus twice-daily use of beclo-methasone dipropionate aqueous nasal spray in the treatment of allergic and non-allergic chronic rhinosinusitis. Eur Arch Otorhinolaryngol 2003;260(3):135–40.

[201] Moller C, Ahlstrom H, Henricson KA, et al. Safety of nasal budesonide in the long-term treatment of children with perennial rhinitis. Clin Exp Allergy 2003;33(6):816–22.

[202] Kaiser HB, Naclerio RM, Given J, et al. Fluticasone furoate nasal spray: A single treatment option for the symptoms of seasonal allergic rhinitis. J Allergy Clin Immunol 2007;119(6):1430–7.

[203] Bielory L. Ocular symptom reduction in patients with seasonal allergic rhinitis treated with the intranasal corticosteroid mometasone furoate. Ann Allergy Asthma Immunol 2008, in press.

[204] Lallemand F, Felt-Baeyens O, Besseghir K, et al. Cyclosporine A delivery to the eye: a pharmaceutical challenge. Eur J Pharm Biopharm 2003;56:307–18.

[205] Fukushima A, Yamaguchi T, Ishida W, et al. Cyclosporin A inhibits eosinophilic infiltration into the conjunctiva mediated by type IV allergic reactions. Clin Experiment Ophthalmol 2006;34(4):347–53.

[206] Kilic A, Gurler B. Topical 2% cyclosporine A in preservative-free artificial tears for the treatment of vernal keratoconjunctivitis. Can J Ophthalmol 2006;41(6):693–8.

[207] Daniell M, Constantinou M, Vu HT, et al. Randomised controlled trial of topical cyclosporin A in steroid dependent allergic conjunctivitis. Br J Ophthalmol 2006;90(4):461–4.

[208] Pucci N, Novembre E, Cianferoni A, et al. Efficacy and safety of cyclosporine eyedrops in vernal keratoconjunctivitis. Ann Allergy Asthma Immunol 2002;89(3):298–303.

[209] Noon L, Cantab B. Prophylactic inoculation against hay fever. Lancet 1911;1572–3.

[210] Alvarez-Cuesta E, Cuesta-Herranz J, Puyana-Ruiz J, et al. Monoclonal antibody-standardized cat extract immunotherapy: risk-benefit effects from a double-blind placebo study. J Allergy Clin Immunol 1994;93(3):556–66.

[211] Lofkvist T, Agrell B, Dreborg S, et al. Effects of immunotherapy with a purified standardized allergen preparation of Dermatophagoides farinae in adults with perennial allergic rhinoconjunctivitis. Allergy 1994;49(2):100–7.

[212] Donovan JP, Buckeridge DL, Briscoe MP, et al. Efficacy of immunotherapy to ragweed antigen tested by controlled antigen exposure. Ann Allergy Asthma Immunol 1996;77(1):74–80.

[213] Lowell F, Franklin W. A double-blind study of the effectiveness and specificity injection therapy in ragweed hay fever. N Engl J Med 1965;273(13):675–9.

[214] Del Prete A, Loffredo C, Carderopoli A, et al. Local specific immunotherapy in allergic conjunctivitis. Acta Ophthalmol Copenh 1994;72(5):631–4.

[215] Gaglani B, Borish L, Bartelson BL, et al. Nasal immunotherapy in weed-induced allergic rhinitis. Ann Allergy Asthma Immunol 1997;79(3):259–65.

[216] Juniper EF, Kline PA, Ramsdale EH, et al. Comparison of the efficacy and side effects of aqueous steroid nasal spray (budesonide) and allergen-injection therapy (Pollinex-R) in the treatment of seasonal allergic rhinoconjunctivitis. J Allergy Clin Immunol 1990;85(3):606–11.

[217] Dreborg S, Agrell B, Foucard T, et al. A double-blind, multicenter immunotherapy trial in children, using a purified and standardized Cladosporium herbarum preparation. I. Clinical results. Allergy 1986;41(2):131–40.

[218] Balda BR, Wolf H, Baumgarten C, et al. Tree-pollen allergy is efficiently treated by short-term immunotherapy (STI) with seven preseasonal injections of molecular standardized allergens. Allergy 1998;53(8):740–8.

[219] Didier A, Malling HJ, Worm M, et al. Optimal dose, efficacy, and safety of once-daily sublingual immunotherapy with a 5-grass pollen tablet for seasonal allergic rhinitis. J Allergy Clin Immunol 2007.

[220] Horak F, Stubner P, Berger UE, et al. Immunotherapy with sublingual birch pollen extract. A short-term double-blind placebo study. J Investig Allergol Clin Immunol 1998;8(3):165–71.

[221] Niggemann B, Jacobsen L, Dreborg S, et al. Five-year follow-up on the PAT study: specific immunotherapy and long-term prevention of asthma in children. Allergy 2006;61(7):855–9.

ELSEVIER
SAUNDERS

Immunol Allergy Clin N Am
28 (2008) 225–234

IMMUNOLOGY
AND ALLERGY
CLINICS
OF NORTH AMERICA

Index

Note: Page numbers of article titles are in **boldface** type.

A

Acantholysis, in pemphigus vulgaris, 128–130

Acne, 141, 158

Acrochordon (skin tags), 140–141, 160–161

Acyclovir
for herpes simplex infections, 157
for herpes zoster, 157–158

Adenovirus infections, 11–12, 171–172

Aeroallergens, dermatitis due to, 153

Allergic conjunctivitis, **43–57**
acute, 6
anatomic considerations in, 43
contact lens wear with, 113–116
diagnostic tests for, 49–50
epidemiology of, 43
examination in, 46–48
history in, 44–46
immunopathology of, 3–5
in pediatric patients, 178–182
late-phase reaction in, 50–51
mast cells in, 34–35
pathophysiology of, 43–44
perennial, 6, 48–49
seasonal, 48. *See also* Vernal conjunctivitis.
symptoms of, 45–46
treatment of, 51–55, **189–224**. *See also specific treatments.*
algorithm for, 193
overview of, 189–192

Allergic contact dermatitis, 149–150

Allergic shiners, 148

Allergy, ocular. *See* Ocular allergy(ies).

Allergy testing, in vernal conjunctivitis, 69

Aminocaproic acid, for urticaria, 159

Amlexanox, for allergic conjunctivitis, 209

Angioedema, 143, 159–160

Antazoline, for allergic conjunctivitis, 51

Antibiotics. *See also specific antibiotics.*
for eyelid infections, 157–158

Antifungal agents, for seborrheic dermatitis, 138

Antihistamines
for allergic conjunctivitis, 51, 180, 191–192, 196–199
for urticaria, 159
for vernal conjunctivitis, 72

Arachidonic acid derivatives, in mast cells, 28–29

Aspirin, for vernal conjunctivitis, 72

Atopic conjunctivitis, 3–8

Atopic dermatitis, 147–149, 156–157

Atopic keratoconjunctivitis, 68

Autoimmune diseases
blistering, **119–136**
experimental uveitis, mast cells in, 36–37

Avoidance
in allergic conjunctivitis, 193
in vernal conjunctivitis, 71

Azelaic acid, for rosacea, 158–159

Azelastine, for allergic conjunctivitis, 53, 180–181, 205–207, 209

B

Bacterial conjunctivitis, 4, 10–11, 170–171, 174–176

Bandage lenses, for dry eye, 113

Basal cell carcinoma, 145, 161

Basement membrane zone, epithelial, autoantibodies to, 119, 121–125

Basophils
in giant papillary conjunctivitis, 91
in vernal conjunctivitis, 67

Beclomethasone, for allergic conjunctivitis, 212

doi:10.1016/S0889-8561(08)00017-9   *immunology.theclinics.com*